Dosage Forms - Emerging Trends and Prospective Drug-Delivery Systems

Edited by Sakthivel Lakshmana Prabu and Appavoo Umamaheswari

Published in London, United Kingdom

Dosage Forms - Emerging Trends and Prospective Drug-Delivery Systems
http://dx.doi.org/10.5772/intechopen.1001773
Edited by Sakthivel Lakshmana Prabu and Appavoo Umamaheswari

Contributors
Achal J. Yeola, Aneri Joshi, Appavoo Umamaheswari, Ayarivan Puratchikody, Dina M. Mahdy, Esraa A. Abd El-Maksod, Gaidaa M. Dogheim, Luca Magagnin, Mohamed Mamdouh M. Elshindidy, Morteza Rabiei, Negar Fouladvari, Neha Verma, Nishant Gaur, Nitin Kumar, Pranav Y. Dave, Rathinasabapathy Thirumurugan, Roberto Bernasconi, Sakineh Shabanpour, Sakthivel Lakshmana Prabu, Seyedeh Sabereh Samavati, Soheil Mehrdadi, Sonam Rai, Vaibhavi Patel, Yousra A. El-Maradny

First published in London, United Kingdom, 2025 by IntechOpen
IntechOpen is the global imprint of INTECHOPEN LIMITED, registered in England and Wales, registration number: 11086078, 167-169 Great Portland Street, London, W1W 5PF, United Kingdom

For EU product safety concerns: IN TECH d.o.o., Prolaz Marije Krucifikse Kozulić 3, 51000 Rijeka, Croatia, info@intechopen.com or visit our website at intechopen.com.

British Library Cataloguing-in-Publication Data
A catalogue record for this book is available from the British Library

Dosage Forms - Emerging Trends and Prospective Drug-Delivery Systems
Edited by Sakthivel Lakshmana Prabu and Appavoo Umamaheswari
p. cm.

This title is part of the Pharmaceutical Science Book Series, Volume 8
Topic: Drug Discovery and Delivery
Series Editor: Rosario Pignatello
Topic Editor: Marilena Vlachou

Print ISBN 978-0-85466-587-7
Online ISBN 978-0-85466-586-0
eBook (PDF) ISBN 978-0-85466-588-4
ISSN 3033-3318

IntechOpen Book Series
Pharmaceutical Science
Volume 8

Aims and Scope of the Series

Pharmaceutical science focuses on the design, synthesis, formulation, targeting, distribution, safety, and efficacy of active compounds as potential therapeutics. It is a large interdisciplinary discipline that aims to integrate the basic principles of physical and organic chemistry, biochemistry, biology, and engineering to discover, develop, and characterize active compounds and to optimize the formulation and delivery of drugs in the body for offering new and improved safe and efficacious therapies against human diseases. The research areas covered by the pharmaceutical sciences range from medicinal chemistry and pharmaceutical technology to pharmacology and toxicology, which represent the preliminary phases of drug development. Medicinal chemistry involves the design and synthesis of pharmaceuticals as well as the isolation of active agents from natural sources. Computer-aided strategies are increasingly involved in this drug discovery process. Pharmaceutics is a multidisciplinary science that examines the relationships between drug formulation, delivery, distribution, and clinical outcomes. Modern clinical approaches are increasingly relying on controlled release strategies and drug delivery and targeting systems, including nanotechnological platforms (nanomedicine). Pharmacology is the science of drug action in biological systems. Pharmacologists also make drugs as tools to explore aspects of cell and tissue functions. Toxicology is the study of the adverse effects of active agents on living organisms and the ecosystem, including the prevention and amelioration of such adverse effects. This book series includes volumes on Drug Discovery, Delivery, and Pharmacology. Their overall aim is to present the latest research in the whole path of drug discovery and development from different points of view of this multidisciplinary and dynamic field.

Meet the Series Editor

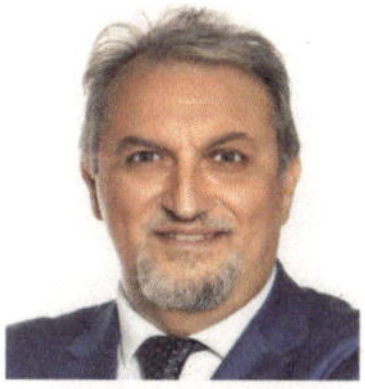

Prof. Rosario Pignatello is a Full Professor of Pharmaceutical Technology and Legislation at the University of Catania, Italy. He is the Director of the Department of Drug and Health Sciences. He has nearly 30 years of experience in the research and development of innovative formulations for the controlled release and targeting of bioactive molecules, through chemical approaches as well as nanotechnological carriers, aimed at treating different disorders. Prof. Pignatello has coauthored about 180 papers and edited a series of textbooks on biomaterials and their application in medicine. The main areas of his research are polymeric and lipid-based micro- and nanoparticles as modified drug delivery systems; vesicular nanocarriers (liposomes, micelles); lipophilic prodrugs and conjugates; synthesis and evaluation of new polymeric biomaterials for drug delivery and tissue regeneration. In particular, Prof. Pignatello works actively in the field of ocular drug delivery, leading the Research Centre for Ocular Nanotechnology, within the NANOMED Centre (Centre for Nanomedicine and Pharmaceutical Nanotechnology) at the University of Catania.

Meet the Volume Editors

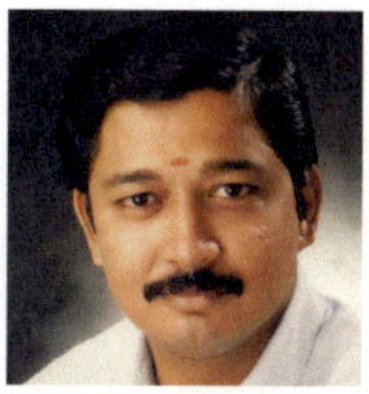

Dr. Sakthivel Lakshmana Prabu has a Ph. D. from Manipal University in Manipal, India. He pursued a postgraduate diploma in IPR law from the National Law School of India University in Bangalore, India. He has been working at Anna University, BIT Campus, Tiruchirappalli, India, since 2009. He has more than 25 years of experience, including both in reputed Pharmaceutical Industries and Academic Institutions. From his research contribution, he has published 125 peer-reviewed publications in reputed international and national journals and authored 40 book chapters. As an editor, he edited seven books and co-authored a book entitled "Pharmaceutical Production Management" by Lambert Academic Publishing. To his credit, he has seven patents. He serves as a reviewer and editorial board member for various reputed journals. Added to his credit, he organized various national and international conferences, hands-on training, workshops and symposiums. He has received funded projects from the Department of Biotechnology, New Delhi, India; the Tamil Nadu State Council for Science and Technology, Tamil Nadu; and the Centre for Sponsored Research and Consultancy, Anna University, Chennai. He has had a strong association with Croatian IntechOpen since 2012.

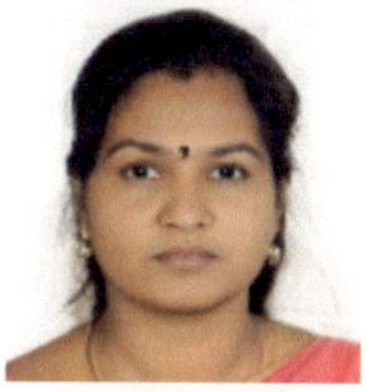

Dr. Appavoo Umamaheswari obtained a Bachelor of Pharmacy from the Tamil Nadu Dr. M. G. R. Medical University in Chennai, India. She received the Thiru Gnana Sebastian Endowment Award in M. Pharmacy and was awarded the Management Gold Medal award as Best Outgoing Student for the Year 2006 by Periyar College of Pharmaceutical Sciences in India. She obtained a Ph.D. in Pharmaceutical Technology from Anna University in India. Since 2006, she has worked at Anna University, BIT Campus, Tiruchirappalli, India. From her research expertise and contribution, she has published over 35 peer-reviewed publications in reputed International and National journals, authored 26 book chapters, and edited four books as an editor. To her credit, she has three patents. She serves as a reviewer and editorial board member for various reputed journals. She has given multiple presentations at national and international conferences and is an active member of many professional and academic bodies. Dr. Umamaheswari serves as a referee for various reputed journals and has worked on projects funded by the Department of Science and Technology, New Delhi, India, and the Centre for Sponsored Research and Consultancy, Anna University, India.

Contents

Preface

Globally, more than half of the population consumes at least one medicine daily in their daily routine. Drug substances are administrated to treat, manage and stop the progress of disease. The desired therapeutic effect of the drug substances is based on different dosage forms. However, both pharmacokinetics and pharmacodynamics play a significant role in producing the desired therapeutic effect. Yet, drugs always have certain limitations, such as drug efficiency, side effects and generating drug resistance on multiple administrations. In addition, drug solubility, stability and drug release at the target sites at the desired rate are key challenging factors in biomedical applications.

In the last few decades, efforts have been made to improve the therapeutic efficacy and reduce the side effects of drug substances. With complimentary knowledge, the development of new drugs and technical advancement have become a good platform for delivering the drug's therapeutic efficiency at the target site by alteration in the structures at the molecular level, thus reducing the dosing frequency and side effects.

Chapter 1, "Introductory Chapter: Innovations in Drug Delivery – Exploring Emerging Trends and Future Directions", by A. Umamaheswari and S. Lakshmana Prabu, outlines the development of drugs from medicinal plants from ancient times therapy to the recent advanced drug delivery system.

Chapter 2, "Advanced Strategy and Future Perspectives in Drug Delivery System" by A.Umamaheswari and team, summarizes the drug discovery and development of new drug molecules and their limitations in the drug delivery system. Also, it highlighted the development of novel drug delivery systems, especially nanoparticles in gene delivery, cancer, disease diagnosis and its biomedical application, lipid-based drug delivery systems, regulatory challenges and artificial intelligence in drug delivery.

Chapter 3, "Emerging Techniques for Herbosomes", by Gaidaa M. Dogheim et al., focuses on various techniques in developing herbosomes and concludes that herbosomes have several advantages over traditional herbal extracts and emerging promising technology in developing new herbal products.

Chapter 4, "A Novel Targeted Drug Delivery Carrier: Herbosomes", by Aneri Joshi et al., focuses on herbosomes and their application in treating different diseases.

Chapter 5, "Phytosome: A Novel Drug Delivery Approach in Herbal Medicine", by Sakineh Shabanpour, describes the structural components of phytosomes, their physicochemical properties, formulation techniques, and merits and demerits.

Chapter 6, "Unlocking the Synergy: Exploring the Solubility Permeability Interplay in Microemulsion-Based Skin Drug Delivery", by Neha Verma and team, focuses on microemulsions, their physicochemical properties and their role in enhancing drug solubility and skin permeability. They concluded that microemulsions can improve patient care, especially in dermatology.

Chapter 7, “Solid Lipid Nanoparticles: A Promising Drug Delivery System and Their Potential for Peptide and Protein Therapeutics”, by Soheil Mehrdadi, deliberates on the potentials of solid lipid nanoparticles, especially in peptide and protein therapeutics.

Chapter 8, “The Application of Nanotechnology in the Pharmaceutical Treatment of Common Diseases”, by Morteza Rabiei and Seyedeh Sabereh Samavati, focuses on the delivery of drugs by nanotechnology in treating different diseases.

Chapter 9, “Smart Drug Delivery for Targeted Therapeutics via Remotely Controlled Microdevices”, by Negar Fouladvari and team, discusses microrobots in drug delivery and the strategies as remotely actuated microcarriers in drug delivery.

Sakthivel Lakshmana Prabu and Appavoo Umamaheswari
Department of Pharmaceutical Technology,
University College of Engineering – BIT Campus,
Anna University,
Tiruchirappalli, Tamil Nadu, India

Section 1

Introduction

Chapter 1

Introductory Chapter: Innovations in Drug Delivery – Exploring Emerging Trends and Future Directions

Appavoo Umamaheswari and Sakthivel Lakshmana Prabu

1. Introduction

Delivering the drug at the desired concentration in the target site has been considered as a major challenge in drug delivery system. To achieve the desired concentration at the target site, more research studies are engaged throughout the world. In the ancient time, people rely medicinal plants for their primary health care purpose. With the development of science and technology, various formulations including solid dosage form as conventional dosage forms are produced. However, the major demerit of these conventional dosage forms is lack of therapeutic efficacy due to poor selectivity and distribution. Gastrointestinal permeability of the drug by solubilization is considered as a primary factor in determining the pharmacokinetic properties as well as the therapeutic efficacy of the drug [1].

There has always been a fascination among researchers to create new chemical entities as new drug substances, composites with novel structures, and specialized functional capability. Most of the approved drugs in the market are poorly water soluble. As per the pharmaceutical marketing scenario, about 30%, 25 and 10% of drugs are categorized under BCS II, BCS III, and BCS IV classification. Further, the majority of the new drug substances in the new drug discovery scheme are water insoluble, which belongs to water insoluble (BCS II/IV) or low permeable (BCS III/IV). Hence, efforts were taken to reformulate the marketed drugs in the aspects of solubility and improved therapeutic efficacy [2–4].

Developing a suitable formulation for these poorly water-soluble drugs has become a great challenging perspective to the formulation scientist, especially its solubility and bioavailability. Numerous research initiatives were taken by both academic as well as pharmaceutical research experts in order to improve the bioavailability. Various solubilization techniques includes drug structural modification, formation of salts, solubilization by incorporating either cosolvents or surfactants, solid dispersion by incorporating water soluble polymers, solubility of basic or acidic drug substances based on pH-dependent, etc. With respect to the drug structural modification, it is considered as a time-consuming process; also, it has shown loss of therapeutic activity. The *eventual effects such as instability,* acceptability, effectiveness and stability *due to its different salt* forms, surfactants and cosolvents have made restriction in the drug development. In addition, scale-up for solid dispersion products in manufacturing process is considered as difficult task [5].

For the past few decades, the recent scientific advances and global initiatives in molecular pharmacology have opened the possibility of delivering the drugs at the molecular level.

In the twenty-first century, the synthesis of nanomaterial by nanotechnology and its application has been recognized extensively as novel drug delivery system in delivering drugs in different diseases. Different nanomaterials include nanocapsules, nanoparticles, nanogels, nanoemulsion, nanosuspension, nanotubes, and dendrimers. These nanomaterial's have unique property such as optical, electrical, mechanical, and magnetic properties; further, their shape, size, surface charge, surface area, etc., have made an interest in the biomedical field, especially in disease diagnosis, drug delivery, and treating different diseases. However, its tiny particle size has a very good interaction with various cells in the biological systems. This interaction increases the Reactive oxygen species production, degrading the membrane integrity by releasing the metal ions into the biological system. As a consequence of the above facts, inhibition of normal cell activity occurs and is considered as nanomaterial toxicity. In addition, these nanomaterials exhibited elevated toxicity, especially in inhalation studies. Therefore, stringent regulatory guidelines were made in nanotoxicity to prove its safety and efficacy [6–8].

Lipid-based drug delivery systems (LBDDS) have been considered as an emerging developed technique in drug delivery systems to solve the low water solubility, Low-oral bioavailability, permeability, toxicity, and bioavailability of these poorly water-soluble drugs. Different lipid-based drug delivery system include liposomes, lipospheres, niosomes, phytosomes, transfersomes, ethosomes, vesosomes, herbosomes, solid lipid nanoparticles, and nanostructure lipid carriers. By varying the composition of the lipids, the developed formulations will have different structural and functional properties. These properties can protect the drug substances from biological degradation, forasmuch as it release the drug molecules into the blood from the lipid matrix, leading to improved bioavailability and, in due course, increased therapeutic activity. Further, this drug delivery system has directed the successful commercialization of the formulation in the market [9–10]. The schematic development of drugs from medicinal plants as ancient time therapy to the recent advanced drug delivery system is shown **Figure 1**.

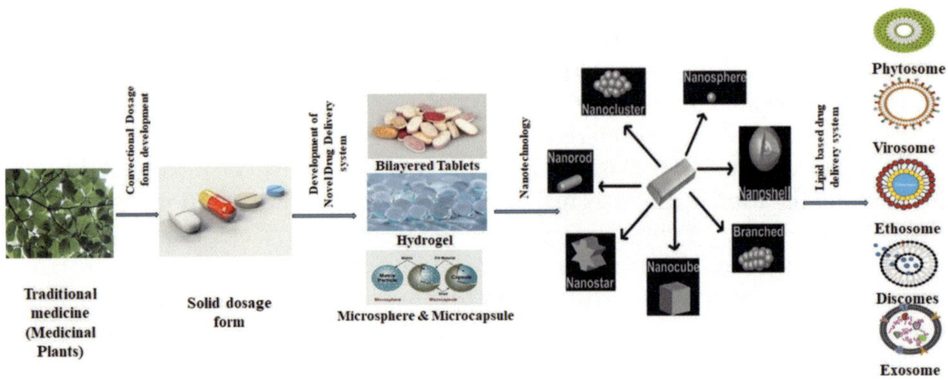

Figure 1.
Development of drugs from medicinal plants to recent advanced drug delivery system.

In conclusion, technological breakthroughs from ancient times to the current development and a better comprehension of drug delivery processes are driving a rapid evolution in the dosage form landscape. New developments in drug delivery systems like nanotechnology and lipid based drug delivery systems are outlined. These developments address various strategies with solubility, stability, and bioavailability in addition to enhancing therapeutic efficacy. Future research in drug delivery system has enormous potential to improve treatment outcomes paving the way for a healthier future and real benefits to the society.

Author details

Appavoo Umamaheswari[†] and Sakthivel Lakshmana Prabu*
Department of Pharmaceutical Technology, University College of Engineering – BIT Campus, Anna University, Tiruchirappalli, Tamil Nadu, India

*Address all correspondence to: slaxmanvel@gmail.com

†Contributed equally to this work.

References

[1] Dahlgren D, Lennernas H. Intestinal Permeability and Drug Absorption: Predictive Experimental, Computational and In Vivo Approaches. Pharmaceutics. 2019;**11**(8):411

[2] Bhalani DV, Nutan B, Kumar A, Singh Chandel AK. Bioavailability Enhancement Techniques for Poorly Aqueous Soluble Drugs and Therapeutics. Biomedicines. 2022;**10**(9):2055

[3] Kalepu S, Nekkanti V. Insoluble drug delivery strategies: review of recent advances and business prospects. Acta Pharmaceutica Sinica B. 2015;**5**(5):442-453

[4] Kumar S, Kaur R, Rajput R, Singh M. Bio Pharmaceutics Classification System (BCS) Class IV Drug Nanoparticles: Quantum Leap to Improve Their Therapeutic Index. Advanced Pharmaceutical Bulletin Pharm Bull. 2018;**8**(4):617-625

[5] Liu X, Zhao L, Wu B, Chen F. Improving solubility of poorly water-soluble drugs by protein-based strategy: A review. International Journal of Pharmaceutics. 2023;**5**(634):122704

[6] Umamaheswari A, Vijayalakshmi M, Sree D, Lakshmana Prabu S, Puratchikody A. A Typical Properties of Nanomaterials for Applications in Drug Delivery: A Review. Bioequivalence & Bioavailability. International Journal. 2021;**5**(2):000155

[7] Umamaheswari A, Jegasubramaniam SN, Harish M, Lakshmana PS. Toxicity Interactions of Nanomaterials in Biological System: A Pressing Priority. Bioequivalence & Bioavailability International Journal. 2022;**6**(2):000173

[8] Umamaheswari A, Jegasubramaniam SN, Harish M, Lakshmana PS. Emerging Approaches and Perception of Toxicity Assessment in Nanomaterials. Bioequivalence & Bioavailability International Journal. 2022;**6**(1):000168

[9] Kesharwani R, Jaiswal P, Patel DK, Yadav PK. Lipid-Based Drug Delivery System (LBDDS): An Emerging Paradigm to Enhance Oral Bioavailability of Poorly Soluble Drugs. Biomedical Materials & Devices. 2023;**1**:648-663

[10] Srivastav AK, Karpathak S, Rai MK, Kumar D, Misra DP, Agarwal V. Lipid based drug delivery systems for oral, transdermal and parenteral delivery: recent strategies for targeted delivery consistent with different clinical application. Journal of Drug Delivery Science and Technology. 2023;**85**:104526

Chapter 2

Advanced Strategy and Future Perspectives in Drug Delivery System

Appavoo Umamaheswari, Ayarivan Puratchikody, Sakthivel Lakshmana Prabu and Rathinasabapathy Thirumurugan

Abstract

One of the main issues with the drug delivery system is delivering the drug to specific target site with anticipated concentration to produce a desired therapeutic potential of the drug. The major drawbacks in the conventional dosage forms are lack of targeted drug delivery, selectivity, non-specific distribution, poor bioavailability, frequent dosage regimen, side effects, first-pass metabolism, solubility for poorly soluble drugs, inability to cross biological barriers, gastrointestinal irritation, drug interaction, and effectiveness. Recent advancements in molecular pharmacology and the drug action in the targeted sites for particular diseases have made a new revolution to develop different novel drug delivery systems. These novel drug delivery systems significantly increase the drug delivery, thus exploiting therapeutic effect and reducing the accumulation of drugs in the off target site. Different novel drug delivery systems include microemulsion and microsphers; nanodrug delivery systems include nanoparticles, nanogels, nanoemulsion, nanosuspension, nanotubes, and dendrimers; and vesicular system includes liposomes, lipospheres, niosomes, phytosomes, transfersomes, ethosomes, vesosomes, herbosomes, solid lipid nanoparticles, and so on. Parameters such as particle size, shape, solubility, surface morphology, charge, solubility, biocompatibility, biodegradability, and drug release play a significant role to deliver the drug to the target site with the desired concentration. This chapter outlines the discovery of new drug molecule, drug development process, limitations of conventional dosage form, current drug delivery system, application of nanoparticles in disease diagnosis, treatment of different diseases like cancer, and regulatory challenges. Further application of artificial intelligence in drug delivery has been outlined as future perspectives in drug delivery system.

Keywords: new drug molecule, drug discovery and development, drug delivery system, nano drug delivery, vesicular drug delivery

1. Introduction

1.1 Drug discovery and development of a new drug molecule

Both drug discovery and its development of new drug molecules run parallel to each other. During the pre-discovery stage in the drug discovery process, relevant information about the illness is identified. Drug discovery and development for a particular disease get initiated based on the pre-discovery stage information, then the target molecular or cellular structure is identified. The next phase is drug discovery phase where 5000 to 10,000 compounds are identified through high-throughput screening and scrutinized for its activity. Subsequent to the identification of the lead molecule, preclinical investigation studies are initiated to assess the drug efficiency. Stages in the pre-discovery and discovery include synthesis, nonclinical testing, nonclinical pharmacology evaluation through *in vitro* techniques, assessment of preliminary animal pharmacokinetics parameters, toxicity studies, and nonclinical pharmacology evaluation through *in vivo* studies and their corresponding *in vitro - in vivo* correlations. Once the drug molecule exhibits the desired efficacy, the pharmaceutical organization files an Investigational New Drug (IND) application to the FDA. Based on approval from the FDA, the organization can begin to investigate the safety and efficacy of new molecule in human beings [1, 2].

During clinical trials, one or more intervention techniques may be adopted to assess the efficacy and safety of the test drug. Clinical trials can be carried out as a treatment trial, prevention trial, diagnostic trial, or screening trial or to assess the quality of life in human beings. In drug discovery and development process, high numbers of failures are observed, specifically in Phase II. If a drug persists in clinical trials, the ultimate new drug approval decision by the FDA will be based upon the data obtained from clinical trial studies [3–6].

1.2 Initial stages in drug delivery systems

In the ancient period, people depended on medicinal plants for their primary health care. These medicinal plants are much beneficial for treating several diseases in lower cost. However, lack of homogenecity, consistency and specificity are the major drawbacks of the same [7].

Previous to the controlled drug delivery system, most of the drug products were produced in capsule or pill formulations. The drug substances are released into the body when they come in contact with gastrointestional fluids and absorbed through blood capillaries and entered into the blood stream. The major drawback of this dosage form is uneven pharmacokinetic profile of the dosage form. In the tenth century, coating technology was developed by Rhazes and Avicemen to mask the bitter taste of the drugs, also alter the drug release. Materaials such as gold and silver were used as coating material; later pearl-coated tablets were developed.

With the advancement of coating technology, in the twentieth century, materials such as shellac and keratin were used for coating. Further, sugar and enteric coating with polymeric cellulose acetate phthalate were also developed during this stage [8]. Based on this controlled release formulation, researchers are motivated to develop several oral as well as transdermal formulations. Lipowski, in 1951, obtained a patent for the slow release of the drug as oral sustained release formulation using enteric polymers [9]. In 1952, a team by Smith, Klein, Beecham, and French developed

Spansule technology to release the drug in a sustained as well as in a controlled manner [10]. In 1955, Jatzkewitz developed polymer-drug conjugate as nanoparticles (NPs) therapeutic. Additionaly, based on this polymer-drug conjugate, in 1960, lipid vesicles as liposome was developed, which made a new revolution as nanocarrier in treating various diseases [11, 12]. Protein-based microsphere was prepared by Scheffel in 1972; later in 1976, microcapsules and NPs were prepared using polymerization technique by Peter Paul Speiser's research group [13]. During this second generation, several new formulations were developed; however, expected clinical results were not obtained for the same [14].

Hence, more research studies were performed based on nanotechnology formulation to get self regulated continuous drug release with long-term depot formulation. As an outcome, long-term depots were developed for peptide/protein drugs [15]. By utilizing various polymers, hydrogel formulation were developed to protect the drug from the physiological changes. More efforts are being made in nanotechnology research by reserachers to develop nanostructured drug delivery system to treat various tumors using several polymers. This nanotechnology drug delivery system has produced high effiency to prevent tumor growth and reduce accumulation of drugs in non-target site in animal models [16, 17].

In the third generation, more research are concentrated to overcome the physicochemical barriers like high molecular weight of proteins and peptides and poor water solubility and biological barriers like systemic distribution of drug related to the earlier drug delivery systems [16, 18]. However, in drug delivery system (DDS), delivering the drug in the target site at the predicted quantity is an utilimate task to provide efficient treatment for various diseases and has become a crucial and major challenge.

1.3 Clinical trials

Clinical trials are a type of research involving human volunteers that aim to determine specific questions about medical intervention or treatment or behavior. These studies help to determine the treatment, either new drug or therapies, is safe and effective to patients. Also, this process beings a new drug molecule or treatment to the market.

The drug discovery and development process includes both preclinical and clinical investigations. Based on the animal pharmacology and toxicology results, clinical trials are initiated in human beings to assess and determine the potential efficacy of the new drug in a specific time period with gradual expansion of human volunteers to the test. The number of subjects involved in clinical trials is based on the nature of the disease or treatment process [19, 20].

1.4 Clinical trial phases include

Comparison of different clinical trial phases is shown in **Table 1** [21].

1.5 Conventional dosge form

For more than a decade, different dosage forms like tablets, capsules, injection, and topical formulation have been utilized entensively as conventional dosage form to deliver the drug for a wide range of therapeutics. However, these conventional dosage form had some limitations.

	Phase I	Phase II	Phase III	Phase IV
Objectives	Determination of pharmacological and metabolic actions and the maximally tolerated dose	Evaluate the effectiveness; determination of the side effects in short-term and to detect common risks for a specific population and disease	Collect additional information related to the effectiveness of outcomes thorugh clinical studies and examine the risk-benefit ratio in a demographically diverse sample	Screen the safety in ongoing studies in large populations and detect other uses of the agents that might be approved by the FDA
Study types	1. Safety & tolerability studies (Single/multiple dose in patients or healthy volunteers) 2. Oncology studies in patients with tolerability / MTD as primary endpoint (efficacy might be a secondary endpoint) 3. Drug-drug interaction & food effects 4. PK in renal or hepatic-impaired patients	1. Proof of concept, efficacy, or mechanism 2. Mechanistic studies 3. Dose range exploration 4. Pilot studies 5. Definite dose finding studies	1. Pivotal studies (vs. placebo/ comparator) 2. Long-term safety studies for registration 3. Local registration studies 4. Post-marketing study commitments 5. Phase IIIA extension studies 6. Studies intended to support publication, claims or to prepare launch, which starts before approval but is not intended for regulatory submissions	1. Post-marketing surveillance studies 2. Studies intended to support publication claims
Factors to be identified	1. ADME 2. Proportionality of the dose 3. Bioavailability 4. Bioequivalence	1. Bioavailability 2. Interaction between drug and disease 3. Interactions between drug and drug 4. Drug-drug interactions 5. Effiect at various dose levels 6. ADME 7. Safety of the patient	1. Interaction between drug and disease 2. Interactions between drug and drug 3. Dosage intervals 4. Details of risk-benefit 5. Safety and effectiveness for subgroups	1. Epidemiological data 2. Safety and effectiveness among large, varied populations 3. Pharmacoeconomics
Data focus	1. Vital signs 2. Levels in serum and plasma 3. Adverse actions	1. Dose response and tolerance 2. Adverse actions 3. Efficiency	1. Data from labtoratory studies 2. Efficiency 3. Adverse actions	1. Efficiency 2. Pharmacoeconomics 3. Epidemiology 4. Adverse actions

DOI: http://dx.doi.org/10.5772/intechopen.1008498

	Phase I	**Phase II**	**Phase III**	**Phase IV**
Design futures	1. Single and rising dose levels 2. Unblinded & Uncontrolled	1. Comparisons of placebo controlled study 2. Comparisons of active controlled study 3. Precise entry criteria	1. Randomized controlled study 2. Two to three treatment techniques 3. Wider eligibility standards	1. Uncontrolled observational study
Duration	1. 1 month	1. Several months	1. Several years	1. Ongoing (after FDA approval)
Population	1. Individuals having specific disease (like HIV and cancer) or healthy volunteers	1. Individuals having specific disease	1. Individuals having specific disease	1. Individuals having specific disease, as well as new age groups, genders
Sample size	1. Between 20 and 80	Between 100 and 200	Between hundreds and thousands	More than a thousand

Table 1.
Comparative structures of different phases in clinical trials.

1.6 Limitations

The limitations of conventional dosage form includes

1. *Lack of targeted drug delivery* – Non-specific distribution, suboptimical targeting and low therapeutic index.

2. *Limited drug delivery to specific sites* – Inability to reach target tissues and difficulty targeting intracellular pathogens

3. *Poor drug bioavailability* – Limited low absorption and variability in absorption

4. *Frequent dosage regimen* – Short half-life of drug, fluctuation in drug levels, and patient inconvenience.

5. *Poor patient compliance* – Complex dosing regimens and invasive administration

6. *First-pass metabolism* – Drug degradation in the liver and formation of inactive metabolites.

7. *Degradation and instability* – Degradation of drug and reduced instability.

8. *Non-specific immune response* – Immune reaction and hypersensitivity.

9. *Poor penetration into certain tissues* – Difficulty in crossing biological barriers like blood brain barrier, tissue penetration, and restricted to local delivery

10. *Drug resistance* - Resistance in cancer and infectious diseases and inability to deliver combination therapies effectively.

11. *Limited control over drug release* – Immediate and uncontrolled release, short-lived therapeutic effect.

12. *Gastrointestinal irritation* – Gastrointestinal side effects and delayed gastric emptying

13. *Challenges with poorly water soluble drugs* – Limited formulation options, precipitation, and degradation.

14. *Challenges in pediatric and geriatric populations* – Difficulty in dosing and compliance issues.

15. *Drug-drug and drug-food interactions* – Interactions with other substances and increased risk of adverse effects [22, 23].

2. Development of novel drug delivery system

In the early days, with the available technological systems, the new drug molecules are formulated and introduced into the body through different dosage forms like oral, sublingual, parental, transdermal, intraocular, conjunctival, intra nasal, rectal, vaginal, intra respiratory, urethral, and so on. The physicochemical properties of the drug play a major responsible role in its therapeutic effect. These limitations of conventional dosage form highlighted the need for continuous research to overcome the issues.

The outcome of their research has become the development of controlled drug delivery system as a new innovation in the drug delivery system. During 1950, the controlled release formulation was approved in the drug delivery system, which showed significant advantage over the conventional dosage form. Over the decades, these controlled release formulation have exhibited improvement in systemic circulation and desired pharmacological effect of the drug [24]. In controlled release formulation, the drugs are released at predetermined time and last for days to months without being affected by the physicological condtions of the body. In addition, this formulation has shown increased solubility of drugs, accumulation of drug in the target site, pharmacokinetic properties, pharmacological activity, efficacy, and patient compliance and further decreased the drug toxicity [25, 26].

2.1 Nanotechnology

Based on this controlled release formulation concept, over the years, various novel DDS have been developed. Among the different DDS, products made by nanotechnology have shown remarkable achievements in all the fields, including in the field of biomedical application. The National Nanotechnology Initiative (NNI) defined nanoparticles as structures with at least one dimension and a size range of 1 to 100 nm. The majority of particles up to several hundred nanometers in size is referred to as "nano" particles.

Nanotechnology is a study of extremely small structures thorugh manipulation of matter on a near-atomic scale to create new structured materials and devices. Through this scientific advancement, this developed product has become a promising tool in various sectors [27]. Nanotechnology not only boosts current technologies, but it can also significantly increase the efficacy of new applications across all industries.

The last few decades have seen a surge in interest in the development of nanotechnology products especially in biomedical applicatons utilizing various classes of biopolymers. Because of their adaptability and the tremendous advancements in nanotechnology, drugs may now be delivered to the intended location, and the appropriate dosage can be administered in the appropriate way at the appropriate time. The materials used to create nanomaterials can be inorganic or organic and can have peculiar characteristic properties with respect to its size, shape, charge, surface area, solubility, chemical property, generation of oxidation potential, agglomeration, electronic, and optical, mechanical, and magnetic properties also to have the ability to permeate the tissues and cell barriers [28, 29]. The developed products have their own uniqueness and modify the various properties, which eventually distress their affinities for various drug substances and show significantly higher solubility, diffusivity, drug release profile, bioavailability, and therapeutic performance than conventional dosage forms. Also, this can provide suitable administration routes, fewer side effects, lower toxicity, and prolonged drug life cycle [30, 31].

Nanoparticle for the drug delivery can be prepared by the following methods:

- Dispersion of preformed polymers includes solvent diffusion method, solvent evaporation method, salting out, and nanoprecipitation

- Polymerization of monomers

- Ionic gelation method for hydrophilic polymers

- Chemical reduction
- Coprecipitation
- Seeding
- Microemulsion and inverse microemulsion
- Hydrothermal method
- Sonoelectrodeposition
- Ball milling
- Electrospinning
- Lithography
- Sputtering
- The arc discharge method
- Laser ablation
- Chemical vapor deposition
- Solvothermal and hydrothermal methods
- The sol-gel method
- Soft and hard templating methods
- Reverse micelle methods [32–34]

Nanostructured materials can deliver the drugs in two ways. They are

1. Passive delivery
2. Self delivery.

In the passive delivery method, the drugs are fused in the inner cavity through hydrophobic effect, then the drugs are released in the targeted site. In self delivery, the drug is conjugated with nanostructure carrier material and released from the carrier at the right time [31].

In targeted drug delivery, the drugs are released

1. Active targeting
2. Passive targeting.

In active targeting, the drugs are linked to suitably designed nanosystems to target the receptors in the target site/tissue. In passive targeting, the complex between the drug and nano carrier will circulate into the blood stream and is delivered into the targeted site/tissue through binding or affinity due to temperature, pH, and molecular size. This passive targeting is used to deliver lipid componets, macrophages, neutrophils, and dendritic cells in the target tissue/site [35].

The major mechanism for its drug release and the rate of drug release are classified as

1. Diffusion
2. Solvent reaction
3. Chemical reaction
4. Stimuli control [36–38].

The mechanism of drug release is shown in **Figure 1**.

Further, this designed products are utilized as biosensors in detection of disease, controlled drug delivery, sustained drug delivery, and targeted drug delivery in different diseases like cancer, AIDS, cardiovascular diseases, and genetic disorders [39].

2.2 Categories of nanoparticle

In drug delivery, the nanoparticles are classified into three categories. They are

1. Polymeric nanoparticle
2. Inorganic nanoparticle
3. Solid lipid nanoparticle

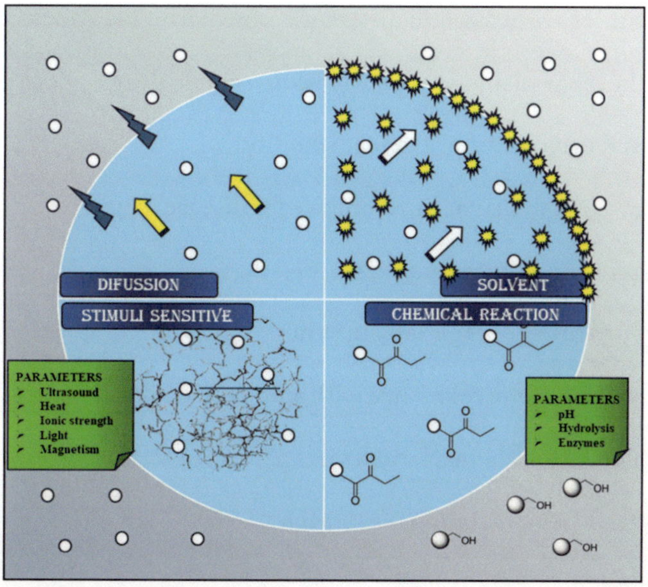

Figure 1.
Mechanism of drug release.

2.2.1 Polymeric nanoparticle

In polymeric nanoparticle, the drugs are surrounded by a polymeric membrane (encapsulated) or trapped in the polymer matrix or adsorbed on the surface of the particle [40].

2.2.2 Dendrimers

Dendrimer are nano-sized polymeric nanoparticles, which are homogenous, well defined, and radially sysmmetic molecules having a monodisperse structure with regular branched structure that possess functional moieties. These unique propertis are suitable for solubilization of drugs and for drug delivery. These dendrimers are preferably utilized in gene delivery. In gene delivery, both dendrimers and DNA are entrapped in water soluble polymer, subsequently packed or deposited in functional polymer film.

Dendrimers are prepared by

1. Divergent method

2. Convergent method.

Other types of dendrimers are

- Amino acid-based dendrimers
- Glycodendrimers
- Hydrophobic dendrimers
- Asymmetric dendrimers [33, 41, 42]

These dendrimers are utilized in different biomedicial fields, including

- Enhance the bioavailability of poorly water soluble drug
- Increase water solubility and higher stability
- As contrast agent in magnetic resonance for disease diagnosis
- Used as a sensor in disease diagnosis
- Treating burn diseases especially in skin
- Electron paramagnetic resonance with spin-labeled dendrimers
- *Antimicrobial and antiviral therapies*
- *Anti-inflammatory and anticancer therapies*
- *Tissue engineering*
- *Gene delivery [43–46]*

2.2.3 Gene delivery system

The term "gene delivery" describes the process of introducing genetic material, such as DNA plasmids, RNA, and siRNA, into target cells either inside or coupled to NPs in order to either express or suppress the production of proteins (a process also known as transfection), which can be used to treat or cure a variety of illnesses.

Gene delivery systems are classified into

1. Viral transduction systems – In this system, virus-mediated transfer of nucleic acid into cells were used as gene delivery

2. Nonviral transfection systems – Genetic materials like DNA, siRNA, RNA, and plasmids are condensed into nanoparticles using a suitable cationic polymer or lipids in this system.

2.2.4 Polymers in gene delivery

Different cationic polymers or lipids are used as polymer in gene delivery. They are classified as

1. *Cationic polymers* – Chitosan, poly L-lysine, polyethyleneimine, branched polyethyleneimine, and dendrimer polyethyleneimine

2. *Cationic Lipids* – DOTMA (N-[1-(2,3-dioleyloxy) propyl]-N,N,N-trimethylammonium chloride), DOTAP [1,2-bis(oleoyloxy)-3-(trimethylammonio) propane and DC-Chol 3β[*N*-(*N*′,*N*′-dimethylaminoethane)-carbamoyl]

3. *Multivalent Cationic Lipids* – DOSPA (2,3-dioleyloxy-N-[2(sperminecarboxamido) ethyl]-N,N-dimethyl-l-propanaminium trifluoroacetate) and DOGS (di-octadecyl-amido-glycyl-spermine)

4. Neutral Lipids – DOPE (dioleoylphosphatidylethanolamine) and DOPC (dioleoylphosphatidylcholine) [41, 42, 47].

2.3 Gums in drug delivery

In the last few decades, gums from natural source material extruded from plants are used in drug delivery system. These gums are polysaccharides containing several sugar units conjugated by a glycosidic bond, leading to form a huge molecule. Because of its non-toxicity, viscosity, adhesive property, cost, availability, interfacial quality, and stability, it receives more attention to do research in DDS via the matrix system, controlled release, buccal drug delivery, film coating, microspheres, hydrogels, and nanoparticle [48, 49].

Gums are classified into three major groups. They are.

Natural gums – Derived from natural sources like trees, hdrocolloids from seweed, and seeds of various legumes. Gum Arabica, guar gum, and tragacanth are examples of natural gums.

Modified gums – Derived by altering its natural property by chemical reaction. Carboxy ethyl cellulose and carboxy methyl cellulose are examples of modified gums.

Synthetic gums – Derived by chemical synthesis. Polyvinyl pyrrolidone and polyethylene oxide are examples of synthetic gums.

Gums are classified as

1. *Based on its source* – Includes marine origin, plant origin, animal origin, and microbial origin.

2. *Based on its charge* – Anionic gums, non-ionic seed gums, cationic polysaccharides, hydrophobic polysaccharides, and amphoteric polysaccharides.

3. *Based on its semi-synthetic property* – Starch and cellulose derivaties.

4. *Based on it shape* – Linear and branched

5. *Based on its chemical structure and its monomeric units* – Homoglycans, heteroglycans, triheteroglycans, tetra-heteroglycans, and penta-heteroglycans.

2.4 Gums in pulmonary drug delivery systems

The following gums are utilized extensively in pulmonary drug delivery systems

- Tamarind gum
- Almond gum
- Cashew gum
- Albizia gum
- Abelmoschus gum
- Ferula gum
- Cordia mucilage [50]

2.5 Biopolymeric nanoparticle disease diagnosis and treatment

Theranostic is a conveyance framework that integrates the diagnosis and treatment in a single portion. Theranostics can be used as imaging agent(s), also as medication in a single portion to resolve the barriers in imaging and treatment [51]. Biopolymeric nanoparticles are used widely for the diease diagnosis and treatment. In disease diagnosis, among the different polymers, chiotsan biopolymer has been utilized extensively due to its unique properties, presence of functional groups, and biocompatibility.

Lee and team coated the oleic acid by FeO nanoparticles (NPs); further, they conjugated the nanoparticles in oleic acid-chitosan. These developed NPs were used to examine the tumor cells by penetrability and holding consequences based on resonance imaging mechanisms and near infrared mechanisms. It was observed that the NPs displayed perceptible signal strength and upgrading in the tumor tissues through a higher EPR consequence [52]. Alginate was physically conjugated with folic acid-modifed chitosan and developed NPs. These developed NPs are utilized to treat colorectal cancer (CC) based on the release of 5-aminolevulinic (5-ALA) in the cells. The study observed that the developed NPs showed improved release of 5-ALA in CC cells [53].

Other than chiotosan, hyaluronic acid (HA) is another biopolymeric material that is glycosaminoglycan, negatively charged, and biocompatible. This HA is present in the extracellular matrix, and it can bind with the CD44 receptor through receptor link interaction. These CD44 receptors are expressed in different cancer cells [54–56]. Dospamine-modified HA was coated on the surface of iron oxide NPs. This developed NP comprises both hydrophilic component in the exterior surface and hydrophobic component in the interior surface containing homocamptothecin as chemotherapeutic agent. Uptake of this NP by cancer cells was examined thorugh MRI and observed that this developed NPs showed improved uptake by tumor cells and eradication of the tumor cells [57]. For earlier detection and to provide effective treatment in colon cancer, NPs were developed by conjugation between polyethylene glycol and HA through the thermostatic system. Subsequently, these developed NPs are chemically conjugated with near-infrared fluorescent dye and then encapsulated in the anticancer drug Irinotecan. The study results demonstrated that the developed NPs with fluorescent dye showed clear images of minute, initial, and liver-embedded colon cancer cells by near infrared (NIR) imaging method. Further, this NP effectively delivered the anticancer drug to the tumor targets and reduced the development of tumors [58].

Alginate is another natural polymer, utilized extensively in biomedical field due to its cost, inert, and tuneful nature and its gelling abilities [59, 60]. Alginate was used to stabilize the perfluorohexane (PFH) nanodroplets, and then the cancer drug doxorubicin was loaded. Further, the nanodroplets are delivered to the target site based on the sensitivity of ultrasound, and then its therapeutic efficacy through imaging is evaluated [61]. Nanogel containing gadolinium was developed and used in MRI imaging as positive contrast agents in different pharmacological applications [62].

Dextran is another neutral polymeric material that is non-toxic, well tolerated, and biodegrable. Dextran NPs are conjugated with Fe_3O_4 nanoparticles by redox-responsive chlorine 6 for MRI and NIR imaging in the determination of cancer [63, 64].

2.6 Nanoparticle in cancer

Nanoparticle has some unique optical, electrical, mechanical, and magnetic properties, as well as size, shape, surface area, and charge. Due to its unique properties and enhanced drug delivery, targeting tumor cells and reduced side effects of nanoparticles have been entensively investigated and utilized in cancer diagnosis as well as treatment. Few nanoparticles in cancer investigation studies are outlined.

Li et al. performed clinical trials by comparing the recurrent ovarian cancer between pegylated liposomal doxorubicin plus carboplastin and paclitaxel plus carboplatin. The study results outlined pegylated liposomal doxorubicin plus carboplastin, which exhibited higher activity than paclitaxel (PAC) plus carboplatin [65]. Lao et al. made a comparative review between doxorubicin and liposomal doxorucin such as myocet, daunoXome, and doxil in the treatment of breast cancer. Myocet is formulated with conventional liposomes; daunoXome has prolonged circulation half life liposomes, and doxil is a liposome made with polyethylene glycol. The side effects of doxorucin include alopecia, cardiotoxicity, mucositis, myelosuppression, emesis, and theoccurrednce of secondary leukemias. Among the different side effects, cardiotoxicity has been considered as a major concern in the treatment of cancer with doxorubicin. The study results demonstrated that liposomal doxorubicin showed decreased cardiotoxicity and higher efficiency in breast cancer. Further, they outlined that liposomal doxorubicin can be used in metastatic and early breast cancer therapy [66].

De Luca et al. examined the activity, safety, and quality of life of metastatic breast cancer (MBC) patients with the treatment of Abraxane (albumin-bound paclitaxel nanoparticle/Nab-paclitaxel), which is a new formulation. The study results demonstrated that Abraxane enhanced the tolerability profile also exhibited an significant effect on metastatic breast cancer. From the study, they concluded that Abraxane can be used as a safe therapeutic compound in treating patients with MBC [67]. Al-Hajeili and team examined the potential of Nab-paclitaxel with gemcitabine against pancreatic cancer. The review results suggested that Nab-paclitaxel with gemcitabine showed improved activity against pancreatic cancer and also suggested to have further investigation for its toxicity [68]. Cancer cells possess low vascular permeability against various anticancer drugs. Kinoshita evaluated the tumor selectivity of Nab-paclitaxel (nab-PTX) with *S*-nitrosated human serum albumin dimer based on the augmention and tumor growth inhibition in B16 murine melanoma subcutaneous inoculation model. The study results demonstrated that nab-PTX with SNO-HAS exhibited higher antitumor activity against pancraetaic cancer [69].

Autio et al. examined the safety and efficacy of prostate-specific membrane antigen (PSMA)-directed docetaxel-containing nanoparticle in patients having metastatic castration-resistant prostate cancer. The study results demonstrated that docetaxel exhibited antitumor activity; they also outlined that the expression levels of PSMA on circulating tumor tissues due to EPR effect may be the reason for its antitumor activity [70]. siRNA nanoparticles (CALAA-01) is a nanoparticle-based therapeutic delivery of siRNA to the tumor cells. This siRNA targets and silences the gene encoding ribonucleotide reductase. This enzyme is responsible for DNA replication in cancer cells. The study results demonstrated that CALAA-01 effectively delivered the gene-silencing molecules into the tumor cells and exhibited antitumor activity [71].

Tak and team examined the lyso-thermosensitive liposomal doxorubicin (ThermoDox) enhancing ability of radiofrequency ablation (RFA) to the patient having hepatocellular carcinoma. The study results highlighted that ThermoDox remained intact in normal body temperataure, whereas it releases the drugs in localized hyperthermia when the heat is applied around 40–42°C. Further, they demonstrated that this heat therapy can be used to release the drug in a controlled maner in the tumor cells as localized drug delivery exhibited significant antitumor activity [72]. A composite nanoparticle consisting of Camptothecin encapsulated with magnetic iron oxide (Fe_3O_4) and β-cyclodextrin as cross-linked with ethylenediaminetetraacetic acid (EDTA) was developed and examined for its antitumor activity against HT29 colon cancer cells and A549 lung cancer cells, and it was outlined that the developed nanoparticle exhibited significant antitumor activity against both cell lines by inducing apoptosis by caspase-3 activation [73].

To overcome the poor solubility of Camptothecin, a polymeric nanoparticle (CRLX101) consisting of cyclodextrin-poly(ethylene glycol) copolymer was developed by cyclodextrin polymeric nanoparticle technology, and its solubility was assessed. The developed nanoparticle showed more than 1000-fold increase in apparent solublity than the parent drug Camptothecin; it also exhibited enhanced pharmacodynamic property [74]. CRLX101 was examined as a radiosensitizer in colorectal cancer cell in xenograft models. The study results demonstrated that CRLX101 sensitized the cancer cells and showed significant antitumor activity by preventing the repairing of DNA and activity of HIF-1α pathway [75].

2.7 Inorganic nanoparticles

Inorganic NPs are hybrids made by association between inorganic NPs and organic compounds. Inorganic NPs include gold, silver, iron, zinc, cerium, copper, selenium, aluminum, cadmium, gadolinium, nickel, titanium, platinum, magnesium, palladium, rhenium, ruthenium, and many are used. Owing to their size, shape, and stability, metal NPs as inorganic NPs are widely utilized in several biomedical applications like biosensor, bioimaging, hyperthermia, drug delivery, and photoablation therapy due to their flexibility and biocompatibility [42, 76–78].

Among these, gold and silver NPs are widely accepted and utilized because of their specific surface plasmon resonance properties. Though these metal NPs are used yet, there is no clear information about their mechanism and toxicity. However, transcytosis and paracellular transport are considered as the proposed mechanisms for their delivery [79].

3. Quantum dots

Quantum dots (QDs) are another category of inorganic nanoparticle, which are semiconductor luminescent nanocrystals with a diameter of 1–10 nm and possess optical property based on their absorbance and photoluminescence [80]. Elements from the group of II to VI like Hg, Cd, Ag, Ln, P, Zn, Pb, Se, and Te are commonly used in the preparation of QDs. These QDs are different from conventional organic compounds. The QDs possess emission in NIR region (<650 nm), increased signal brightness, instantaneous excitation of multiple fluoreence colors, size-tunable light emission, photo bleaching, reduced light scattering, and low absorption by the tissue. Based on the size and laser light source, these QDs exhibit diverse colors like yellow, yellowish green, orange, orange, yellowish orange, maple red-orange, blue, green, greenish blue, and adirondack green. The controlled drug delivery can be accomplished through external stimulation like heat, light, magnetic fields, radio frequency, and so on. Further, the specific properties of QDs are broadly used in biomedical imaging as multiplex imaging, sensors, and theranostics in various cancers as targeted/controlled drug delivery [81–84].

These QDs are spherical semiconductors having three parts like cap, shell, and core. The core part is prepared by CdSe as the semiconductor material and ZnS coat as shell. These core and shell are encapsulated by a double layer [42]. QDs depend on the type of cadmium present in the core as it emits dissimilar wavelengths of radiations. For UV, cadmium sulphide and far – IR and NIR cadmium telluride are used to prepare QDs.

3.1 Biomedical applications

These QDs have unique optical properties, which include good brightness, good quantum yield, good fluorescence signal, and good extinction coefficient. These unique properties are utilized especially in disease diagnosis as imaging based on its emission spectra.

- Fluorescence Imaging – QDs are used as fluorescent probes for imaging tissues, cells, and biomolecules.
- Cancer diagnosis – QDs can be conjugated with antibodies or ligands that target cancer cells as biomarkers to visualize the tumors and metastases.
- Biomarker detection – QDs can be functionalized with different biomolecules such as antibodies, peptides, or nucleic acids to target specific disease biomarkers like cancer proteins.
- Quantum dots in immunoassays – Enhanced ELISA (enzyme-linked immunosorbent assay): QDs are used to improve traditional immunoassays like ELISA. This property has been used to accurately detect the disease-related antigens, such as in HIV, hepatitis, or cancer.
- In vivo imaging and diagnostics – Real-time imaging – It is used to track the progression of disease and growth stage in tumor cells as well as to identify the spread of infections within the body. It is also used in detecting abnormalities within organs or tissues of interest.
- Quantum dots in biosensors – QDs can be incorporated into biosensor platforms as biosensor for detecting different biological fluids like saliva, blood, and urine.
- Detection of genetic mutations as genetic screening – QDs can be used to identify the mutations in DNA or RNA associated with specific diseases like BRCA1/BRCA2 for breast cancer or prenatal diagnostics to detect genetic abnormalities.
- Early detection of neurodegenerative diseases – QDs can be explored to identify the protein aggregates or misfolded proteins like as amyloid-beta or alpha-synuclein. This proteins are attributed to neurodegenerative diseases like Alzheimer's and Parkinson's disease.
- Early detection of infectious diseases – QDs can be conjugate with pathogen-specific probes, which allows the early detection of various infectious dieases like tuberculosis, HIV, and influenza.
- Quantum dot-magnetic nanoparticle hybrids – Incorporation of QDs with magnetic nanoparticles can create a hybrid system that is used for magnetic resonance imaging especially in cardiovascular disease and cancer [85–87].

4. Lipid-based drug delivery system

4.1 Vesicular drug delivery system

In the last few decades, several research studies have been performed in novel drug delivery systems to achieve increased solubility, delivering the drug at the targeted site to improve the bioavailability and extended period of drug release of poorly water-soluble drugs.

During 1965, Bingham used biological origin as vesicle in drug delivery. Vescicular drug delivery system (VDDS) has been considered as one of the outcome of these research studies by the researchers. VDDS are highly ordered assemblies comprising one or more concentric lipid bilayer made with self-assembling of amphiphilic building blocks encountered with water. This drug carrier can be formulated to release the drug at the specific site, and sustained/controlled release leads to prevention of drug loss, increased bioavailablity at the target site, and prevention of drug accumulation and side effects. These lipid-based formulations are generally employed especially to increase the solubility of Class II & IV drugs according to the Biopharmaceutics Classification System (BCS) [88–90].

Lipid-based drug delivery system includes solid lipid nanoparticles and lipid nanoparticles, which are the two major groups of drug delivery. VDDS includes liposome, aquasomes, niosomes, cubosomes, cryptosmes, colloidosomes, discomes, enzymosomes, genosomes, photosomes, virosomes, vesosomes, ethosomes, emulsomes, exosome, eposomes, sphinogosomes, phytosomes, proteasomes, pharmacosomes, transferosomes, ufasomes, and so on.

Lipids like phospholipids, cholesterol, sterols, waxes, oils, and glycerides are preferably used in lipid-based drug delivery systems. These lipids are insoluble in polar solvents and readily soluble in non-polar solvents.

Lipids used in lipid-based drug delivery systems are categoriezed into:

1. Homolipids – Example: Glycerides, cerides, and sterides

2. Heterolipids – Example: Sulfolipids, glycolipids, and phospholipids

3. Complex lipids – Example: Waxes, steroids, and fats [89–94].

Various types of VDDS are shown in **Figure 2**.

4.2 Regulatory challenges in nanoparticle drug delivery

Drug delivery systems based on nanoparticles have shown great potential in improving precision, safety, efficacy, and therapeutic activity. However, these DDS have significant regulatory challenges and ethical concerns due to their unique properties, interaction with biological systems, impact on human health, and the environment. The following issues are considered as major regulatory concerns in the approval of nanoparticle drug delivery systems. The major regulatory concerns are

- Lack of established regulatory frameworks – These nanoparticles do not fit into a class of drugs or devices as undefined regulatory categories; hence, it is difficult to apply any conventional regulatory guidelines and standarrds. U.S. Food and Drug Administration (FDA), European Medicines Agency (EMA), and other agencies are evolving new guidelines for these nanoparticle-based therapies.

- Toxicity and biocompatibility concerns – These nanoparticles have unpredictable interaction with different biological systems and their accumulation in certain organs. Also, they cross the blood-brain barrier. Further, long duration of action and their presence in the body may create non-degrading ability of the nanoparticle in the human being.

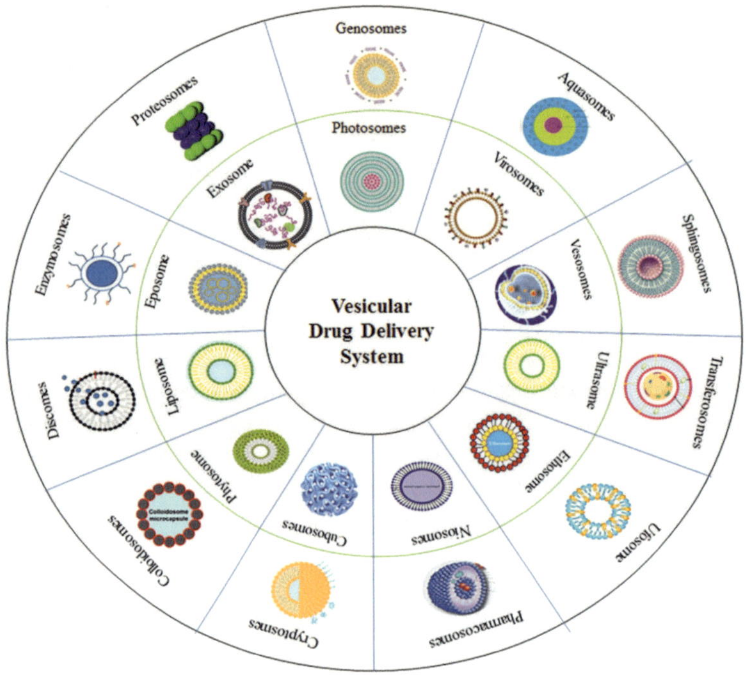

Figure 2.
Various types of vesicular drug delivery systems.

- Challenges in characterization and standardization – Variability in its characterization properties like size, shape, surface charge, and its biological system behavior may show unpredictable therapeutic effect. Further alternation in the synthesis/production process can exhibit significant difference in its properties. So, it is not possible to ensure its batch to batch consistency.

- Uncertain pharmacokinetics and pharmacodynamics – Establishing the relationship between the nanoparticle carrier and active pharmaceutical ingredient is more complex. Also unable to predict the pharmacokinetics (PK) and pharmacodynamics (PD) properties of the drug substances due to its interaction with the biological system. But, established PK and PD details are essential for the approval process.

- Nanoparticle-specific testing requirements – Due to their unique properties, nanoparticle drug delivery systems require specialized technique like advanced imaging method to assess their safety and efficacy during *in vitro* and *in vivo* testing. Further, these nanoparticles may induce immune reactions. In consequence, additional studies are required to determine if any immune response, inflammation, and hypersensitivity are induced.

- Environmental concerns – Due to their unique properties, the great concern in the environmental is how the nanoparticles are inclined/disposed of in manufacturing process as well as how they are excreted by patients.

- Occupational health – Their unique particle size showed health risks to the human being in production and handling of nanoparticle due to their skin exposure and inhalation.

Ethical concerns

- Informed consent and patient safety – These nanoparticles exhbit uncertainties of safety due to their unique sze. Thus, informed consent and their risks should be explained to the patients for better understanding before the treatment therapy.

- Access and equity issues – Cost for the preparation of nanoparticles for treatment is very expensive. Therefore, cost for the equitable access for this therapies in low-resource settings or countries becomes very difficult, and it will be accessable only in the developed countries.

- Long-term health implications – Still, there is a unclear information about their long-term health effects and immediate therapeutic benefits. But, potential adverse effects to patients on treatment have become evident until years later. Further, frequent exposure to the nanoparticle that can accumulate on the tissues may produce unpredicted toxic effect to the tissues.

- Environmental impact – After excretion from the human body, it can enter into the acquatic system. Accumulation in the environment leads to harm the ecosystem. Because of that, the need to balance between nanoparticle benefits and environment cost arises.

Considering the regulatory challenges and environmental concern, regulatory agencies are framing guidelines for safe handling of nanoparticles and their disposal. Ensuring proper safety protocols and regulatory oversight is necessary for approving these nanoparticle drug delivery systems. Also, ensure to prevent potential harm to workers as patient safety and its impact on the environment [95–104].

4.3 Artificial intelligence in drug delivery

Artificial intelligence (AI) is interesting and increasingly playing a transformative role in drug delivery. Also, it is playing a role in drug design, discovery, development, formulation, and delivery to patients.

Role of AI in drug delivery includes

- Predictive modeling for drug formulation – AI algorithms can be used to predict the new drug substance's solubility, stability, and bioavailability during the development process, which can help to improve the development process. Further, it helps to develop a new formulation with higher efficacy and fewer side effects.

- Optimizing nanoparticle design – AI can be used to predict the interaction between nanoparticles and biological environment like tissue/organ and target cells, which can help to design a more suitable and effective drug carrier to deliver the drug at the target sites.

- Nanomedicine drug delivery – AI can help to optimize the nanoparticle size, shape, and surface characteristic property, which can help to deliver the drug to the target site or tissue/organs and reduce the off-target effects in healthy tissues.

- Specific nanoparticle design – AI can help to design the nanoparticle with specific initiates like pH, temperature, enzymes, and so on for targeted drug delivery. It is also used to forecast their release and activity.

- Optimization of route of drug delivery – AI can help to determine the most suitable and effective route of drug delivery based on drug product properties and patient characteristics. Also, it can simulate how the drugs can overcome the difficult-to-penetrate barriers like the blood-brain barrier and gastrointestinal tract.

- Improving controlled and sustained drug release – AI can help to develop the delivery of drugs by optimizing the time, dose, and release of drugs in a controlled manner especially for chronic diseases like diabetes or cancer. Also, it helps to monitor the real-time blood glucose levels and heart rate, accordingly adjusting the delivery of drugs.

- Optimizing drug loading and release in nanocarriers – Based on previous experimental data, AI can help to predict the suitable and best combination of materials for drug loading and release of drugs from nanocarriers to improve the release profile. Further, it helps to modifty the release profile by adjusting the systems for specific therapeutic needs.

- Designing of drug delivery system – AI can help to test different nanocarriers based on their molecular interaction, surface chemistry, and their behavior in biological systems. Subsequently, it can help to predict the suitable drug delivery system as site specific and to produce the desired effect in the body.

- Clinical trial design for drug delivery – AI can help to design more effective and effeicent clinical trials based on the preclinical and clinical data. Also, it helps to predict the populations for study, optimal dosing regimens, and delivery methods to different delivery systems, which can help to reduce the trial and error and length of the clinical trial process.

- Improving drug targeting and precision medicine – Based on the drug molecule profile and genetic, AI can help to predict the most suitable form of targeted drug delivery system especially in treating cancer patients. Also, it helps to modify the surface property of nanoparticles for better cancer cell targeting in cancer therapy.

- Improving biodegradable and biocompatible materials – Based on the earlier data, AI can help to predict the biocompatibility and biodegradable polymers in drug delivery, which can help to identify a suitable material in drug delivery to ensure its safety and effect in the human body. Also, it helps to estimate the degrading ability and clearance from the body to avoid long-term toxicity due to accumulation [105–110].

5. Conclusion

Developing new drug molecules in the drug discovery process depends on the emergency needs and its market potential. A lot of research studies are constantly being performed based on the conventional dosage form in order to provide a desired therapeutic effect. In view of this, as an outcome, novel drug delivery systems were developed as a controlled/sustained release formulation. However, inconsistent delivery of drugs at the targeted site is a drawback of this targeted drug delivery system. Further research studies adopted nanotechnology, and the outcome has been utilized in almost all the fields, especially in biomedical applications where hybrid materials and inorganic and organic materials are used to enhance the solubility of poorly soluble drugs, absorption, and bioavailability. Yet, extending its release rate to targeted drug delivery was a challenging lacuna. Throughout the world, recent advancements in utilization of biopolymers and lipids in nanotechnology as biopolymeric nanoparticle and vesicular drug delivery systems have helped to deliver the drugs in specific tissues/organs as targeted drug delivery is also used as theranostics. This advancement is being effectively adopted to treat cancer, genetic diseases, and many life-threatening diseases. However, there is a lacuna in the regulatory guidelines for the effective utilization of these drug delivery systems. Hence, regulatory agencies are framing different guidelines to ensure its safe utilization and its disposal without affecting the ecosystem. Recently, AI has become a revolutionizing one and is being exploited in drug design, discovery, development, and treatment processes. Still, a lot of research studies are needed in these DDS to overcome the challenges in their usage.

Author details

Appavoo Umamaheswari[1], Ayarivan Puratchikody[1], Sakthivel Lakshmana Prabu[1*] and Rathinasabapathy Thirumurugan[2†]

1 Department of Pharmaceutical Technology, University College of Engineering (BIT Campus), Anna University, Tiruchirappalli, India

2 Department of Pharmaceutical Chemistry, Sree Abirami College of Pharmacy (Affiliated to The Tamil Nadu Dr.M.G.R. Medical University, Chennai), Coimbatore, India

*Address all correspondence to: slaxmanvel@aubit.edu.in

†Rathinasabapthy Thirumurugan contributed equally in this manuscript.

References

[1] Lakshmana Prabu S, Thirumurugan R, Suriyarakash TNK. In: Reedijk J, editor. Elsevier Reference Module in Chemistry, Molecular Sciences and Chemical Engineering. Waltham, MA: Elsevier; 2014. DOI: 10.1016/8978-0-12-409547-2.11400-3

[2] Changxiao L, Panayiotis PC, Yazhuo L. Research and development in drug innovation: Reflections from the 2013 bioeconomy conference in China, lessons learned and future perspectives. Acta Pharmaceutica Sinica B. 2014;**4**(2):112-119

[3] Domenico F. Hypothesis for changing models: Current pharmaceutical paradigms, trends and approaches in drug discovery. PeerJ. 2015;**3**:e813v1

[4] DiMasi JA. Risks in new drug development: Approval success rates for investigational drugs. Clinical Pharmacology and Therapeutics. 2001;**69**:297-307

[5] Arrowsmith J. Phase II failures: 2008-2010. Nature Reviews. Drug Discovery. 2011;**10**:328-329

[6] Arrowsmith J, Miller P. Trial watch: Phase II and phase III attrition rates 2011-2012. Nature Reviews. Drug Discovery. 2013;**12**:569

[7] Akala EO. Oral controlled release solid dosage forms. In: Theory and Practice of Contemporary Pharmaceutics. Florida: CRC Press; 2004. pp. 333-366

[8] Malm CJ, Emerson J, Hiait GD. Cellulose acetate phthalate as an enteric coating material. Journal of the American Pharmacists Association (Scientific Ed.). 1951;**40**:520-525. DOI: 10.1002/jps.3030401014

[9] Hillery A, Park K. Drug Delivery: Fundamentals and Applications. Boca Raton: CRC Press; 2016

[10] Lee PI, Li JX. Evolution of oral controlled release dosage forms. In: Wen H, Park K, editors. Oral Controlled Release Formulation Design and Drug Delivery: Theory to Practice. Hoboken, NJ: John Wiley & Sons, Inc.; 2010. pp. 21-31

[11] Bangham AD, Horne RW. Negative staining of phospholipids and their structural modification by surface-active agents as observed in the electron microscope. Journal of Molecular Biology. 1964;**8**(5):660-668

[12] Bangham AD, Standish MM, Watkins JC. Diffusion of univalent ions across the lamellae of swollen phospholipids. Journal of Molecular Biology. 1965;**8**(1):238-252

[13] Birrenbach G, Speiser PP. Polymerized micelles and their use as adjuvants in immunology. Journal of Pharmaceutical Sciences. 1976;**65**(12):1763-1766

[14] Park K. Drug delivery of the future: Chasing the invisible gorilla. Journal of Controlled Release. 2016;**240**:2-8

[15] Ye M, Kim S, Park K. Issues in long-term protein delivery using biodegradable microparticles. Journal of Controlled Release. 2010;**146**(2):241-260

[16] Zhang W, Zhao Q, Deng J, Hu Y, Wang Y, Ouyang D. Big data analysis of global advances in pharmaceutics and drug delivery 1980-2014. Drug Discovery Today. 2017;**22**(8):1201-1208

[17] Park K. Controlled drug delivery systems: Past forward and future back. Journal of Controlled Release. 2014;**190**:3-8

[18] Yun YH, Lee BK, Park K. Controlled drug delivery: Historical perspective for the next generation. Journal of Controlled Release. 2015;**219**:2-7

[19] RMD K. The clinical development of new drugs. In: Mathieu M, editor. New Drug Development: A Regulatory Overview. 6th ed. Waltham: PAREXEL International Corporation; 2002. pp. 85-110

[20] Friedman LM, Furberg CD, DeMets DL. Introduction to clinical trials. In: Reboussin DM, Granger CB, editors. Fundamentals of Clinical Trials. Switzerland: Springer International Publishing; 2015. pp. 1-18

[21] Comparison of Clinical Trial Phases. Available from: http://gpatindia.com/wp-content/uploads/2010/02/comparison-of-clinical-trial-phases.pdf [Accessed: March 30, 2024]

[22] Adepu S, Ramakrishna S. Controlled drug delivery systems: Current status and future directions. Molecules. 2021;**26**:5905

[23] Laffleur F, Keckeis V. Advances in drug delivery systems: Work in progress still needed? International Journal of Pharmaceutics. 2020;**590**(30):119912

[24] Rajan KV, Sanjay G. Current status of drug delivery technologies and future directions. Pharmaceutical Technology On-Line. 2001;**25**(2):1-14

[25] Keraliya RA, Patel C, Patel P, Keraliya V, Soni TG, Patel RC, et al. Osmotic drug delivery system as a part of modified release dosage form. ISRN Pharmacology. 2012;**2012**:528079

[26] Vargason AM, Anselmo AC, Mitragotri S. The evolution of commercial drug delivery technologies. Nature Biomedical Engineering. 2021;**5**:951-967

[27] Liu Z, Tabakman S, Welsher K, Dai H. Carbon nanotubes in biology and medicine: *in vitro* and *in vivo* detection, imaging and drug delivery. Nano Research. 2009;**2**:85-120

[28] Chen YC, Huang XC, Luo YL, Chang YC, Hsieh YZ, Hsu HY. Non-metallic nanomaterials in cancer theranostics: A review of silica- and carbon-based drug delivery systems. Science and Technology of Advanced Materials. 2013;**14**:404-407

[29] Suri SS, Fenniri H, Singh B. Nanotechnology-based drug delivery systems. Journal of Occupational Medicine and Toxicology. 2007;**2**:16

[30] Faheem A, Abdelkader DH. Novel drug delivery systems. In: Seyfoddin A, Dezfooli SM, Greene CA, editors. Engineering Drug Delivery Systems. Woodhead Publishing Series in Biomaterials. United Kingdom: Elsevier; 2020. pp. 1-16

[31] Rahman HS, Othman HH, Hammadi NI, Yeap SK, Amin KM, Abdul Samad N, et al. Novel drug delivery systems for loading of natural plant extracts and their biomedical applications. International Journal of Nanomedicine. 2020;**15**:2439-2483

[32] Nam NH, Luong NH. Nanoparticles: Synthesis and applications. In: Grumezescu V, Grumezescu AM, editors. Materials for Biomedical Engineering. 2019. pp. 211-240

[33] Umamaheswari A, Vijayalakshmi M, Dhivya Sree M, Lakshmana Prabu S, Puratchikody A. Cogent and strategic

approaches for gene delivery with nanostructures. In: Suresh CA, Rakshit A, editors. The Science of Nanomaterials: Basics and Applications. FL, USA: Apple Academic Press, Inc. Co-published with CRC Press (Taylor & Francis); 2022. pp. 91-121

[34] Baig N, Kammakakam I, Falath W. Nanomaterials: A review of synthesis methods, properties, recent progress, and challenges. Materials Advances. 2021;**2**(6):1821-1871

[35] Kumari A, Kumar V, Yadav S. Nanotechnology: A tool to enhance therapeutic values of natural plant products. Trends in Medical Research. 2012;7:34-42

[36] Joseph RR, Venkatraman SS. Drug delivery to the eye: What benefits do nanocarriers ofer? Nanomedicine. 2017;**12**:683-702

[37] Mirza AZ, Siddiqui FA. Nanomedicine and drug delivery: A mini review. International Nano Letters. 2014;**4**:94

[38] Rudramurthy GR, Swamy MK, Sinniah UR, Ghasemzadeh A. Nanoparticles: Alternatives against drug-resistant pathogenic microbes. Molecules. 2016;**21**:836

[39] Wilczewska AZ, Niemirowicz K, Markiewicz KH, Car H. Nanoparticles as drug delivery systems. Pharmacological Reports. 2012;**64**:1020-1037

[40] Hans ML, Lowman AM. Nanoparticles for Drug Delivery. USA: Taylor & Francis Group, LLC; 2006

[41] Mittal P, Saharan A, Verma R, Altalbawy FMA, Alfaidi MA, Batiha GE, et al. Dendrimers: A new race of pharmaceutical nanocarriers. BioMed Research International. 2021;**2021**:8844030

[42] Lakshmana Prabu S, Ruckmani K. Biopolymers in gene delivery. In: Sabyasachi M, Kalyar KS, editors. Advanced Technology for Delivering Therapeutics. London, UK, Croatia: InTech Publication; 2017. pp. 137-158

[43] Abbasi E, Aval SF, Akbarzadeh A, Milani M, Nasrabadi HT, Joo SW, et al. Dendrimers: Synthesis, applications, and properties. Nanoscale Research Letters. 2014;**9**(1):247

[44] Chis AA, Dobrea C, Morgovan C, Arseniu AM, Rus LL, Butuca A, et al. Applications and limitations of dendrimers in biomedicine. Molecules (Basel, Switzerland). 2020;**25**(17):3982

[45] Wang J, Li B, Qiu L, Yang H. Dendrimer-based drug delivery systems: History, challenges, and latest developments. Journal of Biological Engineering. 2022;**16**:18

[46] Li L, Deng Y, Zeng Y, Yan B, Deng Y, Zheng Z, et al. The application advances of dendrimers in biomedical field. Viewpoints. 2023;**4**(6):20230023

[47] Lakshmana Prabu S, Suriya Prakash TNK, Thirumurugan R. Medicated nanoparticle for gene delivery. In: Sabyasachi M, Kalyar KKS, editors. Advanced Technology for Delivering Therapeutics. London, UK, Croatia: InTech Publication; 2017. pp. 13-29

[48] Bharat T, Yogita C. Gums and mucilages: Excipients for modified drug delivery system. Journal of Advanced Pharmacy Education and Research. 2013;**3**(4):359-367

[49] Lankalapalli S, Sandhala D. A review on natural gums and their use as

pharmaceutical excipients. International Journal of Pharmaceutical Sciences and Research. 2013;**10**(12):5274-5283

[50] Umamaheswari A, Vijayalakshmi M, Barath Raj S, Dinesh Kumar C, Lakshmana PS. Gum based drug delivery systems. In: Harish D, Kamal D, editors. Natural Polymeric Materials Based Drug Delivery Systems in Lung Diseases. Singapore: Springer Nature Singapore Pte Ltd; 2023. pp. 147-166

[51] Xue Y, Gao Y, Meng F, Luo L. Recent progress of nanotechnology-based theranostic systems in cancer treatments. Cancer Biology & Medicine. 2021;**18**(2):336-351

[52] Lee CM, Jang D, Kim J, Cheong SJ, Kim EM, Jeong MH, et al. Oleyl-chitosan nanoparticles based on a dual probe for optical/MR imaging *in vivo*. Bioconjugate Chemistry. 2011;**22**:186-192

[53] Yang SJ, Lin FH, Tsai HM, Lin CF, Chin HC, Wong JM, et al. Alginate-folic acid-modified chitosan nanoparticles for photodynamic detection of intestinal neoplasms. Biomaterials. 2011;**32**:2174-2182

[54] Choi KY, Chung H, Min KH, Yoon HY, Kim K, Park JH, et al. Self-assembled hyaluronic acid nanoparticles for active tumor targeting. Biomaterials. 2010;**31**:106-114

[55] Kamat M, El-Boubbou K, Zhu DC, Lansdell T, Lu X, Li W, et al. Hyaluronic acid immobilized magnetic nanoparticles for active targeting and imaging of macrophages. Bioconjugate Chemistry. 2010;**21**:2128-2135

[56] Arpicco S, Lerda C, Dalla Pozza E, Costanzo C, Tsapis N, Stella B, et al. Hyaluronic acid-coated liposomes for active targeting of gemcitabine. European Journal of Pharmaceutics and Biopharmaceutics. 2013;**85**:373-380

[57] Wang G, Gao S, Tian R, Miller-Kleinhenz J, Qin Z, Liu T, et al. Theranostic hyaluronic acid-iron micellar nanoparticles for magnetic-field enhanced *in vivo* cancer chemotherapy. ChemMed Chem. 2018;**13**:78-86

[58] Choi KY, Jeon EJ, Yoon HY, Lee BS, Na JH, Min KH, et al. Theranostic nanoparticles based on PEGylated hyaluronic acid for the diagnosis, therapy and monitoring of colon cancer. Biomaterials. 2012;**33**:6186-6193

[59] Gombotz WR, Wee S. Protein release from alginate matrices. Advanced Drug Delivery Reviews. 1998;**31**:267-285

[60] Lee KY, Mooney DJ. Alginate: Properties and biomedical applications. Progress in Polymer Science. 2012;**37**:106-126

[61] Baghbani F, Moztarzadeh F, Mohandesi JA, Yazdian F, Mokhtari-Dizaji M. Novel alginate-stabilized doxorubicin-loaded nanodroplets for ultrasounic theranosis of breast cancer. International Journal of Biological Macromolecules. 2016;**93**:512-519

[62] Podgorna K, Szczepanowicz K, Piotrowski M, Gajdosova M, Stepanek F, Warszynski P. Gadolinium alginate nanogels for theranostic applications. Colloids and Surfaces B: Biointerfaces. 2017;**153**:183-189

[63] Moscovici M. Present and future medical applications of microbial exopolysaccharides. Frontiers in Microbiology. 2015;**1012**:6

[64] Ding Z, Liu P, Hu D, Sheng Z, Yi H, Gao G, et al. Redox-responsive dextran based theranostic nanoparticles for

near-infrared/magnetic resonance imaging and magnetically targeted photodynamic therapy. Biomaterials Science. 2017;**5**:762-771

[65] Li XR, Zhu Y, Zhang GN, Huang JM, Pei LX. The impact of pegylated liposomal doxorubicin in recurrent ovarian cancer: An updated meta-analysis of randomized clinical trials. Journal of Ovarian Research. 2021;**14**:42

[66] Lao J, Madani J, Puertolas T, Álvarez M, Hernández A, Pazo-Cid R, et al. Liposomal doxorubicin in the treatment of breast cancer patients: A review. Journal of Drug Delivery Science and Technology. 2013;**2013**:456409

[67] De Luca R, Profita G, Cicero G. Nab-paclitaxel in pretreated metastatic breast cancer: Evaluation of activity, safety, and quality of life. Oncotargets and Therapy. 2019;**12**:1621-1627

[68] Al-Hajeili M, Azmi AS, Choi M. Nab-paclitaxel: Potential for the treatment of advanced pancreatic cancer. Oncotargets and Therapy. 2014;**7**:187-192

[69] Kinoshita R, Ishima Y, Chuang VT, Nakamura H, Fang J, Watanabe H, et al. Improved anticancer effects of albumin-bound paclitaxel nanoparticle via augmentation of EPR effect and albumin-protein interactions using S-nitrosated human serum albumin dimer. Biomaterials. 2017;**140**:162-169

[70] Autio KA, Dreicer R, Anderson J, Garcia JA, Alva A, Hart LL, et al. Safety and efficacy of BIND-014, a docetaxel nanoparticle targeting prostate-specific membrane antigen for patients with metastatic castration-resistant prostate cancer: A phase 2 clinical trial. JAMA Oncology. 2018;**4**(10):1344-1351

[71] Hattab D, Gazzali AM, Bakhtiar A. Clinical advances of siRNA-based nanotherapeutics for cancer treatment. Pharmaceutics. 2021;**13**(7):1009

[72] Tak WY, Lin SM, Wang Y, Zheng J, Vecchione A, Park SY, et al. Phase III HEAT study adding lyso-thermosensitive liposomal doxorubicin to radiofrequency ablation in patients with unresectable hepatocellular carcinoma lesions. Clinical Cancer Research. 2018;**24**(1):73-83

[73] Krishnan P, Rajan M, Kumari S, SakinahS, PriyaSP, AmiraF, et al. Efficiency of newly formulated camptothecin with β-cyclodextrin-EDTA-Fe_3O_4 nanoparticle-conjugated nanocarriers as an anti-colon cancer (HT29) drug. Scientific Reports. 2017;**7**:10962

[74] Svenson S, Wolfgang M, Hwang J, Ryan J, Eliasof S. Preclinical to clinical development of the novel camptothecin nanopharmaceutical CRLX101. Journal of Controlled Release. 2011;**153**(1):49-55

[75] Tian X, Nguyen M, Foote HP, Caster JM, Roche KC, Peters CG, et al. CRLX101, a nanoparticle-drug conjugate containing Camptothecin, improves rectal cancer chemoradiotherapy by inhibiting DNA repair and HIF1α. Cancer Research. 2017;**77**(1):112-122

[76] McNamara K, Tofail SA. Nanosystems: The use of nanoalloys, metallic, bimetallic, and magnetic nanoparticles in biomedical applications. Physical Chemistry Chemical Physics. 2015;**17**:27981-27995

[77] McNamara K, Tofail SA. Nanoparticles in biomedical applications. Advances in Physics. 2017;**2**:54-88

[78] Kudr J, Haddad Y, Richtera L, Heger Z, Cernak M, Adam V, et al. Magnetic nanoparticles: From design and synthesis to real world applications. Nanomaterials. 2017;**7**:243

[79] Choi SJ, Lee JK, Jeong J, Choy JH. Toxicity evaluation of inorganic nanoparticles: Considerations and challenges. Molecular & Cellular Toxicology. 2013;**9**:205-210

[80] Vengala P, Dasari A, Yeruva N. Quantum dots for drug delivery and therapy international. Journal of Pharmacy Technology. 2012;**4**(2):2055-2074

[81] Cheki M, Moslehi M, Assadi M. Marvelous applications of quantum dots. European Review for Medical and Pharmacological Sciences. 2013;**17**:1141-1148

[82] Ozkan M. Quantum dots and other nanoparticles: What can they offer to drug discoveryμ. Drug Discovery Today. 2004;**9**:1065-1071

[83] Volkov Y. Quantum dots in nanomedicine: Recent trends, advances and unresolved issues. Biochemical and Biophysical Research Communications. 2015;**468**:419-427

[84] Xu G, Zeng S, Zhang B, Swihart MT, Yong K-T, Prasad PN. New generation cadmium-free quantum dots for biophotonics and nanomedicine. Chemical Reviews. 2016;**116**:12234-12327

[85] Abdellatif AAH, Younis MA, Alsharidah M, Al Rugaie O, Tawfeek HM. Biomedical applications of quantum dots: Overview, challenges, and clinical potential. International Journal of Nanomedicine. 2022;**17**:1951-1970

[86] Cotta MA. Quantum dots and their applications: What lies ahead? ACS Applied Nano Materials. 2020;**3**(6):4920-4924

[87] Nguyen AT, Baucom DR, Wang Y, Heyes CD. Compact, fast blinking Cd-free quantum dots for super-resolution fluorescence imaging. Chemical & Biomedical Imaging. 2023;**1**(3):251-259

[88] Ravi B, Sreekanth N, Bhargavi S, Babu RC, Arun K, Jaya Kishore BC, et al. Vesicular drug delivery system - an over view. Research Journal of Pharmaceutical, Biological and Chemical Sciences. 2013;**4**(3):462-474

[89] Puri A, Loomis K, Smith B, Lee JH, Yavlovich A, Heldman E, et al. Lipid-based nanoparticles as pharmaceutical drug carriers: From concepts to clinic. Critical Reviews in Therapeutic Drug Carrier Systems. 2009;**26**(6):523-580

[90] Attama AA, Momoh MA, Builders PF. Lipid nanoparticulate drug delivery systems: A revolution in dosage form design and development. In: Sezer AD, editor. Recent Advances in Novel Drug Carrier Systems. InTech: Croatia; 2012. pp. 107-140

[91] Jain S, Jain V, Mahajan SC. Lipid based vesicular drug delivery systems. Advance Pharmaceutical. 2014;**1**:574673

[92] Alenzi AM, Albalawi SA, Alghamdi SG, Albalawi RF, Albalawi HS, Qushawy M. Review on different vesicular drug delivery systems (VDDSs) and their applications. Recent Patents on Nanotechnology. 2023;**17**(1):18-32

[93] Bhupinder K, Reena G, Monica G, Sachin Kumar S, Rubiya K, Mukta G. The why, where, who, how, and what of the vesicular delivery systems. Advances in Colloid and Interface Science. 2019;**271**:101985

[94] Mohammad AR, Soma M, Yousof M, Faezeh A, Mohammad HN, Akram N, et al. A comprehensive and updated review on the applications of vesicular drug delivery systems in treatment of

brain disorders: A shelter against storms. Journal of Drug Delivery Science and Technology. 2023;**89**:105011

[95] Desai N. Challenges in development of nanoparticle-based therapeutics. The AAPS Journal. 2012;**14**(2):282-295

[96] Mühlebach S. Regulatory challenges of nanomedicines and their follow-on versions: A generic or similar approach? Advanced Drug Delivery Reviews. 2018;**131**:122-131

[97] Pasut G. Grand challenges in nano-based drug delivery. Frontiers in Medical Technology. 2019;**1**:1

[98] Csoka I, Ismail R, Jojart-Laczkovich O, Pallagi E. Regulatory considerations, challenges and risk-based approach in nanomedicine development. Current Medicinal Chemistry. 2021;**28**(36):7461-7476

[99] Foulkes R, Man E, Thind J, Yeung S, Joy A, Hoskins C. The regulation of nanomaterials and nanomedicines for clinical application: Current and future perspectives. Biomaterials Science. 2020;**8**(17):4653-4664

[100] Patra JK, Das G, Fraceto LF, Campos EVR, Rodriguez-Torres MP, Acosta-Torres LS. Nano based drug delivery systems: Recent developments and future prospects. Journal of Nanbiotechnology. 2018;**16**:71

[101] Ali F, Neha K, Parveen S. Current regulatory landscape of nanomaterials and nanomedicines: A global perspective. Journal of Drug Delivery Science and Technology. 2023;**80**:104118

[102] Wasti S, Lee IH, Kim S, Lee JH, Kim H. Ethical and legal challenges in nanomedical innovations: A scoping review. Frontiers in Genetics. 2023;**14**:1163392

[103] Souto EB, Dias-Ferreira J, Shegokar R, Durazzo A, Santini A. Ethical issues in research and development of nanoparticles. In: Ranjita S, editor. Drug Delivery Aspects. USA: Elsevier; 2020. pp. 157-168

[104] Sheng J, Wu L, Ding H, Zhang Y, Gu N. Ethics of nanomedicine. In: Gu N, editor. Nanomedicine. Micro/Nano Technologies. Singapore: Springer; 2022. pp. 1-11

[105] Vora LK, Gholap AD, Jetha K, Thakur RRS, Solanki HK, Chavda VP. Artificial intelligence in pharmaceutical technology and drug delivery design. Pharmaceutics. 2023;**15**(7):1916

[106] Gholap AD, Uddin MJ, Faiyazuddin M, Omri A, Gowri S, Khalid M. Advances in artificial intelligence in drug delivery and development: A comprehensive review. Computers in Biology and Medicine. 2024;**178**:108702

[107] Paul D, Sanap G, Shenoy S, Kalyane D, Kalia K, Tekade RK. Artificial intelligence in drug discovery and development. Drug Discovery Today. 2021;**26**(1):80-93

[108] Visan AI, Negut I. Integrating artificial intelligence for drug discovery in the context of revolutionizing drug delivery. Life. 2024;**14**(2):233

[109] Ali KA, Mohin S, Mondal P, Goswami S, Ghosh S, Choudhuri S. Influence of artificial intelligence in modern pharmaceutical formulation and drug development. Future Journal of Pharmaceutical Sciences. 2024;**10**:53

[110] Vidhya KS, Sultana A, Ayesha S, Naveen Kumar M, Harish R. Artificial intelligence's impact on drug discovery and development from bench to bedside. Cureus. 2023;**15**(10):e47486

Section 2

Vesicular or Lipid Drug Delivery System

Chapter 3

Emerging Techniques for Herbosomes

Gaidaa M. Dogheim, Esraa A. Abd El-Maksod, Yousra A. El-Maradny, Mohamed Mamdouh M. Elshindidy and Dina M. Mahdy

Abstract

Herbosomes are a relatively new technology that involves encapsulating herbal extracts in liposomes, which are tiny spheres made of phospholipids. This allows for better absorption of the herbal compounds into the body. Herbosomes have a higher bioavailability compared to traditional herbal extracts, improved stability and can be designed to target specific areas of the body, as well as reduced side effects as they can be delivered in smaller doses. The production of herbosomes involves the use of various techniques including solvent injection, thin-film hydration, and sonication. The production of herbosomes involves the use of various techniques that aim to create stable and effective nanocarriers for herbal extracts. There is limited research available on the safety and toxicity of herbosomes specifically, but studies have been conducted on the safety of lipid-based nanoparticles in general. It is important to note that the safety and toxicity of herbosomes may vary depending on the specific herbal extract and lipid used in their formulation. Further research is needed to fully understand the potential risks and benefits of using herbosomes as a drug delivery system. In conclusion, herbosomes offer several advantages over traditional herbal extracts, making them a promising technology for the development of new herbal products.

Keywords: herbosomes, solvent evaporation, thin film hydration, toxicity, safety

1. Introduction

Extensive research and clinical trials have focused on natural products and secondary metabolites as potential treatments for various human diseases. Medicinal plants and their bioactive components have long been utilized in the food and pharmaceutical industries and for treating diverse ailments [1]. The increased use of herbal drugs can be attributed to several significant factors, including the limitations of modern medicine in addressing all human pathologies, concerns regarding the reliability and safety of synthetic drugs, and the demonstrated efficacy of many natural products in yielding superior outcomes compared to synthetic drugs, without accompanying adverse effects [2]. However, their utilization in pharmaceutical and food sectors is constrained by challenges such as poor water solubility and stability concerns. The inadequate absorption of active phytochemicals arises from factors such as the large, multi-ring structures of polyphenols hindering their passive absorption mechanisms and the limited solubility of active compounds in water or lipids impeding their passage across the outer membrane of gastrointestinal cells [1, 3]. Moreover, upon ingestion, they may undergo various reactions during the digestion process, potentially resulting in significant modifications to their molecular structure and consequently affecting their bioactive properties [4].

In response to these challenges, pharmaceutical research has focused on developing lipid-based drug delivery systems to improve bioavailability while preserving therapeutic efficacy [5]. One such approach involves integrating standardized herbal extracts into phospholipids, forming complexes known as "herbosomes" or "phytosomes." These vesicular drug delivery systems, engineered to enhance the absorption and bioavailability of poorly soluble drugs, consist of phospholipids and natural active phytochemicals forming complexes through interactions with plant extracts in a solvent without protons [6]. Phospholipids, crucial for constructing cell membranes, serve as natural digestive aids and carriers for nutrients in both fat and water. They demonstrate compatibility with aqueous and lipid environments, allowing for effective oral absorption. The primary phospholipid utilized in phytosome formation is phosphatidylcholine, sourced from soybeans (*Glycine max*). Phospholipids, being lipophilic substances, are capable of forming complexes with polyphenolics, facilitating their absorption [7, 8].

Herbosomes, formed by loading phytoconstituents into phospholipids, exhibit improved physical stability due to the formation of hydrogen bonds between phospholipids and phytoconstituents. This enhances the absorption of hydrophilic polar phytoconstituents, leading to increased bioavailability and greater therapeutic benefits [9]. Herbosomes represent an innovative formula of botanicals and phytoconstituents, exhibiting enhanced absorption through both oral and transdermal routes when encapsulated with phosphatidylcholine. This technology serves as a bridge between conventional phytoconstituent delivery systems and emerging drug delivery methodologies [8, 10]. Demonstrating enhanced pharmacological and pharmacokinetic properties compared to conventional preparations, herbosomes have the lipid-soluble phosphatidyl component enveloping the hydrophilic phytoconstituent-choline complexes entirely [11]. Several methodologies, including solvent evaporation, rotatory evaporation, anti-solvent precipitation, freeze-drying, and solvent ether injection, are utilized for herbosome preparation. Evaluation of herbosomes involves techniques such as UV-spectra analysis, differential scanning calorimetry (DSC), assessment of drug entrapment and loading capacity, measurement of surface tension activity, and in vitro/in vivo studies [12]. Notable advantages include high drug encapsulation, stability attributed to chemical bonding, flexibility in administration routes, and increased bioavailability, including enhanced absorption, minimized side effects, controlled release, and targeted delivery, necessitating lower dosages of active constituents for biological effects, even for polar phytoconstituents [13, 14].

2. Structure of a phytosome

The four essential components required to produce herbosomes are phospholipids, phytoactive ingredients, solvents, and a specific ratio relationship involved in the creation of herbosome as shown in **Figure 1**.

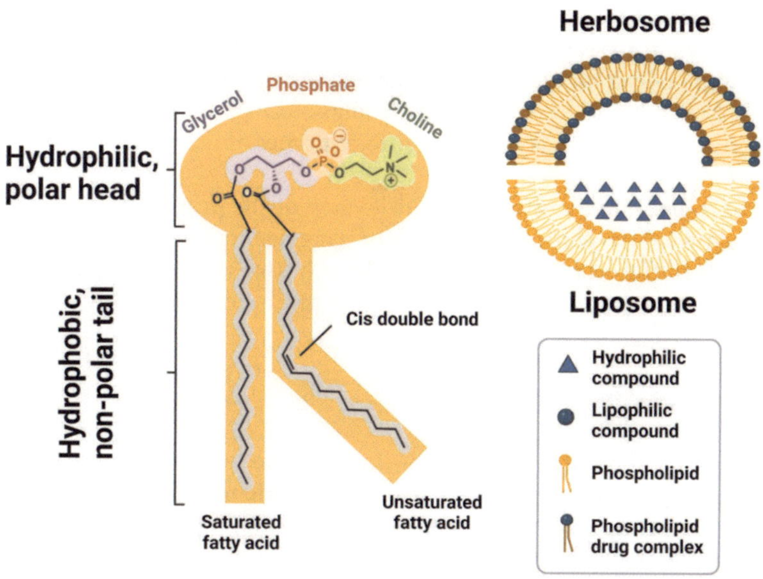

Figure 1.
Principle of herbosome formation.

1. *Phospholipids*: they mainly constitute egg yolk and plant seeds that are considered the most prevalent natural sources of phospholipids. Phospholipids produced in an industrial setting are available for commercial purposes. Phosphatidyl choline is the most used phospholipid in the formation of phospholipid complexes. Phosphatidylcholine has a moderate solubility in both aqueous and lipid environments. In addition to its amphipathic properties, it is considered as an essential component of cell membranes and exhibits high biocompatibility and low toxicity. Phospholipids are used as a vehicle-creating component in the creation of phytosomes [14].

2. *Phytoactive constituents*: the phytoactive constituents are typically selected based on significant in vitro pharmacological effects. Water-soluble flavonoids, such as quercetin, catechin, and silybin, are unable to cross biological membranes, unlike lipophilic curcumin and rutin, which are insoluble in aqueous gastrointestinal fluids. In the aqueous phase, phytosome complexes enhance the water solubility of lipophilic flavonoids and the membrane permeability of hydrophilic flavonoids. Furthermore, flavonoids can be shielded from external impacts, such as hydrolysis, photolysis, and oxidation, by forming complexes [13].

3. *Solvents*: different solvents are used for complexation, mainly aromatic hydrocarbons, halogen derivatives, methylene chloride, ethyl acetate, and cyclic ethers have all been employed in the past to form phytophospholipid complexes. Protonic solvents, such as ethanol and methanol, have recently been used successfully to form phospholipid complexes. Ethanol is a useful and popular solvent because it leaves behind fewer residues and causes minimal damage [13].

4. *Stoichiometric ratio*: phyto-phospholipid complexes are formed by reacting a synthetic or natural phospholipid with the active components in a molar ratio

ranging from 0.5 to 2.0 in many cases. A stoichiometric ratio of 1:1 is considered the most efficient for creating phytosome complexes because it enhances interaction between the two components. The stoichiometric ratio of active components and phospholipids should be experimentally adjusted for various purposes, such as achieving maximal drug loading, in different types of pharmaceuticals [14].

5. *pH maintenance*: to maintain the consistency of the preparation's pH, a buffering agent is used. Two commonly used buffering agents are 7% (v/v) saline phosphate buffer at pH 6.5 and ethanol tris buffer at pH 6.5. The purpose of using a buffer is to maintain the hydration of phytosomes [14].

3. Preparation of phytosomes

The process of producing phytosomes involves the following steps: step 1: phospholipids and herbal compounds are present in aprotic media, such as dioxane and acetone; step 2: hydrogen bond formation; step 3: wrapping the non-polar tail around the polar complex.

Traditional methods: there are mainly three methods available for the preparation of phytosome; solvent evaporation method, rotary evaporation method, and anti-solvent precipitation method as summarized in **Figure 2** [5].

Anti-solvent precipitation technique: involves combining a fixed amount and quantity of phospholipid with herbal extract in a suitable ratio in a 100 mL round bottom flask. The mixture is then refluxed with 20 mL of dichloromethane for 2 hours at a specific temperature.

Rotary evaporation: is a technique in which a specified amount of herb extract is mixed with phospholipids dissolved in 30 mL of tetrahydrofuran at a specific temperature.

The solvent evaporation technique: involves mixing the specified quantity of herbal extract with phospholipids in a 100 mL round-bottom flask. The solution was refluxed with 20 mL of acetone for 2 hours at a temperature ranging from 50–60°C. The mixture was then concentrated to 5–10 mL, filtered to collect the precipitate, and the formed complex was finally stored in an amber-colored glass bottle at 25°C.

Ether-injection technique: dissolve the drug-lipid complex in an organic solvent. Inject this mixture slowly into a heated aqueous solution to form amphiphilic vesicles with different structures.

Sonication technique: place the appropriate amount of phospholipid and cholesterol in a flat-bottomed flask, dissolved in 10 mL of chloroform. Subsequently, sonicate the mixture in a bath sonicator using a rotating evaporator at 40°C, while reducing the pressure to remove organic solvents [14].

Traditional methods exhibit several drawbacks, including multistep processes, difficulty in extraction, and time consumption [13].

Non-traditional methods: supercritical fluid methods can be used to alter the size, shape, and morphology of materials of interest, in addition to other benefits such as high product purity, control of crystal polymorphism, the ability to process thermolabile substances in a single step, and eco-friendly technology (**Figure 3**).

Supercritical fluids techniques: utilize a supercritical fluid, typically CO_2, as an antisolvent to reduce the solute's solubility in the solvent.

Gas anti-solvent technique (*GAS*): it is not necessary for the CO_2 gas used as an antisolvent to be in a supercritical state. The substance is injected into the solution within a closed chamber, ideally from the bottom, to ensure uniform mixing. As a result

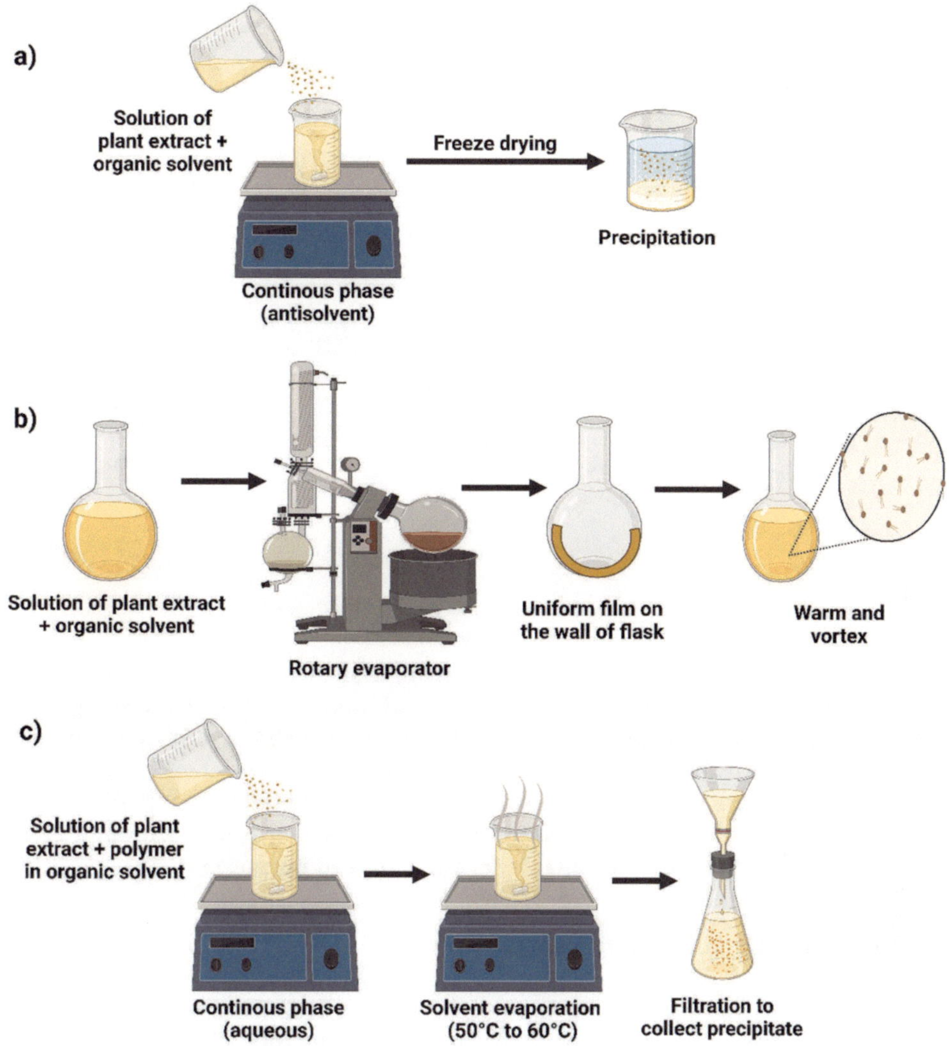

Figure 2.
Traditional methods for the preparation of herbosome: (a) antisolvent precipitation technique; (b) rotary evaporation technique; (c) solvent evaporation technique.

of CO_2 gas dissolving, the organic solvent's ability to dissolve solutes is reduced, leading to the precipitation of solutes. The particles are washed with extra antisolvent to eliminate any remaining solvent. In comparison to the solvent-antisolvent technique, the GAS technique yields superior results when scaled up to industrial levels [13].

4. Evaluation, characterization, and stability

4.1 Introduction

A variety of nanoparticles, differing in both quantity and materials, are currently being developed. These materials exist in various chemical forms, such as micelles,

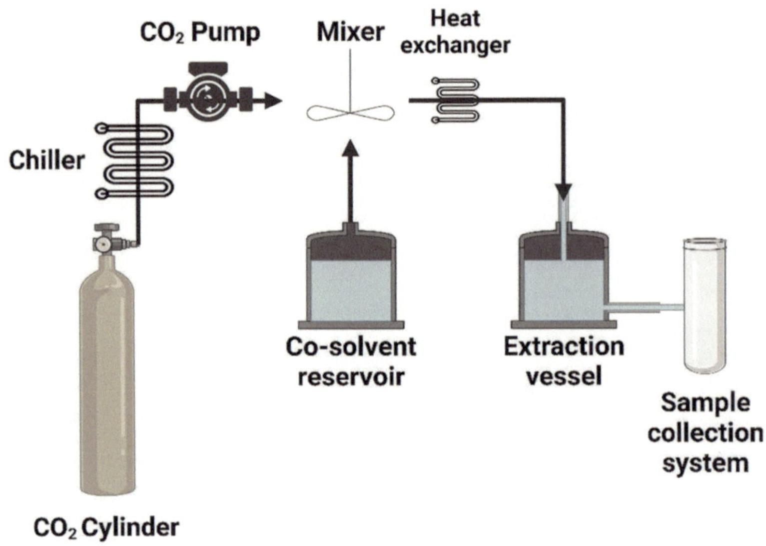

Figure 3.
Preparation of herbosomes by non-traditional methods using supercritical fluid technique.

metal oxides, or large biomolecules. This diversity underscores the need for the development of enhanced characterization methods and protocols that provide greater precision and increased credibility. However, each characterization technique has its own set of advantages and limitations (**Figure 4**). To overcome these constraints, it is advisable to use a combination of methods to effectively characterize individual nanoparticles. When choosing these methods of characterization, it is essential to ensure that they are suitable for the intended purpose [15, 16].

4.2 Characterization of herbosomes

1. *Entrapment efficiency*: to evaluate the efficiency of drug entrapment within planterosomes, we employ the ultracentrifugation method [1]. This method aids in the determination of the percentage of the drug present within the phospholipid mesh. In all phytosome formulations, approximately 100% of the drug is present [17]. The entrapment efficacy is calculated using the following formula:

$$\%\text{entrapment efficacy} = (\text{amount of drug in sediment} / \text{total amount of drug added}) \times 100 \quad (1)$$

1. *Drug content*: the quantity of drug in herbosomes is typically determined using a modified high-performance liquid chromatography method or by UV analysis. One way to measure the drug content is to dissolve a known quantity of phyto-phospholipid dispersion in 10 mL of methanol. The drug concentration of the phyto-phospholipid complex is then determined. After appropriate dilution, the absorbance is measured using spectroscopic techniques at a specific wavelength, and the drug content is calculated using the formula:

$$\%\text{drug content} = (\text{actual drug content in phyto} - \text{phospholipid complex} / \text{theoretical yield}) \times 100 \quad (2)$$

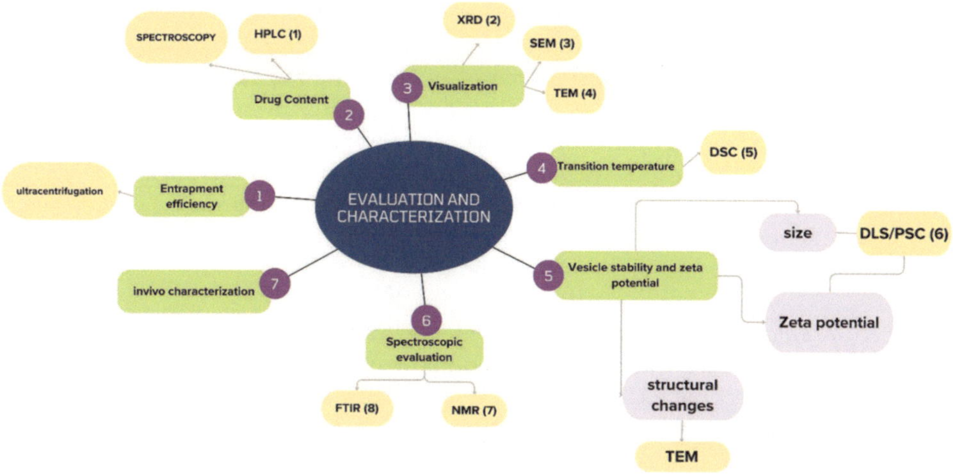

Figure 4.
Methods employed for characterization: (1) high performance liquid chromatography, (2) X-ray diffraction analysis, (3) scanning electron microscopy, (4) transmission electron microscopy, and (5) differential scan.

1. *In vitro drug release studies*: we utilize the Franz diffusion cell method or dialysis bag in combination with various kinetic models. These methods help to identify the mechanisms involved in the release of drug content. Furthermore, an in vitro dissolution test is conducted to understand the drug release process [14].

2. *Visualization*: the most commonly used visualization methods are transmission electron microscopy (TEM) and scanning electron microscopy (SEM). Additionally, when the SEM analysis of nanoparticles (NPs) does not yield clear results regarding the size and shape of the NPs due to its very high resolution, field emission scanning electron microscopy (FESEM) is used [18].

3. *X-ray diffraction analysis (XRD)*: can provide valuable assistance in analyzing various particles. This method is utilized for identifying crystalline compounds [19] and for determining particle roughness, topography, surface area, and surface chemistry.

4. *Transition temperature*: a thermoanalytical method, such as differential scanning calorimetry (DSC), can be employed to assess the transition temperature of vesicular lipid systems. DSC plays a crucial role in elucidating changes in material properties in response to temperature variations. This tool is valuable for determining the crystal structure of the active pharmaceutical ingredient (API). Several phenomena are observed, including temperature transitions, the disappearance of endothermic peaks, alterations in relative peak areas, and the emergence of new peaks. These observations provide valuable insights into the melting and crystallization behavior of the sample being investigated [20].

5. *Vesicle stability and zeta potential*: the stability of vesicles can be assessed over an extended period through comprehensive measurements that include size, zeta

potential, and structural characteristics. Zeta potential, which is the surface charge, is defined as the difference in electric potential (ΔV) between the dispersion medium and the stationary fluid layer on the surface of the dispersed phase [21]. A zeta potential of ± 30 mV or $\pm$ 20 mV is preferred for high physical stability. For the determination of both size and zeta potential, dynamic light scattering (DLS) coupled with a computerized inspection system and photon correlation spectroscopy (PCS) proves to be a valuable approach [21]. Simultaneously, transmission electron microscopy (TEM) is used to observe structural changes, as mentioned earlier.

6. *Spectroscopic techniques*: to confirm the formation of a complex or investigate the interaction between the plant-based component and the phospholipids, scientists utilize spectroscopic techniques such as nuclear magnetic resonance (NMR), Fourier transform infrared spectroscopy (FTIR), and X-ray diffraction (XRD). This involves comparing the outcomes of the individual elements with those of the complexes [5].

5. Applications of herbosomes

The utilization of phytochemicals in pharmaceutical products is constrained by several factors, including solubility, bioavailability, and stability. The large molecular size of most phytochemicals, along with their high lipophilicity or hydrophilicity, affects their absorption and bioavailability and, consequently, their therapeutic effectiveness [1, 4]. Moreover, the stability of phytochemicals depends on temperature, pH, and enzymes. Degradation of phytoconstituents through hydrolysis, oxidation, or enzymatic activity during processing, storage, or after administration can limit their effectiveness. Furthermore, phytochemicals are recognized by the host immune system as foreign antigens, eliciting an immune response that leads to rapid clearance and reduced clinical effects. The use of phytochemicals in nanocarriers, such as herbosomes, presents an appealing strategy for overcoming their in vivo limitations and enhancing their therapeutic effects [22, 23]. Herbosomes are drug delivery systems that have several therapeutic effects, including anticancer, hepatoprotective, and wound healing properties. The details of their applications are discussed in the following section and summarized in **Table 1**.

5.1 Anticancer effects

Current cancer therapy strategies, such as chemotherapy, radiotherapy, immunotherapy, and surgery, have numerous limitations and can cause systemic adverse effects. Furthermore, complete remission and full recovery are not always attained in cancer patients. Various plant-based compounds have inherent anticancer activity through various mechanisms, including antioxidant effects, interference with signaling pathways, and inhibition of chemoresistance. Several studies have demonstrated the efficacy and safety of herbosomes as a form of anticancer therapy [87, 88].

5.1.1 Breast cancer

Murugesan and team [24] prepared an *Aloe vera*-based herbosome gel as an anticancer nanosystem against breast cancer. The herbosome gel showed enhanced

Study	Phospholipid	Herbal component	Application	Therapeutic outcomes
Murugesan et al. [24]	Milk phospholipids	*Aloe vera*	Breast cancer	• Cytotoxicity on the MCF-7 cell line
Wanjiru et al. [25]	Soy phosphatidylcholine	*Moringa oleifera*		• Cytotoxicity on the 4 T1 breast cancer cell line • Induction of apoptosis and cell proliferation
Alhakamy et al. [26]	Soybean phosphatidylcholine	Quercetin		• Cytotoxicity against the MCF-7 cell line • Induction of apoptosis and necrotic cell death
Sabzichi et al. [27]	Phosphatidylcholin, phosphatidyletanolamine, and phosphatidylserin	Luteolin		• Cytotoxicity against MDA-MB231 • Enhance sensitivity of doxorubicin
Talaat et al. [28]	Soy phosphatidylcholine	Fisetin		• Cytotoxicity against MDA-MB231 • Induction of apoptosis • Inhibition of the activity of TGF-β and MMP-9 • Enhance E-cadherin expression levels
Komeil et al. [29]	Soy phosphatidylcholine	Genistein		• Significant reduction in tumor size • Significant reduction in levels of CEA and CA15.3
Kumar et al. [30]	Soy lecithin	Taxifolin		• Cytotoxicity against the MCF-7 cell line • Radical scavenging activity (H_2O_2, NO, and DHHP)
Hashemzehi et al. [31]	N/A	Curcumin		• Cytotoxicity against MCF-7 cell lines • Reduction in cell invasion • Increased expression of E-cadherin and MMP-9 • Reduced levels of MDA and thiol • Inhibition of mTOR and Wnt/β-catenin signaling
El-Far et al. [32]	Soy phosphatidylcholine	Monascin, ankaflavin, and resveratrol		• Cytotoxicity on the MCF-7 cell line • Decrease tumor weight and volume • Reduce levels of VEGF, NF-κB, and CD1 • Induce apoptosis and necrosis

Study	Phospholipid	Herbal component	Application	Therapeutic outcomes
Xu et al. [33]	Lecithin	Diosgenin	Lung cancer	• Cytotoxicity against A549 and PC9 cell lines • Induction of apoptosis
Al-Rabia et al. [34]	Soy phosphatidylcholine	Curcumin	Prostate cancer	• Cytotoxicity against the PC3 cell line • Induction of apoptosis and necrosis • Disrupt the mitochondrial membrane potential
Pastorelli et al. [35]	Phosphatidylcholine	Curcumin		• Increase in disease control rate and overall survival rate • Reduced levels of IL-6, sCD40L, and CRP
Li et al. [36]	Soy phosphatidylcholine	Mitomycin C	Cervical cancer	• Cytotoxicity on HeLa cell lines • Reduction in tumor weight and volume
Komeil et al. [37]	Phosphatidylcholine solubilized in medium-chain and long-chain TGs	Genistein	Liver cancer	• Cytotoxicity on HepG2 cells • Induction of apoptosis • Reduced the levels of VEGF and MMP-9
Teng et al. [38]	Phosphatidylcholine	Curcumin		• Cytotoxicity against the Huh-7 cell line • Reduced tumor volume • Decreased lipid and leukocyte accumulation
Mazumder et al. [39]	Soy phosphatidylcholine	Sinigrin	Skin cancer	• Cytotoxicity against the A375 cell line
Mukherjee et al. [40, 41]	Phosphatidylcholine	Curcumin	Glioblastoma	• Improved survival of mice • Reduced the number of CD68 high GBM tumor cells • Increased the level of iNOS • Reduced the level of ARG1 • Induced polarization of M2-TAMs into the M1 phenotype • Induced the expression of monocyte chemotactic protein-1
Singh et al. [42]	Phosphatidylcholine	Silibinin	Colorectal cancer	• Enhanced antitumor activity • Inhibition of angiogenesis • Reduced the expression of VEGF, COX, iNOS, and HIF-1α

DOI: http://dx.doi.org/10.5772/intechopen.1005232

Study	Phospholipid	Herbal component	Application	Therapeutic outcomes
Marjaneh et al. [43]	N/A	Curcumin		• Cytotoxicity on the CT26 cell line • Induced cell death • Reduced cell invasion • Reduced the levels of cyclin-D1 • Increased the level of E-cadherin and beclin • Increase in CAT, and SOD activity • Reduced the level of MDA
Karekar et al. [44]	Soy phosphatidylcholine	*Andrographis paniculata*	Hepatoprotective effect	• Reduced the levels of hepatic enzymes • Antioxidant activity
Chi et al. [45]	Soy phosphatidylcholine	Silybin		• Reduced the levels of hepatic enzymes • Reduced hepatocyte denaturation, inflammation, and fibrosis
Naik and Panda [46]	Soy phospholipids	*Gingko biloba*		• Reduced the levels of hepatic enzymes • Antioxidant activity
Shriram et al. [47]	Soy phosphatidylcholine	Silymarin		• Reduced the levels of hepatic enzymes • Antioxidant activity
El-Gazayerly et al. [48]	• Soy phosphatidylcholine • Egg yolk phosphatidylcholine	Silymarin		• Reduced the levels of hepatic enzymes • Antioxidant activity
Mahmoudabad et al. [49]	Soy phosphatidylcholine	Silymarin		• Reduced liver enzymes and lipid peroxidation • Antioxidant activity
Al-Kahtani et al. [50]	Soy phosphatidylcholine	Curcumin		• Reduced liver enzymes and lipid peroxidation • Antioxidant activity • Downregulated caspase-3 expression • Upregulated anti-apoptotic protein Bcl-2
Bui et al. [51]	Phosphatidylcholine	Curcumin		• Reduced liver enzymes and lipid peroxidation • Antioxidant activity
Jain et al. [52]	Soy phosphatidylcholine	Mangiferin		• Antioxidant and hepatoprotective activity
Sharma et al. [53]	Soy phosphatidylcholine	*Abutilon indicum* and *Piper longum*		• Reduced the levels of hepatic enzymes • Antioxidant activity

Study	Phospholipid	Herbal component	Application	Therapeutic outcomes
Telange et al. [54]	Hydrogenated soy phosphatidylcholine	Apigenin		• Reduced liver enzymes and lipid peroxidation • Antioxidant activity
Mangrulkar et al. [55]	Hydrogenated soy phosphatidylcholine	Caffeic acid		• Antihyperlipidemic and hepatoprotective activity • Reduced liver enzyme levels and fat deposition
Mazumder et al. [39]	Hydrogenated soy phosphatidylcholine	Sinigrin	Wound healing	• Wound healing properties on the HaCaT cell line
Varadkar and Gadgoli [56]	Phosphatidylcholine	Corcetin		• Improved wound healing in rats • Improved % of contraction and the breaking strength of the wounds • Reduction in granulation tissue formation
Tafish et al. [57]	• Soybean phosphatidylcholine • Hydrogenated soy phosphatidylcholine	Carvacrol		• Enhanced skin permeation • Increase % of wound closure • Reduced wound area • Increased collagen deposition, tissue remodeling, and wound healing capacity
Lim et al. [58]	Soybean lecithin	*Moringa oleifera*		• Improved wound closure
Jeeja et al. [59]	Soybean lecithin	*Onosma echioides*		• Improved breaking and tensile strength • Increased wound inhibition • Reduced lipid peroxidation
Refai et al. [60]	L α-phosphatidylcholine	Spirulina platensis		• Improved contraction rate • Complete wound closure • Improved skin appearance • Reduced the expression of HMGB1, TLR-4, and NF-κB • Increased NRF-2 and HO-1 levels • Autophagy and anti-apoptotic properties • Increased VEGF and collagen deposition

Study	Phospholipid	Herbal component	Application	Therapeutic outcomes
Rajamma et al. [61]	Soy phosphatidylcholine	*Geophila repens*	Alzheimer's disease	• Inhibition of cholinesterase
Habbu et al. [62]	L α-phosphatidylcholine	*Bacopa monnieri*		• Reduced transfer latency • Reduced the escape latency time and TSTQ • Improved the mice's response to shock • Reduced the activity of acetylcholinesterase
Naik et al. [63]	N/A	*Ginkgo biloba*		• Increased the levels of SOD and CAT • Enhanced the activity of glutathione peroxidase and glutathione reductase
Naik et al. [64]	Soy phospholipids	*Ginkgo biloba*	Cognitive Impairment and Neuronal Damage	• Reduced the phenobarbital-induced sleeping time • Increased spontaneous motor activity • Reduced the recovery time from convulsions • Reduction in transfer latency • Antiamnesic properties • Reduced mobility time
Mancini et al. [65]	Phosphatidylcholine	*Annona muricata* L.		• Enhanced translocation into hCMEC/D3 cells • Inhibited MAO activity (antidepressant activity) • Hydrogen peroxide scavenging activity
Ullah et al. [66]	Soy phosphatidylcholine	Curcumin		• Reduced neuroinflammation
Sbrini et al. [67, 68]	N/A	*Centella asiatica* L.		• Increased mRNA levels of Bdnf and its receptor TRKB • Increased local proteins peEF2 Thr56 and OPHN-1 • Improved performance in rats
Ahmad et al. [69]	Egg phosphatidylcholine	Rutin	Cerebral ischemia	• Neuroprotective activity • Increased level of GSH • Decreased level of MDA • Reduced the infarction area
Ahmad et al. [70]	Hydrogenated soy phosphatidylcholine	NMITLI118RT+		• Increased GSH levels • Decreased MDA levels • Decreased neurological deficit score • Reduced the infarction area

Study	Phospholipid	Herbal component	Application	Therapeutic outcomes
Hatamipour et al. [71]	• Phosphatidylcholine • Phosphatidylserine	Curcumin	Atherosclerosis	• Significant reduction in atherosclerotic plaque area
Panda et al. [72]	Soy phospholipids	*Ginkgo biloba*	Myocardial infarction	• Reduced the serum levels of AST, LDH, and CPK • Antioxidant effect
Riva et al. [73]	N/A	Artichoke Bergamot	Hypercholesterolemia	• Reduced the levels of total cholesterol and LDL • Increased level of HDL • Combination reduced glycated hemoglobin levels
Singh et al. [74]	Soy lecithin	Lawson	Skin conditions (antifungal and anti-inflammatory)	• Enhanced antifungal activity • Enhanced skin permeation • Reduction of edema
Djekic et al. [75]	N/A	Escin β-sitosterol	Skin conditions (anti-hyperalgesic)	• Potent anti-hyperalgesic as compared to ibuprofen gel
Kalita et al. [76]	Phosphatidylcholine	Resveratrol	Skin conditions (anti-inflammatory)	• Enhanced skin permeation • Reduced edema
Baradaran et al. [77]	Soy phospholipids	Curcumin		• Increased activity of CAT and SOD • Reduced latency times
Maramaldi et al. [78]	Phosphatidylcholine	Quercetin	Skin conditions (soothing and anti-itch effect)	• Reduced erythema • Photoprotective effect • Decrease in wheal diameter and itching • Increased skin hydration levels • Reduced TEWL values
Antiga et al. [79]	Phosphatidylcholine	Curcumin	Skin conditions (psoriasis)	• Reduction in PASI values • Decrease in the level of IL-22
Yu et al. [80]	Dipalmitoyl phosphatidylcholine	Naringenin	Respiratory tract diseases	• Reduced edema and fluid exudation • Reduced the levels of total proteins in BALF • Increased the levels of SOD • Inhibited the expression of COX-1 and ICAM-1
Singh et al. [81]	Soya Lecithin	Gingerol		• Antioxidant and scavenging properties • Antimicrobial activity against *S. aureus* and *E. coli* • Reduced RBC membrane lysis and albumin denaturation

Study	Phospholipid	Herbal component	Application	Therapeutic outcomes
Abd El-Fattah et al. [82]	Phosphatidylcholine	Quercetin	Metabolic syndrome	• Decrease in the levels of TNF-α and MDA • Increased levels of GSH • Reduced the body weight of rats • Reduced the levels of bone biomarkers (ACP and ALP) • Increased the levels of calcium and phosphorus in bones • Decreased levels of TG, TC, LDL-C, and VLDL-C • Increased the level of HDL-C • Decreased blood glucose level
Kim et al. [83]	• Phosphatidylcholine • Egg phospholipid	Chrysin		• Enhanced glucose uptake effect in C2C12 cell lines • Upregulation of PPAR γ and GLUT4
Poruba et al. [84]	N/A	Silymarin		• Reduced the levels of TG and (TC) • Increased the level of HDL-C • Increased levels of ABCG5 and ABCG8 • Increased levels of CYP7A1 and CYP4A
Palachai et al. [85]	Phosphatidylcholine	Mulberry and ginger		• Reduced body weight • Decreased levels of TG, TC, and LDL-C • Increased the level of HDL-C • Reduce insulin resistance • ACE gene expression • Reduction in MDA levels • Increased levels of SOD, CAT, and GSH • Reduced levels of HDAC3 • Increased level of PPAR γ • Reduction in IL-6 and TNF-α
Yu et al. [86]	Soybean phosphatidylcholine	Berberin		• Reduction in fasting blood glucose levels • Reduced the level of TGs

Table 1.
Summary of herbosome-based studies included.

concentration-dependent cytotoxicity on the MCF-7 cell line. The mechanism by which the system induces the anticancer effect is through *Aloe vera*'s antioxidant properties. The cytotoxic effects of polyphenolic compounds from *Moringa oleifera* leaves were explored against breast cancer [25]. *Moringa oleifera* herbosomes (Mop) showed enhanced dose-dependent cytotoxicity on the 4 T1 breast cancer cell line as compared to doxorubicin. Mop was found to induce apoptosis in 4 T1 cell lines and thus have an antiproliferative effect on cancer cells. A novel scorpion venom-decorated phytosomes encapsulating quercetin (QRT-PHM-SV) were developed by Alhakamy et al. [26] QRT-PHM-SV exhibited significantly high cytotoxicity against the MCF-7 cell line as compared to the free drug. The nanosystem could induce apoptosis and necrotic cell death more significantly than the free drug as demonstrated by increased levels of caspase-9, Bax, and p53, while levels of Bcl2 decreased. Furthermore, the level of TNF-α was significantly increased after treatment with QRT-PHM-SV, while the level of NF-κB decreased confirming the induction of apoptosis. Sabzichi and colleagues [27] investigated the combination of luteolin-loaded phytosomes (Nano-lut) with doxorubicin in the MDA-MB231 cell line. Nano-lut in combination with doxorubicin had enhanced cytotoxicity against MDA-MB231 as compared to doxorubicin alone. Nano-lut was shown to inhibit the Nrf2 signaling pathway and its downstream genes HO1 and MDR1 resulting in enhanced sensitivity of MDA-MB231 to doxorubicin. The anticancer effect of self-assembled fisetin phytosomes (FIS-PHY) against the MDA-MB-231 cell line was studied by Talaat et al. [28]. The FIS-PHY formulation exhibited increased cytotoxicity with a lower IC50 value than the free drug. The phytosome could induce apoptosis and necrosis in a time-dependent manner. FIS-PHY was shown to inhibit the activity of TGF-β and MMP-9 by interfering with NF-κB and ERK1/2 signaling pathways. Furthermore, the phytosome system may enhance E-cadherin expression levels, leading to the inhibition of tumor progression. A pegylated, hyaluronic acid-CD44 targeting genistein phytosome (G-PHA) was formulated by Komeil et al. [29]. G-PHA demonstrated enhanced deposition in mammary glands and a significant reduction in tumor size compared to the free drug. Levels of CEA and CA15.3 biomarkers significantly decreased after treatment with G-PHA. Taxifolin phytosomes (PC3) were developed, and their antioxidant and cytotoxic effects on the MCF-7 cell line were studied [30]. PC3 exhibited an antioxidant effect that was dependent on its concentration, as demonstrated by its ability to scavenge radicals such as H_2O_2, NO, and DHHP. Cell viability studies showed a concentration-dependent cytotoxicity of PC3 against the MCF-7 cell line. Hashemzehi and team [31] investigated the antitumor effects of curcumin-loaded phytosomes (CUR-PHY) both independently and in conjunction with fluorouracil (FU). CUR-PHY exhibited concentration-dependent cytotoxicity against MCF-7 cell lines, as well as a reduction in cell invasion. The antitumor activity of CUR-PHY was found to be associated with increased expression of E-cadherin and MMP-9, which was further enhanced after combination with FU. The combination showed increased cytotoxicity in vivo compared to each treatment alone. Moreover, the antioxidant activity of CUR-PHY + FU was superior to that of either treatment alone, as demonstrated by the reduced levels of MDA and thiol, while catalase activity was significantly enhanced. The antitumor activity of curcumin is attributed to the activation of the AMPK signaling pathway, which in turn inhibits mTOR and Wnt/β-catenin signaling, resulting in cell cycle arrest through the inhibition of cyclin D1 (CD1). A multi-reservoir nanosystem comprising casein micelles incorporated into resveratrol phytosomes (PC-CAS MCs) was developed by El-Far et al. [32] PC-CAS micelles demonstrated significant cytotoxicity on the MCF-7 cell line compared to casein/resveratrol micelles and free drugs. Furthermore, the phagosomal-nano micelle system was able to decrease tumor weight and volume in vivo. The levels of tumor biomarkers, including aromatase, VEGF, NF-κB, and CD1, showed significant reductions following treatment with PC-CAS MCs. The phytosomal nanomicelles were found to induce apoptosis and necrosis, as evidenced by elevated levels of caspase-3 and % necrosis in histopathological analysis.

5.1.2 Lung cancer

Xu et al. [33] developed a diosgenin derivative-based herbosome (P2P) as an anticancer nanosystem for treating lung cancer. P2P exhibited cytotoxicity against A549 and PC9 cell lines that was both time- and dose-dependent, in comparison to the free drug. P2P demonstrated anticancer activity by inducing apoptosis through G0/G1 cell cycle arrest.

5.1.3 Prostate cancer

A new nanoplatform, CUR-PL-SV was formulated by conjugating scorpion venom with curcumin phytosomes by to combat prostate cancer effectively Al-Rabia et al. [34]. CUR-PL-SV exhibited increased cytotoxicity against the PC3 cell line compared to curcumin and scorpion venom-conjugated phytosomes. CUR-PL-SV cytotoxicity was demonstrated through the induction of apoptosis and necrosis, as evidenced by increased levels of Bax, p53, and caspase-3, while levels of Bcl-2, NF-κB, and TNF-α were significantly reduced. Furthermore, the nanophytosome disrupted the mitochondrial membrane potential, leading to further induction of apoptosis. A Phase II clinical trial conducted by Pastorelli and colleagues [35] investigated the antitumor activity of curcumin phytosomes as a combination therapy with gemcitabine in prostate cancer. Complementary administration of curcumin phytosomes increased the efficacy of gemcitabine, as evidenced by an increase in disease control rate (DCR) and overall survival rate (OS). Furthermore, there was a decrease in hematological and neurotoxic adverse events associated with the gemcitabine-curcumin phytosome combination. Analysis of tumor markers, such as IL-6, sCD40L, and CRP, showed reduced levels after treatment with complementary therapy, highlighting the role of curcumin in reducing inflammation and inhibiting tumor progression and metastasis.

5.1.4 Cervical cancer

Li and team [36] developed folic acid-decorated pegylated mitomycin C phytosomes (FA-PEG-MMC) as a targeted anticancer nanoplatform for cervical cancer. The specific nanosystem exhibited enhanced cytotoxicity on HeLa cell lines in a concentration and time-dependent manner compared to non-targeted NPs. In vivo studies demonstrated preferential accumulation in tumor tissue and enhanced antitumor activity, as evidenced by a reduction in tumor weight and volume.

5.1.5 Liver cancer

The antitumor activity of oral medium-chain (GP) and long-chain (GPL) phosphatidylcholine, genistein-loaded phytosomes was investigated by Komeil et al. [37] against hepatocellular carcinoma (HCC). GP demonstrated a time-dependent increase in cellular uptake compared to the genistein solution and GPL. The cytotoxicity in

HepG2 cells demonstrated increased toxicity of genistein-loaded phytosomes compared to free genistein. The in vivo antitumor activity of GP and GPL was found to be enhanced through the induction of apoptosis, as indicated by increased levels of AIF, caspase-3, and caspase-8. Furthermore, genistein-loaded phytosomes reduced the levels of VEGF and MMP-9, which are crucial factors in cancer advancement and metastasis. In another study, the antitumor impact of curcumin phytosomes on hepatitis B virus-induced HCC was investigated [38]. Phytosomal curcumin NPs showed enhanced time-dependent cytotoxicity against the Huh-7 cell line. The cytotoxic effect was achieved through the activation of PPARγ and the inhibition of mTOR and NF-κB signaling pathways. The in vivo study demonstrated that phytosomal curcumin significantly reduced tumor volume and also decreased lipid and leukocyte accumulation compared to free curcumin.

5.1.6 Skin cancer

Sinigrin phytosomes (sin-phy) were developed by Mazumder et al. [39] to study their antitumor activity against skin cancer. Sin-phy exhibited concentration-dependent cytotoxicity against the A375 cell line but not the HaCat cell line.

5.1.7 Brain tumors

Mukherjee and colleagues [40, 41] investigated the anticancer effects of phytosomal curcumin (CCP) in glioblastoma. CCP significantly improved the survival of mice compared to the control and reduced the number of CD68 high GBM tumor cells. CCP significantly increased the level of iNOS and reduced the level of ARG1, as demonstrated by histopathology and flow cytometry analysis. In addition, CCP enhanced the activation of NF-κB to p65 NF-kB and the activation of STAT1 to its phosphorylated form (P-STAT1). CCP induces polarization of M2-TAMs into the M1 phenotype, as evidenced by a reduction in the level of IL-10 and an increase in the level of IL-12. Finally, curcumin phytosomes induced the expression of monocyte chemotactic protein-1 (MCP-1), leading to the recruitment of M1-TAMs and activated NK cells.

5.1.8 Colorectal cancer

Silibinin phytosomes' (SP) anticancer activity against colorectal cancer was investigated in an HT29 xenograft model [42]. In comparison to free silibinin, SP exhibited enhanced antitumor activity, as demonstrated by a decrease in tumor weight and volume. The mechanism by which silibinin produced its antitumor activity was found to be through its antiproliferative and pro-apoptotic effect demonstrated by a reduction in PCNA+ and CD-1+ cells. Furthermore, silibinin inhibited ERK1/2 and Akt signaling which play a role in tumor progression. Furthermore, it inhibited angiogenesis by reducing the expression of VEGF, COX, iNOS, and HIF-1α in tumor cells. Marjaneh et al. [43] investigated the antitumor activity of curcumin phytosomes against colitis-induced colorectal cancer. Phytosomal curcumin showed a concentration and time-dependent cytotoxicity on the CT26 cell line. The tumor spheroids model showed the ability of curcumin phytosomes to induce cell death as compared to control. The preparation also reduced cell invasion and reduced the levels of cyclin-D1 while increasing the level of E-cadherin and beclin. Curcumin phytosomes induced cell cycle arrest as demonstrated by increased cell population in the G0/G1 phase as compared to control. In vivo studies showed that the nanophytosomes significantly reduced tumor numbers, area, and disease activity. The antioxidant effects of curcumin phytosomes were demonstrated through an increase in CAT and SOD activity, while the level of MDA was reduced significantly. Furthermore, the nanophytosome inhibited the Wnt/β-catenin signaling pathway as shown by reduced CD-1 and p-Gsk-3a/b expression levels.

5.2 Hepatoprotective effects

Herbal remedies have been long used in the management of liver diseases such as hepatitis, fatty liver, and acute liver injury. Medicinal plants contain a plethora of phytoconstituents that possess inherent hepatoprotective activities [89]. Bioactive molecules are classified into phenols, flavonoids, monoterpenes, coumarins, alkaloids, and glycosides. There are several mechanisms by which phytoconstituents produce their hepatoprotective effects. Phytochemicals regulate gastrointestinal and liver functions, boost the immune system, scavenge free radicals, and reduce lipid peroxidation. Moreover, they suppress the activity of cytochrome P450 enzymes which in some cases are responsible for the conversion of drugs/compounds into toxic products. Furthermore, phytochemicals shield the structure of the mitochondrial membrane and augment the activity of ATPase enzymes. Incorporation of phytochemicals into phospholipids to form phytosomes enhanced their hepatoprotective effects as phosphatidylcholine which is the most commonly used phospholipid and has inherent hepatoprotective properties. Phosphatidylcholine enhances the activity of collagenase enzyme which prevents liver fibrosis. The most commonly used phytochemicals are silymarin, eugenol, silybin, piperidine, and caffeine, among others.

Karekar and team [44] developed a nanophytosome incorporating *Andrographis paniculata* extract (APP) and studied its hepatoprotective activity. APP successfully reduced the levels of hepatic enzymes (ALT, AST, ALP, and total bilirubin). Serum biochemistry showed that APP could reduce the levels of gamma-glutamyl transferase (GGT) and lactate dehydrogenase (LDH) which are biomarkers of liver damage. APP could significantly enhance the levels of superoxide dismutase (SOD) and glutathione (GSH), while decreasing the level of malondialdehyde (MDA) highlighting the antioxidant activity of the nanophytosome. Silybin-phospholipid complex loaded nanosuspension (SPC-NPs) was formulated by Chi et al. [45] as a hepatoprotective nanosystem. SPC-NPs could significantly reduce the levels of ALT, AST, and AKP as compared to free silybin. Histopathological analysis showed the ability of SPC-NPs to reduce hepatocyte denaturation, inflammation, and fibrosis. *Gingko biloba* phytosomes (GBP) were investigated by Naik and Panda [46] as hepatoprotective nanosystems in carbon tetrachloride-induced (CCl4) liver injury. GBP was shown to reduce hepatic enzyme levels (ALT, AST, and ALP) while increasing the levels of albumin and total protein. Analysis of the antioxidant effect of GBP which is a measure of its hepatoprotective activity showed the ability of the nanosystem to enhance the activity of catalase (CAT), SOD, and GSH in addition to reducing lipid peroxidation demonstrated by reduced levels of TBARS. Shriram et al. [47] and El-Gazayerly et al. [48] demonstrated the hepatoprotective ability of silymarin phytosomes in CCl4-induced liver damage. Silymarin phytosomes reduced the levels of hepatic enzymes and enhanced the levels of antioxidant enzymes. Furthermore, the nanophytosomes could reduce lipid peroxidation evidenced by reduced levels of MDA. Another study by Mahmoudabad and colleagues [49] also investigated silymarin phytosomes hepatoprotective activity in ethanol-induced hepatotoxicity which demonstrated an enhanced ability to reduce liver enzymes and lipid peroxidation while enhancing the activity of antioxidant enzymes. Curcumin phytosomes' (CP) ability to reverse aluminum chloride (AlCl3)-induced hepatotoxicity was investigated by Al-Kahtani et al. [50]. CP successfully reversed hepatotoxicity shown by reduced levels of hepatic and antioxidant enzymes. The ability of CP to reduce oxidative stress was demonstrated by decreased levels of nitric oxide (NO) and lipid peroxidase (LPO) expression. On the other hand, CP enhanced the activity of SOD and GSH. Immunohistochemistry assessment showed that treatment with CP downregulated caspase-3 expression while upregulated the anti-apoptotic protein Bcl-2. A similar approach has been developed by Tung et al. [51] proving the hepatoprotective ability of curcumin phytosomes in paracetamol-induced liver toxicity. Mangiferin phytosomal preparation was developed by Jain et al. [52] and demonstrated antioxidant and hepatoprotection in ethanol-induced liver damage. A combination of ethanolic extracts of *Abutilon indicum* and *Piper longum* was incorporated in a nanophytosome [53]. The combination nanophytosome significantly reduced liver enzymes (ALT, AST, and APL) and bilirubin levels (total and direct) as compared to combined ethanolic extracts. The potential of apigenin phytosome to produce antioxidant effects and thus reverse liver damage was studied by Telange et al. [54]. The nanophytosome enhanced antioxidant enzymes levels (SOD, CAT, and GSH) and reduced lipid peroxidation (reduced MDA levels). Caffeic acid phytosome (CA-PC) formulated by Mangrulkar and team [55] showed its potential use as an antihyperlipidemic and hepatoprotective nanosystem in non-alcoholic fatty liver disease (NAFLD). CA-PC reduced the levels of total cholesterol, low-density lipoprotein (LPL), triglycerides, very low-density lipoprotein (VLDL), and enhanced levels of high-density lipoprotein (HDL). Furthermore, the nanophytosome reduced liver enzyme levels and fat deposition demonstrated by histopathological analysis.

5.3 Wound healing properties

Wound healing is a complex and dynamic process that involves multiple sequential steps, including homeostasis, inflammation, proliferation, and remodeling [90]. In acute wounds, the healing process progresses smoothly until the wound is completely resolved. On the other hand, chronic wounds result from an impaired wound healing process, leading to complications such as fibrosis and non-healing ulcers. The use of herbal medicine in wound healing has emerged as a promising strategy because of the pleiotropic effects of phytochemicals. Phytochemicals possess antioxidant, anti-inflammatory, angiogenic, and cell synthesis-modulating properties. Several studies provide evidence of the wound-healing properties of herbal medicine. Incorporating phytochemicals into phytosomes has been shown to enhance their wound-healing properties by improving absorption and bioavailability at the wound site.

Sinigrin phytosomes demonstrated enhanced wound healing properties on the HaCaT cell line compared to free sinigrin [39]. Varadkar and Gadgoli [56] investigated the wound healing properties of corcetin phytosomes (F2) gel preparation. F2 showed improved wound healing in rats demonstrated by an increase of the level of hydroxyproline. Furthermore, excision and incision wounds showed that F2 improved both the percentage of contraction and the breaking strength of the wounds. Histopathological analysis revealed a significant reduction in granulation tissue formation, confirming the wound healing properties of the nanophytosome. Carvacrol-loaded phytosomes (CAR-PHY) were developed by Tafish and team [57] to investigate their potential for wound healing activity. CAR-PHY demonstrated enhanced permeation across the skin with sustained release, indicating that the skin can act as a reservoir for the phytosomal preparation. In vivo wound healing showed the ability of CAR-PHY hydrogel to increase the percentage of wound closure and reduce wound area. Histopathological examination revealed increased collagen deposition, tissue remodeling, and wound healing capacity. *Moringa oleifera* extract phytosomes (MOPCT) were developed as a potential platform for wound dressing [58]. MOPCT showed rapid and improved wound closure in the NHDF cell line compared to the control and free MO extract. Phytosomal gel loaded with *Onosma echioides* extract was evaluated for its wound healing effects by Jeeja et al. [59]. The phytosomal gel exhibited improved breaking and tensile strength compared to the control group. Moreover, the percentage of wound inhibition was significantly higher in the group treated with the phytosomal gel compared to control. The analysis of hydroxyproline and collagen deposition demonstrated the enhanced effect of the gel on wound healing. Furthermore, the gel reduced lipid peroxidation, as demonstrated by an increased level of catalase, while the level of MDA was reduced. Refai and colleagues [60] investigated an intriguing nanophytosomal gel containing Spirulina platensis extract (SPNP-gel). The SPNP-gel markedly improved contraction rate compared to the control and standard treatment demonstrated by complete wound closure and improved skin appearance. The analysis of inflammatory markers revealed that SPNP-gel exhibited anti-inflammatory properties by reducing the expression of HMGB1, TLR-4, and NF-κB. Furthermore, SPNP-gel increased NRF-2 and HO-1 levels, demonstrating its antioxidant capability. Moreover, histopathological analysis of TNF-α demonstrated enhanced reduction after treatment with the gel, further confirming its anti-inflammatory effects. SPNP-gel possess autophagy and anti-apoptotic properties, as evidenced by increased levels of LC3BII/I and Beclin-1 and reduced levels of caspase-3 and AIF. Furthermore, the levels of VEGF and collagen deposition markedly increased after treatment with the phytosomal gel, demonstrating its ability to promote wound healing through several mechanisms.

5.4 Nervous system conditions

5.4.1 Alzheimer's disease

Alzheimer's disease (AD) is a progressive neurodegenerative disease that accounts for 60% of all cases of dementia worldwide in people aged 65 years and older [91]. Alzheimer's disease (AD) is associated with memory loss and cognitive deficits, including aphasia, agnosia, and apraxia. The exact cause of the disease is still unclear. However, the deposition of β-amyloid and τ-proteins, loss of synapses, and cholinergic neuron apoptosis appear to be the most common factors. Pharmacological treatment of Alzheimer's disease mainly includes acetylcholinesterase inhibitors (AChE) and N-methyl-D-aspartate (NMDA) receptor antagonists. However, pharmacological treatment is not entirely effective and is often accompanied by several adverse effects. The efficacy of phytoconstituents like huperzine-A, ginkgolides, and asiaticosides in treating AD has been investigated in a number of studies proving their efficacy. Yet, their effectiveness is hindered by their low solubility and bioavailability, as well as their ability to pass through the blood-brain barrier (BBB). Therefore, incorporating phytochemicals into phytosomes offers a way to enhance their therapeutic effects.

Rajamma et al. [61] studied the therapeutic effects of *Geophila repens* phytosomal gel (MEGR-PG) for intranasal delivery in Alzheimer's disease (AD). MEGR-PG demonstrated good intranasal permeation, which was further enhanced by the addition of

1% transcutol as a permeation enhancer. The in vitro cholinesterase inhibition assay demonstrated that MEGR-PG has the ability to inhibit cholinesterase compared to the control. *Bacopa monnieri*-loaded phytosomes (BPC) were studied for their antiamnesic effects in AD [62]. BPC could reduce transfer latency in the elevated plus maze test compared to control. In addition, in the Morris water maze test, BPC significantly reduced the escape latency time (ELT) and TSTQ as compared to the control groups. BPC also improved the mice's response to shock (step-through latency time) and significantly reduced the activity of acetylcholinesterase. *Ginkgo biloba* phytosomes were formulated and assessed for their antioxidant effects to enhance cognitive function in AD [63]. The nanophytosomes significantly increased the levels of superoxide dismutase (SOD) and (CAT) enzymes in rat brains compared to the free *Ginkgo biloba* and control groups. Furthermore, the phytosomal system enhanced the activity of both glutathione peroxidase and glutathione reductase, confirming the antioxidant properties of *Ginkgo biloba* phytosomes.

5.4.2 Cognitive impairment and neuronal damage

A study by Naik and team [64] assessed the central nervous system (CNS) activity of *Ginkgo biloba* (GB) phytosomes in Wistar rats. The phytosomal preparation reduced the phenobarbital-induced sleeping time in a concentration-dependent manner compared to the control. In addition, the phytosomes increased spontaneous motor activity (SMA) for up to 60 minutes at concentrations of 50 and 100 mg/kg. GB phytosomes did not alter the duration of convulsions, but they reduced the recovery time compared to control. There was a significant reduction in transfer latency after treatment with GB phytosomes in the elevated plus maze. On the other hand, in the scopolamine-induced amnesia test, the phytosomes prolonged the transfer latency time, demonstrating the preparation's antiamnesic properties. Finally, the phytosomes reduced the rats' mobility time and prolonged their swimming time in the forced swimming test. The antidepressant activity of mApoE-decorated phytosomes loaded with *Annona muricata* L. extract (mApoE-P-AE) was investigated by Mancini et al. [65]. mApoE-P-AE demonstrated enhanced translocation into hCMEC/D3 cells, indicating the system's ability to cross the BBB. The phytosomes significantly inhibited MAO activity compared to the free extract, demonstrating its antidepressant activity. Moreover, mApoE-P-AE exhibited strong hydrogen peroxide scavenging activity compared to the free extract. The anti-inflammatory effect of curcumin phytosomes (MC) on chronic glial activation was studied by Ullah and colleagues [66]. MC demonstrated the ability to reduce neuroinflammation, as evidenced by a decrease in Iba-1 + microglia, TSPO+ microglial cells/macrophages, and GFAP+ astrocytes in the hippocampus and cerebellum of GFAP-IL6 mice. Two studies by Sbrini et al. [67, 68] investigated the potential of *Centella asiatica* L. phytosomes, with or without *Curcuma longa* L., to enhance cognitive function by promoting Bdnf expression. Phytosomes increased the mRNA levels of Bdnf and its receptor TRKB. Moreover, the levels of local proteins peEF2 Thr56 and OPHN-1 increased significantly. The novel object recognition test demonstrated improved performance in rats following chronic treatment with phytosomes.

5.4.3 Cerebral ischemia

Ahmad and team [69] investigated the neuroprotective effect of rutin phytosomes (RU-PLC) in ischemic stroke. RU-PLC exhibited high and preferential accumulation in the brain compared to free rutin. The neuroprotective activity of the phytosomes was demonstrated by an increased level of GSH, while the level of MDA was significantly decreased. Furthermore, RU-PLC reduced the infarction area at a dose less than half of free rutin, demonstrating its neuroprotective role in ischemic stroke. Another study by Ahmad et al. [70] evaluated the neuroprotective activity of NMITLI118RT+ loaded phytosomes (NIMPLC). NIMPLC significantly increased GSH levels and decreased MDA levels. The neurological deficit score significantly decreased after treatment with NIMPLC. Moreover, the infarction area was also reduced compared to the free extract at 1 and 6 hours post-injury.

5.5 Cardiovascular disease

Cardiovascular disease (CVD) is a widespread health issue that causes the death of one-third of the global population. CVD encompasses a plethora of conditions, including atherosclerosis, coronary artery disease, diabetes mellitus, and cerebrovascular diseases. Although pharmacological treatment has advanced, it has improved symptoms and survival but does not cure the disease. Herbal medicine has been utilized in the treatment of various cardiovascular diseases, with many therapies derived from plant sources. For example, digoxin is derived from *Digitalis purpurea*, aspirin from *Salix alba*, and lovastatin from *Monascus purpureus*, among others. Currently, researchers are exploring the use of traditional herbs such as ginseng, *Ginkgo biloba*, and *Gynostemma pentaphyllum* incorporated in phytosomes.

5.5.1 Atherosclerosis

Hatamipour et al. [71] investigated the anti-atherosclerotic effects of curcumin phytosomes by formulating curcumin-phosphatidylcholine (curcumin-PC) and curcumin-phosphatidylserine phytosomes (curcumin-PS). Curcumin-PC/PS had no significant effect on lipid profile (TC, TG, LDL, VLDL, and HDL) or CRP levels as compared to the control. However, curcumin-PS (100 mg/kg) demonstrated a significant reduction in atherosclerotic plaque area compared to curcumin-PC and the control group.

5.5.2 Myocardial infarction

The study by Panda and colleagues [72] studied the cardioprotective effects of *Ginkgo biloba* phytosomes (GBP) in rats with isoproterenol-induced myocardial necrosis. GBP could reduce the serum levels of AST, LDH, and CPK in a concentration-dependent manner compared to the control. The antioxidant effect of GBP was demonstrated by a decrease in the level of MDA, yet an increase in GSH, CAT, GPx, and GR levels.

5.5.3 Hypercholesterolemia

An RCT investigating the efficacy of a combination of Artichoke Phytosomes and Bergamot Phytosomes in patients with mild hypercholesterolemia was conducted by Riva et al. [73]. Supplementation with both phytosomal preparations reduced the levels of total cholesterol and LDL, while the level of HDL was significantly increased. Furthermore, the combination reduced glycated hemoglobin levels compared to the control group, but there was no significant change in glycemia, insulin resistance, or triglyceride levels.

5.6 Inflammatory skin conditions

Singh et al. [74] evaluated the antifungal and anti-inflammatory properties of Lawson phytosomes. The phytosomes exhibited enhanced antifungal activity compared to the plant drug and standardized ketoconazole. The phytosomes exhibited enhanced skin permeation abilities compared to the free drug. The nanophytosome's anti-inflammatory properties were demonstrated by the significant reduction of edema in rat paws compared to the free plant drug. An escin β-sitosterol phytosome (ES) investigated the anti-hyperalgesic effects of topical hydrogel preparation [75]. ES exerted a more potent anti-hyperalgesic effect in vivo compared to the control and ibuprofen gel. Resveratrol phytosomes embedded in a polymeric patch (RSVP) were developed, and their anti-inflammatory properties were investigated [76]. RSVP polymeric patch showed enhanced skin permeation compared to the free drug. The in vivo anti-inflammatory effect of RSVP was investigated using carrageenan-induced paw swelling, and the study showed that the phytosomes significantly reduced edema compared to the control group. A study by Baradaran et al. [77] examined the anti-inflammatory impact of curcumin phytosomes on carrageenan-induced inflammation. Curcumin phytosomes exhibited antioxidant properties, as evidenced by the increased activity of CAT and SOD enzymes compared to the control. Behavioral responses of the mice were evaluated using the tail pinch and hot plate tests, which revealed that mice treated with curcumin phytosomes exhibited reduced latency times compared to the control group. A single-blind study was conducted by Maramaldi and team [78] to evaluate the soothing and anti-itch effects of phytosomal quercetin on healthy volunteers. Quercetin phytosomes reduced erythema caused by UV irradiation, demonstrating a photoprotective effect. Additionally, they led to a significant decrease in wheal diameter and itching after a histamine prick test. Furthermore, quercetin phytosomes increased skin hydration levels and reduced TEWL values compared to the control. Antiga et al. [79] conducted a phase III, double-blind, placebo-controlled randomized controlled trial (RCT) to investigate the effectiveness of oral curcumin as a supplementary treatment to topical methylprednisolone aceponate 0.1% ointment in psoriasis. Curcumin phytosomes, when combined with topical methylprednisolone, resulted in a reduction in PASI values compared to methylprednisolone alone. The combination therapy resulted in a decrease in the level of IL-22 compared to the placebo, but it had no effect on IL-17.

5.7 Respiratory tract diseases

5.7.1 Anti-inflammatory

Yu and team [80] investigated the use of naringenin-loaded phytosomes as a dry powder inhalation (NPDPI) treatment for acute lung injury. NPDPI significantly reduced edema and fluid exudation resulting from acute lung injury compared to the control group. The mechanism by which the preparation exerts its effect is through the inhibition of MAPK phosphorylation, leading to p38 MAPK. NPDPI reduced the levels of total proteins in bronchoalveolar lavage fluid (BALF) compared to the positive control. In addition, the phytosomal preparation significantly increased the levels of SOD compared to the positive control. RT-PCR analysis showed that NPDPI inhibited the expression of COX-1 and ICAM-1 compared to the positive control, demonstrating its anti-inflammatory effect.

5.7.2 Anti-microbial

Gingerol-loaded phytosomes complexed with chitosan (GLPC4) were investigated for their antimicrobial and anti-inflammatory properties in lung infections [81]. GLPC4 exhibited antioxidant and scavenging properties by inhibiting free radicals (DPPH and H_2O_2). The study demonstrated that GLPC4 exhibited greater antimicrobial activity against *S. aureus* and *E. coli* compared to free gingerol, effectively inhibiting bacterial growth. Furthermore, GLPC4 demonstrated anti-inflammatory properties by reducing RBC membrane lysis and albumin denaturation compared to free gingerol.

5.8 Metabolic syndrome

Abd El-Fattah et al. [82] investigated the antiestrogenic activity of quercetin-loaded phytosomes (QP) in ovariectomized rats (Ovx). The QP compound exhibited antioxidant properties, as evidenced by a decrease in the levels of TNF-α and MDA, while the levels of GSH increased compared to the Ovx group. The phytosomes also significantly reduced the body weight of rats in a concentration-dependent manner. QP reduced the levels of bone biomarkers (ACP and ALP) compared to the Ovx group and consequently increased the levels of calcium and phosphorus in bones. Furthermore, QP had a significant impact on the lipid profile by decreasing levels of TG, TC, LDL-C, and VLDL-C, while increasing the level of HDL-C. Furthermore, the phytosomal preparation significantly decreased blood glucose levels compared to the Ovx group. Chrysin-loaded phytosomes using soy phosphatidylcholine (CSP) and egg phospholipid (CEP) were developed to investigate their glucose uptake-promoting activity [83]. CEP demonstrated an enhanced glucose uptake effect in C2C12 cell lines compared to the control in a dose-dependent manner. The mechanism by which CEP produces its activity has been shown to be through the upregulation of peroxisome proliferator-activated receptor γ (PPAR γ) and glucose transporter type 4 (GLUT4). The study by Poruba and team [84] investigated the anti-hyperlipidemic activity of silymarin phytosomes (PS) in metabolic syndrome. PS reduced the levels of triglycerides (TG) and total cholesterol (TC) compared to the control, while the level of high-density lipoprotein (HDL) was significantly increased. The levels of ABCG5 and ABCG8 transporters involved in cholesterol metabolism were enhanced in the group treated with PS. In addition, the levels of CYP7A1 and CYP4A were significantly increased in the PS group compared to control. Another study investigated the effectiveness of phytosomes containing a combination of mulberry and ginger extracts (PMG) in treating metabolic syndrome [85]. PMG reduced body weight and levels of triglycerides (TG), total cholesterol (TC), and low-density lipoprotein cholesterol (LDL-c) compared to the positive control, while increasing the level of high-density lipoprotein cholesterol (HDL-c). In addition, the homeostasis model assessment of insulin resistance (HOMA-IR) indicated that PMG could reduce insulin resistance in a dose-dependent manner. The level of ACE gene expression was also reduced in the group treated with PMG compared to the positive control. Furthermore, PMG exhibited antioxidant effects as demonstrated by the reduction in MDA levels, while the levels of SOD, CAT, and GSH were significantly increased in a dose-dependent manner. The expression levels of HDAC3 were significantly reduced, while PPARγ

was significantly increased in the group treated with PMG compared to the control group. Furthermore, the PMG group showed a dose-dependent reduction in the expression of inflammatory cytokines (IL-6 and TNF-α). Berberine phytosomes encapsulated within microparticles (microparticles@P-BER) were developed, and their anti-diabetic properties were studied [86]. Microparticles containing berberine (P-BER) exhibited anti-diabetic activity, as evidenced by a reduction in fasting blood glucose levels compared to free berberine and the positive control (db/db mice). However, there was no difference in insulin levels. Moreover, Microparticles@P-BER reduced the level of TGs in the liver significantly as compared to free berberine and positive control.

6. Future perspectives

Phytosomes have been demonstrated to be an effective drug delivery system for phytochemicals. However, there are still several limitations that hinder their clinical application and commercialization in the market. While phytosomes are complexes of naturally occurring phospholipids and herbal constituents, safety concerns still arise because of their nanoscale size. Some parameters, such as biocompatibility, bioaccumulation, metabolism, and excretion, should be carefully assessed before their release to the market [92, 93]. Another limitation is their biological effectiveness and safety, which is related to their ability to cross biological barriers and reach target cells. The complete pharmacokinetic and pharmacodynamic profile of phytosomes should be assessed in vivo and in clinical trials. The selection of the dosage form is a crucial aspect that should be taken into consideration during the manufacturing and scaling-up process. Post-marketing surveillance and quality control of commercial phytosomes are necessary to ensure their safety and efficacy. Currently, herbal medicine has gained tremendous popularity worldwide, and many people are shifting toward natural remedies instead of relying on chemical drugs. Several phytosomes are already on the market, including Siliphos®, Ginkgoselect®, Centevita®, and Soyselect®. Further optimization of phytosomal preparations will facilitate their seamless transition from the laboratory to clinical use.

7. Conclusion

Phytochemicals have recently garnered significant interest in the prevention and management of various disease conditions due to people's increasing inclination toward natural products. Phytochemicals comprise a range of compounds, including flavonoids, tannins, glycosides, carotenoids, phytosterols, and saponins, among others. They exhibit various biological activities, including antioxidant, antimicrobial, anticancer, hepatoprotective, cardioprotective, anti-hyperlipidemic, anti-inflammatory, and neuroprotective actions. However, they suffer from poor solubility in water, low permeability, biotransformation, and the formation of insoluble complexes in the gastrointestinal tract (GIT), which results in low bioavailability and reduced efficacy. As a result, integrating these phytochemicals into delivery systems has become a critical factor in enhancing their therapeutic activity. Phytosomes are lipid-based nanoparticles formed by complexing phospholipids with phytochemicals. Phytosomes address the limitations of phytochemicals by enhancing their solubility, improving bioavailability, providing sustained and controlled release, enabling targeted delivery, reducing toxic effects, and enhancing stability. Numerous studies have investigated the biological activities of phytosomes and have demonstrated their superiority to free phytochemicals. Phytosomes have been studied in various ailments such as cancer, CNS diseases (including neurodegenerative diseases), liver diseases, skin conditions and wound healing, respiratory tract conditions, and metabolic syndromes. Several phytosomes are currently available in the market. However, further optimization of phytosomes is necessary to ensure safety and efficacy and to facilitate their clinical translation on a larger scale.

Author details

Gaidaa M. Dogheim[1], Esraa A. Abd El-Maksod[2], Yousra A. El-Maradny[3,4], Mohamed Mamdouh M. Elshindidy[3] and Dina M. Mahdy[3,5]*

1 Faculty of Pharmacy, Pharmaceutics Department, Alexandria University, Alexandria, Egypt

2 Cancer Nanotechnology Research Laboratory (CNRL), Faculty of Pharmacy, Alexandria University, Alexandria, Egypt

3 Pharmaceutics Department, College of Pharmacy, Arab Academy for Science, Technology and Maritime Transport (AASTMT), El-Alamein, Egypt

4 PFIDC, SRTA-City, New Borg El-Arab, Alexandria, Egypt

5 Pharmaceutical and Fermentation Industries Development Center (PFIDC), The City of Scientific Research and Technological Applications (SRTA-City), New Borg El-Arab, Alexandria, Egypt

*Address all correspondence to: dina.mahdy@alexu.edu.eg

References

[1] Barani M, Sangiovanni E, Angarano M, et al. Phytosomes as innovative delivery systems for phytochemicals: A comprehensive review of literature. International Journal of Nanomedicine. 2021;**16**: 6983-7022. DOI: 10.2147/ijn.s318416

[2] Bhise JJ, Bhusnure OG, Jagtap SR, et al. Phytosomes: A novel drug delivery for herbal extracts. Journal of Drug Delivery and Therapeutics. 2019;**9**: 924-930. DOI: 10.22270/jddt.v9i3-s.2863

[3] Alharbi WS, Almughem FA, Almehmady AM, et al. Phytosomes as an emerging nanotechnology platform for the topical delivery of bioactive phytochemicals. Pharmaceutics. 2021;**13**: 1475. DOI: 10.3390/pharmaceutics13091475

[4] Martins-Gomes C, Souto EB, Silva AM. Nanophytosomes: A novel approach for the delivery of herbal drugs. Chapter 15. In: Nayak AK, Hasnain MS, Aminabhavi TM, Torchilin VP, editors. Systems of Nanovesicular Drug Delivery. United Kingdom: Academic Press; 2022. pp. 239-257. DOI: 10.1016/B978-0-323-91864-0.00015-2

[5] Lu M, Qiu Q, Luo X, et al. Phyto-phospholipid complexes (phytosomes): A novel strategy to improve the bioavailability of active constituents. Asian Journal of Pharmceutical Sciences. 2019;**14**:265-274. DOI: 10.1016/j.ajps.2018.05.011

[6] Kafle A, Timilsina A, Gautam A, et al. Phytoremediation: Mechanisms, plant selection and enhancement by natural and synthetic agents. Environmental Advances. 2022;**8**:100203. DOI: 10.1016/j.envadv.2022.100203

[7] Manach C, Scalbert A, Morand C, et al. Polyphenols: Food sources and bioavailability. The American Journal of Clinical Nutrition. 2004;**79**:727-747. DOI: 10.1093/ajcn/79.5.727

[8] Semalty A, Semalty M, Rawat MS, et al. Supramolecular phospholipids-polyphenolics interactions: The phytosome strategy to improve the bioavailability of phytochemicals. Fitoterapia. 2010;**81**:306-314. DOI: 10.1016/j.fitote.2009.11.001

[9] Dash D, Sahu A, Tripathi V, et al. Herbosomes: A potent drug carrier. Journal of Pharmaceutical and Biological Sciences. 2022;**10**:44-46. DOI: 10.18231/j.jpbs.2022.008

[10] Divakar MC, Nikethen GS, Vishwapal SS, et al. Evaluation of the cytotoxic and anti-cancer activities of polyscias fruticosa (l) harms root phytosome on neuroblastoma cell line. Journal of Population Therapeutics and Clinical Pharmacology. 2024;**31**:22-29. DOI: 10.53555/jptcp.v31i1.3839

[11] Gaurav V, Paliwal S, Singh A, Pandey S, Aqil M. Phytosomes: Preparation, evaluation and application. International Journal of Research in Engineering Science. 2021;**9**(2):35-39

[12] Susilawati Y, Chaerunisa AY, Purwaningsih H. Phytosome drug delivery system for natural cosmeceutical compounds: Whitening agent and skin antioxidant agent. Journal of advanced Pharmaceutical Technology & Research. 2021;**12**:327-334. DOI: 10.4103/japtr.JAPTR_100_20

[13] Dewan N, Dasgupta D, Pandit S, et al. Review on-herbosomes, a new arena for drug delivery. Journal of

Pharmacognosy and Phytochemistry. 2016;5(4):104-108

[14] Nsairat H, Khater D, Odeh F, et al. Phytosomes: A modernistic approach to the delivery of herbal drugs. Chapter 12. In: Nayak AK, Hasnain MS, Laha B, Maiti S, editors. Advanced and Modern Approaches for Drug Delivery. San Diego: Academic Press; 2023. pp. 301-355. DOI: 10.1016/B978-0-323-91668-4.00029-0

[15] Pandey V, Barve K, Londhe V. Chapter 9—Synthesis and characterization of nanoherbal formulations for topical wound healing applications. In: Thomas S, Oyedeji AO, Oluwafemi OS, Jaquilin PJR, editors. Nanotechnology in Herbal Medicine. Cambridge, MA: Woodhead Publishing; 2023. pp. 255-278. DOI: 10.1016/B978-0-323-99527-6.00012-4

[16] Fadeel B. Nanomaterial characterization: Understanding nano-bio interactions. Biochemical and Biophysical Research Communications. 2022;**633**:45-51. DOI: 10.1016/j.bbrc.2022.08.095

[17] Patel P, Modi C, Patel H, et al. Phytosome: An emerging technique for improving herbal drug delivery. The Journal of Phytopharmacology. 2023;**12**: 51-58. DOI: 10.31254/phyto.2023.12108

[18] Perrie Y, Ali H, Kirby DJ, et al. Environmental scanning electron microscope imaging of vesicle systems. Methods in Molecular Biology. 2017; **1522**:131-143. DOI: 10.1007/978-1-4939-6591-5_11

[19] Ghanbarzadeh B, Babazadeh A, Hamishehkar H. Nano-phytosome as a potential food-grade delivery system. Food Bioscience. 2016;**15**:126-135. DOI: 10.1016/j.fbio.2016.07.006

[20] Mondal R, Bobde Y, Ghosh B, et al. Development and characterization of a phospholipid complex for effective delivery of capsaicin. Indian Journal of Pharmaceutical Sciences. 2019;**81**: 1011-1019. DOI: 10.36468/pharmaceutical-sciences.598

[21] Anwana U, Eghianruwa Q. Herbosomes in the delivery of phytotherapeutics and nutraceuticals: Concepts, applications and future perspective. Covenant Journal of Physical and Life Sciences. 2015;**3**:10-22

[22] Ting Y, Jiang Y, Ho C-T, et al. Common delivery systems for enhancing in vivo bioavailability and biological efficacy of nutraceuticals. Journal of Functional Foods. 2014;**7**:112-128. DOI: 10.1016/j.jff.2013.12.010

[23] Shakeri A, Sahebkar A. Opinion paper: Phytosome: A fatty solution for efficient formulation of phytopharmaceuticals. Recent Patents on Drug Delivery & Formulation. 2016; **10**:7-10. DOI: 10.2174/187221130966 6150813152305

[24] Murugesan MP, Venkata Ratnam M, Mengitsu Y, et al. Evaluation of anti-cancer activity of phytosomes formulated from aloe vera extract. Materials Today: Proceedings. 2021;**42**:631-636. DOI: / 10.1016/j.matpr.2020.11.047

[25] Wanjiru J, Gathirwa J, Sauli E, et al. Formulation, optimization, and evaluation of *Moringa oleifera* leaf polyphenol-loaded phytosome delivery system against breast cancer cell lines. Molecules. 2022;**27**:4430. DOI: 10.3390/molecules27144430

[26] Alhakamy NA, Fahmy UA, Eldin SMB, et al. Scorpion venom-functionalized quercetin phytosomes for breast cancer management: In vitro response surface optimization and

anticancer activity against MCF-7 cells. Polymers. 2022;**14**:93. DOI: 10.3390/polym14010093

[27] Sabzichi M, Hamishehkar H, Ramezani F, et al. Luteolin-loaded phytosomes sensitize human breast carcinoma MDA-MB 231 cells to doxorubicin by suppressing Nrf2 mediated signalling. Asian Pacific Journal of Cancer Prevention. 2014;**15**:5311-5316. DOI: 10.7314/apjcp.2014.15.13.5311

[28] Talaat SM, Elnaggar YSR, El-Ganainy SO, et al. Self-assembled fisetin-phospholipid complex: Fisetin-integrated phytosomes for effective delivery to breast cancer. European Journal of Pharmaceutics and Biopharmaceutics. 2023;**189**:174-188. DOI: 10.1016/j.ejpb.2023.06.009

[29] Komeil IA, Abdallah OY, El-Refaie WM. Surface modified genistein phytosome for breast cancer treatment: In-vitro appraisal, pharmacokinetics, and in-vivo antitumor efficacy. European Journal of Pharmaceutical Sciences. 2022;**179**:106297. DOI: 10.1016/j.ejps.2022.106297

[30] Kumar S, Baldi A, Sharma DK. In vitro antioxidant assay guided ex vivo investigation of cytotoxic effect of phytosomes assimilating taxifolin rich fraction of *Cedrus deodara* bark extract on human breast cancer cell lines (MCF7). Journal of Drug Delivery Science and Technology. 2021;**63**:102486. DOI: /10.1016/j.jddst.2021.102486

[31] Hashemzehi M, Behnam-Rassouli R, Hassanian SM, et al. Phytosomal-curcumin antagonizes cell growth and migration, induced by thrombin through AMP-kinase in breast cancer. Journal of Cellular Biochemistry. 2018;**119**:5996-6007. DOI: 10.1002/jcb.26796

[32] El-Far SW, Helmy MW, Khattab SN, et al. Phytosomal bilayer-enveloped casein micelles for codelivery of monascus yellow pigments and resveratrol to breast cancer. Nanomedicine. 2018;**13**:481-499. DOI: 10.2217/nnm-2017-0301

[33] Xu L, Xu D, Li Z, et al. Synthesis and potent cytotoxic activity of a novel diosgenin derivative and its phytosomes against lung cancer cells. Beilstein Journal of Nanotechnology. 2019;**10**:1933-1942. DOI: 10.3762/bjnano.10.189

[34] Al-Rabia MW, Alhakamy NA, Rizg WY, et al. Boosting curcumin activity against human prostatic cancer PC3 cells by utilizing scorpion venom conjugated phytosomes as promising functionalized nanovesicles. Drug Delivery. 2022;**29**:807-820. DOI: 10.1080/10717544.2022.2048133

[35] Pastorelli D, Fabricio ASC, Giovanis P, et al. Phytosome complex of curcumin as complementary therapy of advanced pancreatic cancer improves safety and efficacy of gemcitabine: Results of a prospective phase II trial. Pharmacological Research. 2018;**132**:72-79. DOI: 10.1016/j.phrs.2018.03.013

[36] Li Y, Wu H, Jia M, et al. Therapeutic effect of folate-targeted and pegylated phytosomes loaded with a mitomycin c–soybean phosphatidyhlcholine complex. Molecular Pharmaceutics. 2014;**11**:3017-3026. DOI: 10.1021/mp5001873

[37] Komeil IA, El-Refaie WM, Gowayed MA, et al. Oral genistein-loaded phytosomes with enhanced hepatic uptake, residence and improved therapeutic efficacy against hepatocellular carcinoma. International Journal of Pharmaceutics. 2021;**601**:120564. DOI: 10.1016/j.ijpharm.2021.120564

[38] Teng C-F, Yu C-H, Chang H-Y, et al. Chemopreventive effect of phytosomal curcumin on hepatitis b virus-related hepatocellular carcinoma in a transgenic mouse model. Scientific Reports. 2019;**9**: 10338. DOI: 10.1038/s41598-019-46891-5

[39] Mazumder A, Dwivedi A, du Preez JL, et al. In vitro wound healing and cytotoxic effects of sinigrin–phytosome complex. International Journal of Pharmaceutics. 2016;**498**: 283-293. DOI: 10.1016/j.ijpharm.2015.12.027

[40] Mukherjee S, Fried A, Hussaini R, et al. Phytosomal curcumin causes natural killer cell-dependent repolarization of glioblastoma (GBM) tumor-associated microglia/macrophages and elimination of GBM and GBM stem cells. Journal of Experimental & Clinical Cancer Research. 2018;**37**:168. DOI: 10.1186/s13046-018-0792-5

[41] Mukherjee S, Baidoo J, Fried A, et al. Curcumin changes the polarity of tumor-associated microglia and eliminates glioblastoma. International Journal of Cancer. 2016;**139**:2838-2849. DOI: /10.1002/ijc.30398

[42] Singh RP, Gu M, Agarwal R. Silibinin inhibits colorectal cancer growth by inhibiting tumor cell proliferation and angiogenesis. Cancer Research. 2008;**68**:2043-2050. DOI: 10.1158/0008-5472.can-07-6247

[43] Marjaneh RM, Rahmani F, Hassanian SM, et al. Phytosomal curcumin inhibits tumor growth in colitis-associated colorectal cancer. Journal of Cellular Physiology. 2018;**233**: 6785-6798. DOI: 10.1002/jcp.26538

[44] Karekar P, Killedar S, More H. Nanophytosomes Loading Andrographis paniculata Hydroalcoholic Extract: Promising Drug Delivery for Hepatoprotective Efficacy. Journal of Pharmaceutical Innovation. Sep 2023; **18**(3):1084-1099. DOI: 10.1007/s12247-023-09712-x

[45] Chi C, Zhang C, Liu Y, et al. Phytosome-nanosuspensions for silybin-phospholipid complex with increased bioavailability and hepatoprotection efficacy. European Journal of Pharmaceutical Sciences. 2020;**144**: 105212. DOI: 10.1016/j.ejps.2020.105212

[46] Naik SR, Panda VS. Antioxidant and hepatoprotective effects of Ginkgo biloba phytosomes in carbon tetrachloride-induced liver injury in rodents. Liver International. 2007;**27**: 393-399. DOI: 10.1111/j.1478-3231.2007.01463.x

[47] Shriram RG, Moin A, Alotaibi HF, et al. Phytosomes as a plausible nano-delivery system for enhanced oral bioavailability and improved hepatoprotective activity of silymarin. Pharmaceuticals. 2022;**15**:790. DOI: 10.3390/ph15070790

[48] El-Gazayerly ON, Makhlouf AIA, Soelm AMA, et al. Antioxidant and hepatoprotective effects of silymarin phytosomes compared to milk thistle extract in CCl4 induced hepatotoxicity in rats. Journal of Microencapsulation. 2014;**31**:23-30. DOI: 10.3109/02652048.2013.805836

[49] Mahmoudabad AG, Gheybi F, Mehrabi M, et al. Synthesis, characterization and hepatoprotective effect of silymarin phytosome nanoparticles on ethanol-induced hepatotoxicity in rats. BioImpacts: BI. 2023;**13**:301-311. DOI: 10.34172/bi.2023.24128

[50] Al-Kahtani M, Abdel-Daim MM, Sayed AA, et al. Curcumin phytosome modulates aluminum-induced hepatotoxicity via regulation of antioxidant, Bcl-2, and caspase-3 in rats. Environmental Science and Pollution Research. 2020;**27**:21977-21985. DOI: 10.1007/s11356-020-08636-0

[51] Bui Thanh T, Nguyen H, Phan KS. Hepatoprotective effect of Phytosome curcumin against paracetamol-induced liver toxicity in mice. Brazilian Journal of Pharmaceutical Sciences. 2017;**53**: e16136. DOI: 10.1590/s2175-97902017000116136

[52] Jain PK, Kharya M, Gajbhiye A. Pharmacological evaluation of mangiferin herbosomes for antioxidant and hepatoprotection potential against ethanol induced hepatic damage. Drug Development and Industrial Pharmacy. 2013;**39**:1840-1850. DOI: 10.3109/03639045.2012.738685

[53] Sharma S, Sahu AN. Development, characterization, and evaluation of hepatoprotective effect of *Abutilon indicum* and *Piper longum* phytosomes. Pharmacognosy Research. 2016;**8**:29-36. DOI: 10.4103/0974-8490.171102

[54] Telange DR, Patil AT, Pethe AM, et al. Formulation and characterization of an apigenin-phospholipid phytosome (APLC) for improved solubility, in vivo bioavailability, and antioxidant potential. European Journal of Pharmaceutical Sciences. 2017;**108**: 36-49. DOI: 10.1016/j.ejps.2016.12.009

[55] Mangrulkar S, Shah P, Navnage S, et al. Phytophospholipid complex of caffeic acid: Development, in vitro characterization, and in vivo investigation of antihyperlipidemic and hepatoprotective action in rats. AAPS PharmSciTech. 2021;**22**:28. DOI: 10.1208/s12249-020-01887-7

[56] Varadkar M, Gadgoli C. Preparation and evaluation of wound healing activity of phytosomes of crocetin from Nyctanthes arbor-tristis in rats. Journal of Traditional and Complementary Medicine. 2022;**12**:354-360. DOI: 10.1016/j.jtcme.2021.10.002

[57] Tafish AM, El-Sherbiny M, Al-Karmalawy AA, et al. Carvacrol-loaded phytosomes for enhanced wound healing: Molecular docking, formulation, doe-aided optimization, and in vitro/in vivo evaluation. International Journal of Nanomedicine. 2023;**18**:5749-5780. DOI: 10.2147/IJN.S421617

[58] Lim A-W, Ng P-Y, Chieng N, et al. *Moringa oleifera* leaf extract–loaded phytophospholipid complex for potential application as wound dressing. Journal of Drug Delivery Science and Technology. 2019;**54**:101329. DOI: 10.1016/j.jddst.2019.101329

[59] Jeeja P, Chhaya G. Phytosomes of naphthoquinone enriched extract of root bark of onosma echioides exhibit wound healing activity in rats. Indonesian Journal of Pharmacy. 2021;**32**:474-483. DOI: 10.22146/ijp.2351

[60] Refai H, El-Gazar AA, Ragab GM, et al. Enhanced wound healing potential of spirulina platensis nanophytosomes: Metabolomic profiling, molecular networking, and modulation of HMGB-1 in an excisional wound rat model. Marine Drugs. 2023;**21**:149. DOI: 10.3390/md21030149

[61] Rajamma SS, Krishnaswami V, Prabu SL, et al. Geophila repens phytosome-loaded intranasal gel with improved nasal permeation for the effective treatment of Alzheimer's disease. Journal of Drug Delivery Science and Technology. 2022;**69**:103087. DOI: 10.1016/j.jddst.2021.103087

[62] Habbu P, Madagundi S, Kulkarni R, et al. Preparation and evaluation of Bacopa–phospholipid complex for antiamnesic activity in rodents. Drug Invention Today. 2013;**5**:13-21. DOI: 10.1016/j.dit.2013.02.004

[63] Naik SR, Pilgaonkar VW, Panda VS. Evaluation of antioxidant activity of Ginkgo biloba phytosomes in rat brain. Phytotherapy Research. 2006;**20**: 1013-1016. DOI: 10.1002/ptr.1976

[64] Naik SR, Pilgaonkar VW, Panda VS. Neuropharmacological evaluation of Ginkgo biloba phytosomes in rodents. Phytotherapy Research. 2006;**20**: 901-905. DOI: 10.1002/ptr.1973

[65] Mancini S, Nardo L, Gregori M, et al. Functionalized liposomes and phytosomes loading *Annona muricata* L. aqueous extract: Potential nanoshuttles for brain-delivery of phenolic compounds. Phytomedicine. 2018;**42**: 233-244. DOI: 10.1016/j.phymed. 2018.03.053

[66] Ullah F, Liang H, Niedermayer G, et al. Evaluation of phytosomal curcumin as an anti-inflammatory agent for chronic glial activation in the GFAP-IL6 mouse model. Original research. Frontiers in Neuroscience. 2020;**14**: 512270. DOI: 10.3389/fnins.2020.00170

[67] Sbrini G, Brivio P, Sangiovanni E, et al. Chronic treatment with a phytosomal preparation containing *Centella asiatica* L. and *Curcuma longa* L. affects local protein synthesis by modulating the BDNF-mTOR-S6 pathway. Biomedicine. 2020;**8**:544. DOI: 10.3390/biomedicines8120544

[68] Sbrini G, Brivio P, Fumagalli M, et al. *Centella asiatica* L. phytosome improves cognitive performance by promoting Bdnf expression in rat prefrontal cortex. Nutrients. 2020;**12**: 355. DOI: 10.3390/nu12020355

[69] Ahmad H, Arya A, Agrawal S, et al. Rutin phospholipid complexes confer neuro-protection in ischemic-stroke rats. RSC Advances. 2016;**6**:96445-96454. DOI: 10.1039/C6RA17874J

[70] Ahmad H, Arya A, Agrawal S, et al. Phospholipid complexation of NMITLI118RT+: Way to a prudent therapeutic approach for beneficial outcomes in ischemic stroke in rats. Drug Delivery. 2016;**23**:3606-3618. DOI: 10.1080/10717544.2016.1212950

[71] Hatamipour M, Jamialahmadi T, Ramezani M, et al. Protective effects of curcumin phytosomes against high-fat diet-induced atherosclerosis. Advances in Experimental Medicine and Biology. 2021;**1308**:37-44. DOI: 10.1007/978-3-030-64872-5_4

[72] Panda VS, Naik SR. Cardioprotective activity of *Ginkgo biloba* Phytosomes in isoproterenol-induced myocardial necrosis in rats: A biochemical and histoarchitectural evaluation. Experimental and Toxicologic Pathology. 2008;**60**:397-404. DOI: 10.1016/j.etp.2008.03.010

[73] Riva A, Petrangolini G, Allegrini P, et al. Artichoke and bergamot phytosome alliance: A randomized double blind clinical trial in mild hypercholesterolemia. Nutrients. 2022; **14**:108. DOI: 10.3390/nu14010108

[74] Singh RP, Singh RP, Ramakant N. Preparation and evaluation of phytosome of lawsone. International Journal of Pharmaceutical Sciences and Research (IJPSR). 2015;**6**:5217-5226. DOI: 10.13040/IJPSR.0975-8232

[75] Djekic L, Čalija B, Micov A, et al. Topical hydrogels with escin β-sitosterol

phytosome and escin: Formulation development and in vivo assessment of antihyperalgesic activity. Drug Development Research. 2019;**80**: 921-932. DOI: 10.1002/ddr.21572

[76] Kalita B, Das MK, Sarma M, et al. Sustained anti-inflammatory effect of resveratrol-phospholipid complex embedded polymeric patch. AAPS PharmSciTech. 2017;**18**:629-645. DOI: 10.1208/s12249-016-0542-y

[77] Baradaran S, Hajizadeh Moghaddam A, Khanjani Jelodar S, et al. Protective effects of curcumin and its nano-phytosome on carrageenan-induced inflammation in mice model: Behavioral and biochemical responses. Journal of Inflammation Research. 2020; **13**:45-51. DOI: 10.2147/jir.s232462

[78] Maramaldi G, Togni S, Pagin I, et al. Soothing and anti-itch effect of quercetin phytosome in human subjects: A single-blind study. Clinical, Cosmetic and Investigational Dermatology. 2016;**9**:55-62. DOI: 10.2147/ccid.s98890

[79] Antiga E, Bonciolini V, Volpi W, et al. Oral Curcumin (Meriva) Is Effective as an Adjuvant Treatment and Is Able to Reduce IL-22 Serum Levels in Patients with Psoriasis Vulgaris. BioMed Research International. 2015;**2015**: 283634. DOI: 10.1155/2015/283634

[80] Yu Z, Liu X, Chen H, et al. Naringenin-loaded dipalmitoylphosphatidylcholine phytosome dry powders for inhaled treatment of acute lung injury. Journal of Aerosol Medicine and Pulmonary Drug Delivery. 2020;**33**:194-204. DOI: 10.1089/jamp.2019.1569. Epub 2020 Mar 16

[81] Singh RP, Gangadharappa HV, Mruthunjaya K. Phytosome complexed with chitosan for gingerol delivery in the treatment of respiratory infection: In vitro and in vivo evaluation. European Journal of Pharmaceutical Sciences. 2018;**122**:214-229. DOI: 10.1016/j.ejps.2018.06.028

[82] Abd El-Fattah AI, Fathy MM, Ali ZY, et al. Enhanced therapeutic benefit of quercetin-loaded phytosome nanoparticles in ovariectomized rats. Chemico-Biological Interactions. 2017; **271**:30-38. DOI: 10.1016/j.cbi.2017.04.026

[83] Kim S-M, Jung J-I, Chai C, et al. Characteristics and glucose uptake promoting effect of chrysin-loaded phytosomes prepared with different phospholipid matrices. Nutrients. 2019; **11**:2549. DOI: 10.3390/nu11102549

[84] Poruba M, Kazdová L, Oliyarnyk O, et al. Improvement bioavailability of silymarin ameliorates severe dyslipidemia associated with metabolic syndrome. Xenobiotica. 2015;**45**:751-756. DOI: 10.3109/00498254.2015.1010633

[85] Palachai N, Wattanathorn J, Muchimapura S, et al. Antimetabolic syndrome effect of phytosome containing the combined extracts of mulberry and ginger in an animal model of metabolic syndrome. Oxidative Medicine and Cellular Longevity. 2019; **2019**:5972575. DOI: 10.1155/2019/5972575

[86] Yu F, Li Y, Chen Q, et al. Monodisperse microparticles loaded with the self-assembled berberine-phospholipid complex-based phytosomes for improving oral bioavailability and enhancing hypoglycemic efficiency. European Journal of Pharmaceutics and Biopharmaceutics. 2016;**103**:136-148. DOI: 10.1016/j.ejpb.2016.03.019

[87] Tao F, Zhang Y, Zhang Z. The Role of Herbal Bioactive Components in Mitochondria Function and Cancer Therapy. Evid Based Complement Alternative Medicine. 2019;**2019**: 3868354

[88] Mateti T, Aswath S, Vatti AK, et al. A review on allopathic and herbal nanofibrous drug delivery vehicles for cancer treatments. Biotechnology Reports. 2021;**31**:e00663. DOI: 10.1016/j.btre.2021.e00663

[89] Saini V, Bala R, Arora S, et al. Phyto-phospholipids complexes as a potential carrier for bioactives having hepatoprotective activity. Plant Archives. 2020;**20**:3835-3844

[90] Kumar M, Keshwania P, Chopra S, et al. Therapeutic potential of nanocarrier-mediated delivery of phytoconstituents for wound healing: Their current status and future perspective. AAPS PharmSciTech. 2023; **24**:155. DOI: 10.1208/s12249-023-02616-6

[91] Breijyeh Z, Karaman R. Comprehensive review on alzheimer's disease: Causes and treatment. Molecules. 2020;**25**:5789. DOI: 10.3390/molecules25245789

[92] Kaur IP, Kakkar V, Deol PK, et al. Issues and concerns in nanotech product development and its commercialization. Journal of Controlled Release. 2014;**193**: 51-62. DOI: 10.1016/j.jconrel.2014.06.005

[93] Agarwal A, Chakraborty P, Chakraborty DD, et al. Phytosomes: Complexation, utilisation and commercial status. Journal of Biologically Active Products from Nature. 2012;**2**:65-77. DOI: 10.1080/22311866.2012.10719111

Chapter 4

A Novel Targeted Drug Delivery Carrier: Herbosomes

Aneri Joshi, Vaibhavi Patel, Achal J. Yeola and Pranav Y. Dave

Abstract

Herbosomes have been modified liposomes that can encapsulate botanical extracts and medicinal substances, improving stability, bioavailability, and targeted administration in herbal medicine. A ribosome or similar drug delivery system can improve the absorption rate and amount of drug that cross the lipoidal biofilm, thus overcoming bioavailability issues. Herbosomes, which are herbal drugs based on phospholipids, offer better stability and absorption profiles than other drug delivery systems. Many critical hepatoprotective phytoconstituents, including xanthones, terpenes, and flavones, play roles in effective medication delivery. To achieve therapeutic purposes, such as cardiovascular, antibacterial, dermatological, neurological, anti-inflammatory, chemotherapy for cancer, and health as nutraceuticals, herbosomes can be produced. Twelve characterization procedures and analytical techniques can be adjusted for innovative formulation through particle size evaluation, membrane permeability, percentage entrapped solutes, and drug release. Herbosomes can be used in dentifrices, medicinal gels, and other local delivery methods. In light of rising concerns about medication dependency and safety, and where modern medicine fails to address complex illnesses, people choose traditional treatments with modern technology, such as nano-formulation, for better outcomes with no side effects and a goal to target spot.

Keywords: nano-formulation, carrier, drug delivery, herbosome, herbal formulations

1. Introduction

Our country's rich knowledge base of ayurvedic medicine has recently garnered attention. However, the current approach to delivering herbal medicine to patients is antiquated and traditional, leading to a decrease in drug efficacy. The integration of innovative drug delivery technology into natural medicine is a pivotal concept that can significantly enhance the potency and reduce the adverse effects of various herbs and plants used in natural medicine [1]. Herbosomes have improved pharmacological and pharmacokinetic properties, making them effective for treating acute and chronic liver disorder [2]. Phytomedicines have been used to treat various diseases since ancient times, and different plant materials have been shown to exhibit multiple biological activities, such as immunomodulatory activity, antilipidemic activity, hepatoprotective activity, and others [3]. *In vitro*, numerous plant extracts display remarkable bioactivity. However, due to their inadequate molecular size and low lipid solubility, the constituents of the plant extract are often poorly absorbed and have low bioavailability. Additionally, when taken orally, gastric fluids can destroy these constituents [2]. This leads to increased bioavailability of herbosomes compared to noncomplex plant extracts. Herbosomes are innovative herbal products that combine phospholipids, resulting in a better absorption and utilization profile in the body. This improves therapeutic efficacy compared to conventional herbal extracts or individual molecules [4]. Herbosomes can help overcome the limitations of traditional therapies [5]. Phospholipids in herbosomes have proven health benefits and demonstrate better pharmacokinetic and pharmacodynamic profiles than conventional herbal extracts [6]. Traditional medicine systems, such as African, Chinese, and Indian systems, usually involve crude extracts of various herbs, which may contain unwanted and sometimes toxic principles and active ingredients [7]. Specific or groups of similar plant ingredients are extracted, isolated, and tested for their therapeutic properties using photo and analytical chemistry methods [8].

2. Herbosomes and liposomes: A comparison

Using appropriate methods, liposomes can be created by combining water-soluble phytoconstituents with phosphatidylcholine in a specific ratio. This process does not involve the formation of chemical bonds; instead, the water-soluble phytoconstituents are held in place by the phosphatidylcholine, resulting in the drug molecule being surrounded by hundreds or even thousands of phosphatidylcholine molecules (**Figure 1**). Regarding her bosoms, the phosphatidylcholine and plant constituents join together in a 1:1 or 2:1 ratio, and the phagosome process involves the formation of chemical bonds. In contrast, liposomes do not form chemical bonds between the phosphatidylcholine molecule and the phytoconstituents. Pyrosomes are more bioavailable than liposomes since they have a lower phospholipid content and are absorbed more effectively [9].

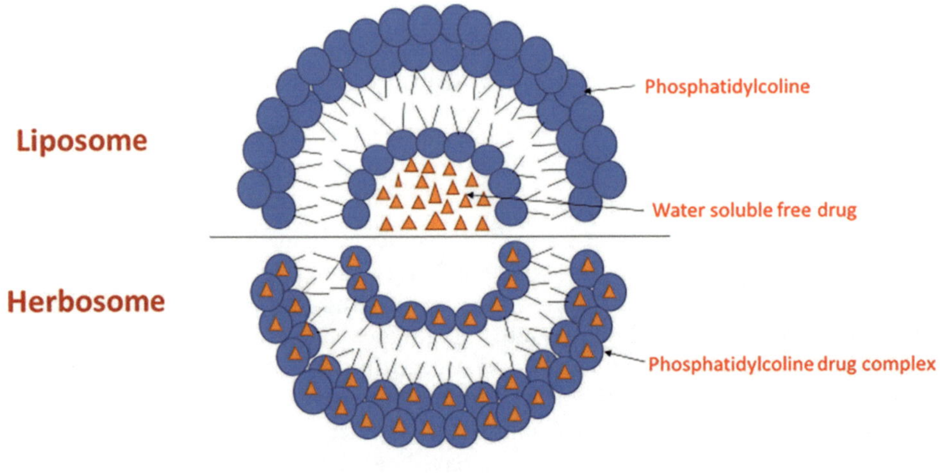

A Comparision: Liposomes and Herbosomes

Figure 1.
Schematic diagram of the liposome and herbosome.

3. Properties of herbosomes

3.1 Physical properties

- Herbosomes are made up of lipophilic compounds that have specific melting points.
- The size of these bosoms usually varies between 50 nm to a few 100 μm.
- When herbosomes come in contact with water, they form liposomal-like structures with a micellar shape [10].

3.2 Chemical properties

- Ribosomes are complexes between the phospholipid's polar head and the substrate's water-soluble functional group [11].
- They formed hydrogen bonds between the polar head of the phospholipid and a polar portion of the substrate [12].
- Herbosomes develop micelle-like liposomes when exposed to water [13].

3.3 Genetic properties

- Phytosomes are novel complexes that are highly absorbed and used. Hence, they manufacture additional bioavailability and higher results than the standard natural herb or non-complexed extracts established by pharmacokinetic studies or pharmacodynamic tests in experimental animals and human subjects.
- Phytosomes categorize their behavior in a physical or biological system based on their physical size, membrane porosity, percentage entrapment, chemical composition, and the amount and purity of the materials used [14].

3.4 Physio-chemical properties

- Phytosomes can be produced by reacting to a stoichiometric amount of phospholipid with phytoconstituents in an aprotic solvent.
- The size of phytosomes can range from 50 nm to a few 100 μm.

When exposed to water, phytosomes take on a micellar shape similar to liposomes, and photon correlation spectroscopy (PCS) can reveal these liposomal structures formed by phytosomes [15].

4. Mechanism

The binding of polyphenolic components in plant extracts directly to phosphatidylcholine has been well-established. When combined with standard extracts or polyphenolic components, such as simple flavonoids, in an aprotic solvent, phospholipids

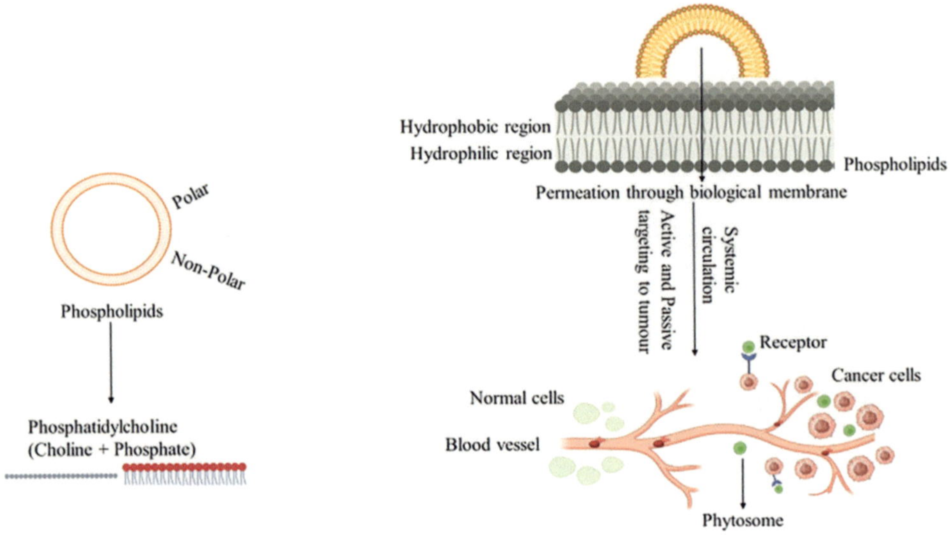

Figure 2.
Mechanism of phytosome complex formation (herbosome).

like soy phosphatidylcholine produce herbosomes. Phosphatidylcholine is a bifunctional molecule, comprising a lipophilic phosphatidyl moiety and a hydrophilic choline moiety. These chemicals are primarily bound by the choline head of phosphatidylcholine, and the lipid-soluble phosphatidyl section, consisting of the body and tail, surrounds the choline-binding substance. The outcome is the formation of the phyto-phospholipid complex, a lipid-soluble molecular complex between the phytomolecules and phospholipids. The polar head of phospholipids is where phytomolecules are chemically bonded, as shown by spectroscopic methods. However, according to the chemical study, the herbosome unit usually comprises at least one phosphatidylcholine molecule and one or more flavonoid molecules (**Figure 2**) [16].

The fundamental mechanism responsible for the formation of herbosomes, in dependent of the manufacture technique, is the interplay between hydrophobic and hydrophilic lipid-lipid and lipid-water molecules. It has been suggested that symmetric membranes need energy to curve because they desire to be flat (spontaneous curvature: CO = 0). Membrane curvature is determined by several factors, including the kind of lipids utilized and the presence or lack of sterols. Lipid-water systems with a cylindrical shape, which constitute bilayer sheet structures, can take on curves and become liposomes [17].

5. Excellence of herbosomes

1. *Enhanced delivery to the target site, systematic absorption, and bioavailability*: As herbosomes are likely to pass through the lipophilic environment of cell membranes, enter the cell, and ultimately enter the circulation, they offer a natural way to improve the usage of herbal formulations. The extracts are better absorbed by the intestinal lumens and more effectively penetrate the skin for dermal and transdermal administration. Because of increased bioavailability, a lower phytoconstituent dose is needed to achieve the intended result. There is

also an increase in the action's duration. Herbosomes withstand the activity of gut microorganisms and are more stable in the stomach environment. Additionally, because the complex is biodegradable, drug entrapment is not an issue with herbosomes [18, 19].

2. *Safety*: The herbosome technique is noninvasive and passive. Herbosome components can be used in cosmetic and medicinal products and are nontoxic and nonmutagenic [20, 21]. Hydrophilic solvent ethanol has now primarily replaced hazardous organic solvents such as tetrahydrofuran and dichloromethane, which are used in conventional procedures to generate herbosome complexes, enhancing their safety and potential for clinical applications.

3. *Additional advantages*: No complex technological investments are needed, and the production of herbosomes is a relatively straightforward procedure. Since the toxicological profiles of the components of herbosome technology are well-documented in scientific literature, there is little risk associated with developing new drugs [21]. In addition to their physiologically acceptable pharmacokinetic and toxicological profiles, the phospholipids used in creating herbosomes have several important medicinal qualities for humans. Phospholipids, such as phosphatidylserine, which functions as food for brain cells, increase the nutritional value of the plant extract.

4. Phospholipids are an excellent source of choline and phosphatidylcholine, which melt fat deposits in the liver, such as in fatty liver or hepatic steatosis. Research has demonstrated the hepatoprotective properties of soy phospholipids, which work in concert to protect the liver from toxins, alcohol, and other medications. Additionally, they have been shown to raise plasma levels of circulating HDL and help with blood cholesterol clearance [20]. Phospholipids with a particular affinity for biological membranes include phosphatidylcholine. Phosphatidylcholine has been demonstrated to be integrated into the cell membrane in place of cellular phospholipids, altering the membrane's flexibility and helping to nourish and preserve the skin. Additionally, because herbosomes are poorly soluble in aqueous solutions, the creation of stable emulsions and creams is made possible by the limited solubility of herbosomes in aqueous environments.

5. Drug delivery platform for numerous drug groups such as peptides and molecular proteins [22].

6. Phytoconstituent dose is lowered due to enhanced bioavailability of plant-based constituents in complex form [23].

7. The herbosomes formulation looks at strengthened phytoconstituent permeability across biological membranes. It is simple to formulate as there is no specific issue in drug entrapment.

8. They increase bioavailability and systematic absorption and ensure distribution to the target site. They can be carried across lipophilic cell membrane environments and improve extract absorption in the intestinal lumen and permeation through the skin for dermal and transdermal application [22].

9. Phytoconstituents generate a small cell that protects the critical components of herbal extracts from deterioration by gut bacteria and digestive secretions [24].

10. The dosage needed is lowered because the significant ingredient enhances absorption. They can also contribute smaller amounts to attain the desired outcomes [25].

11. The vesicular system is apathetic, non-intrusive, and ready for commercialization immediately [26].

12. The dosage needed is lowered because of enhanced absorption of the primary ingredient. They can also contribute smaller amounts to attain the desired outcomes [27].

6. Failing of herbosomes

1. Complicated manufacturing process: The intricate manufacturing procedure needed to create herbosomes is one of their disadvantages. In this procedure, active plant components are extracted and then bound to phospholipids. The several steps in this process might make production more expensive and make it more difficult to scale up production for commercial usage.

2. Leaching of the phytoconstituents off the "some," which lowers the intended medication concentration and suggests their unstable nature, maybe the chief drawback of herbosome [28].

3. Plant constituents in herbosomes are rapidly removed and have a short half-life [27].

4. Because of their increased size, complications will arise while attempting to focus on the various tissues [23].

5. There is a high cost of manufacture and a typical predominance of aversions to ribosomal components.

7. Application

- Herbosomes are also used as an anti-inflammatory, lipolytic, isokinetic, anti-edema, cicatrizing, trophodermic, nutraceutical immunomodulator, antioxidant for skin and liver, cardioprotective, anti-wrinkle, and UV protectant [7].

- Grape seed, for example, is employed as an antineoplastic and inhibitor. It is used to treat benign prostatic dysplasia and as a cancer chemopreventive medication.

- A phytosome in grape seeds comprises phospholipid-complexed oligomeric polyphenols with different molecular sizes. Procyanidin flavonoids from grape seeds have several key characteristics, including a significant protective effect against atherosclerosis, a boost to the human body's natural antioxidant defenses, an increase in total antioxidant capacity, and protection against heart damage caused by ischemia and reperfusion. These actions are achieved through complicated mechanisms that go beyond the flavonoids' higher antioxidant potency [29].

- Green tea's long-term health benefits include its antioxidant, antimutagenic, anticarcinogenic, antiatherosclerotic, hypocholesterolemic, cardioprotective, and antibacterial properties. Green tea polyphenols have very low oral bioavailability from standard preparations, notwithstanding their potential activity. Their combination with phospholipids significantly improves their low oral bioavailability [30].

- By preserving glutathione in the parenchyma cells, silybin shields the liver, while parenchyma cells (PC) aid in cell membrane replacement and repair. These ingredients probably have the combinatorial effect of protecting liver cells from oxidative damage [31].

- They are used to treat hyperlipidemia and vascular and skin problems.

- They are also used to treat high blood pressure.

- It aids in treating heavy metal toxicity through chelation therapy.

- Useful for safe gene therapy.

- Any fundamental nano-formulation must have a specific target, site avoidance administration, and intracellular drug delivery [32].

8. Characterization and evaluation

8.1 Characterization

8.1.1 Visualization

Transmission electron microscopy (TEM) can visualize herbosomes, revealing their internal composition and characteristics, such as morphology, crystallization, stress, and magnetic domains [7].

8.1.2 Vesicle size and zeta potential

Vesicle size and shape over time can be used to evaluate vesicle stability. Dynamic light scattering (DLS) measures size and TEM monitors structural changes [4]. Zeta potential for herbosomes may also be measured using a computerized inspection system and photon correlation spectroscopy (PCS).

8.1.3 Entrapment efficiency

The ultracentrifugation technique may assess the entrapment efficiency of herbal medicine formulations using herbosomes. Liposomes were centrifuged at 2000 rpm for 1 hour at a regulated temperature of 4°C. The supernatant containing unentrapped medication was removed, and UV spectrophotometrically evaluated against phosphate-buffered saline pH 7.4 [32].

8.1.4 Transition temperature

Differential scanning calorimetry may be used to assess the transition temperature of vesicular lipid systems [4].

8.1.5 Surface tension activity measurement

Using a Du Nouy ring tensiometer and the ring technique, it is possible to determine the surface tension activity of medication in an aqueous solution [23].

8.1.6 Stability studies

The capacity of vesicles to hold the medication was determined by maintaining liposomal solutions at 4–8°C for 60 days. The physical examination, drug content, and particle size distribution investigations for liposomal suspension were conducted regularly [32].

8.1.7 Drug content

Quantifying the quantity of medication can be done using a modified high-performance liquid chromatographic (HPLC) method or an appropriate spectroscopic approach [23].

8.2 Spectroscopic evaluation

8.2.1 In vitro and In vivo evaluation

The selection of *in vitro* and *in vivo* assessment models is based on the potential therapeutic effectiveness of physiologically active phytoconstituents present in herbosomes. For instance, the compound's stability can be evaluated by comparing its emission spectrum at different time points in the solid state with a spectrum of a dispersion in water made up of small particles. To assess the stability of phytosomal gels of meconazole, an optimized gel formulation of meconazole was kept at 40 and 4°C for 90 days and then examined for pH, thickness, and drug content modification. The *in vitro* anti-hepatotoxic activity is often determined by evaluating the ribosomes' antioxidant and free radical scavenging activity [33].

8.2.1.1 In vitro drug release

Investigating different pH levels using commonly available dissolving equipment is *in vitro* drug release. The outcomes are evaluated based on the active ingredients therapeutic action [27].

8.2.1.2 In vitro permeation study

For an *ex vivo* permeation investigation of the phytosome compound gel of legal substance measuring 1.5 cm^2, an improved Franz diffusion cell with a capacity of 7 ml was utilized. To ensure accuracy, a literature review was conducted and a diffusion medium of phosphate buffer saline pH 7.4 was employed. The dermal surface of rat skin/cellulose acetate membrane measuring 0.5 cm^2 was treated with a phytosome compound gel containing a legal substance and a plant drug gel. A needle-shaped magnetic stirrer was used to continuously mix the diffusion medium at a rate of around 300–350 revolutions per minute (rpm). The use of hot water helped to keep the temperature at 32 ± 0.5°C. For 6 hours, the diffusion was passed. The 0.5 ml sample was removed at predetermined intervals (0.5, 1, 2, 4, and 6 hours) and replaced with an equivalent volume of freshly made phosphate buffer saline with a pH of 7.4. The solutions' absorbance was determined at 227 nm using UV spectrophotometry. How much medicine permeated the phytosome compound gel of lawsone and the plant drug gel was determined cumulatively [13].

8.2.1.3 In vivo anti-inflammatory study

Four male Wistar rats formed teams for management, inflammation, phytosome gel, and plant medication gel. Every rat was given regular food and kept on a 12-hour light/dark cycle. Furthermore, rats became used to the daily anti-inflammatory activities for a week. Rats were given 0.2 ml injections of a substance known as (1% w/v) under their right and left paw's planter regions to cause inflammation. The present-day 01 orchid scientifics, India digital paleothermometer, was used to measure the anti-inflammatory activity [34].

8.2.2 H-NMR

In polar solvents, a modification is noticeable in the 1H-NMR signal of (+)-catechin and its stoichiometric complex with distearoylphosphatidylcholine. This alteration is due to the atoms that participate in the formation of the complex and is not the outcome of any aggregation of the signal characteristic of the individual molecules. It is necessary to broaden the signals from the flavonoid's protons to prevent the proton's discharge. In the case of phospholipids, all signals become broader, while the singlet corresponding to N-(CH3)3OF choline shifts higher. When the sample is heated to 60°C, extra broad bands appear, primarily related to the resonance of the flavonoid moiety [23].

8.2.3 C-NMR

The carbons of the phytoconstituents were not visible when recording the C-NMR of both the phytoconstituents and the stoichiometric compound with phosphatidylcholine. However, the signals associated with the glycerol and choline portions were amplified and shifted some [7]. Nuclear resonance study of umbelliferone H-NMR. The samples of umbelliferone and composition were dissolved within the solvent dimethyl sulphoxide and analyzed with a Bruker Avance II 400 NMR spectroscope. The spectrum was obtained and compared for the drug and composition. The 13C-NMR spectrum was taken to confirm the interaction between the drug and lipoid and, therefore, the formation of the composition. The sample of umbelliferone and composition was dissolved within the solvent dimethyl sulphoxide and then analyzed with a Bruker Avance II 400 NMR spectroscope (SAIF, Panjab University, Chandigarh). The spectrum was obtained and compared for the drug and complex [35].

8.2.4 FTIR

Comparing the spectrum of the complex and the individual components to that of the mechanical mixes can be done using FTIR to support the spectroscopic evaluation of the produced complex. Determining the stability of the ribosomal complex can also be achieved through FTIR, which is a valuable tool. To validate the strength of the complex in solid form, the spectra of the complex in solid form can be compared with the spectrum of micro-dispersion in water after lyophilization at various intervals, which is a practical approach [4]. In a laboratory setting, the stability will be verified by comparing the spectrum of the compound in the solid form (herbosomes) with the spectrum of its micro-dispersion in water after lyophilization, at entirely different times. For basic formulations, the spectrum of the excipients (blank) must be subtracted from the spectrum of the cosmetic type at entirely different times, and the remaining spectrum of the compound itself must be compared [27].

The meconazole phytosome FTIR spectrum analysis indicates any interactions between the various functional groups present in the drug and excipients. This study used the FTIR peak matching technique to assess the compatibility between the drug, SRE, lipid, and alternative excipients. The FTIR spectra of meconazole, SRE, and MP1B were compared several times. All of the characteristic peaks of MCZ and SRE of C-Cl, C=C, C-O, C-N, -O H, and C=O were maintained within the formulation and were detected multiple times at 638.46 cm^{-1}, 1612.54 cm^{-1}, 1089.82 cm^{-1}, 1375.58 cm^{-1}, 3400 cm^{-1}, and 1734.06 cm^{-1}, respectively. No physicochemical interaction between MCZ, SRE, and Soya lecithin was found, and MCZ and SRE were present within the pure type within the formulation [36].

8.2.5 DSC differential scanning measuring

DSC may be a rapid and dependable tool for analyzing the interaction of various components and medication excipient compatibility. The absence of an endothermic peak characterizes these interactions, the appearance of the most recent peak, changes in peak shape, onset temperature, relative peak space, or total heat. The sample was weighed (2.00–10.00 ± 5 mg) and put into a sealed aluminum crimp cell. The sample was scanned in a N2 environment at 100°C per minute up to 3500°C. Temperatures at which peak transitions begin were noted [27].

DSC can be utilized to accurately and promptly investigate phytosome drug excipient compatibility and multiple element interaction in citrus lemon. The presence of these interactions can be detected by observing the disappearance of the endothermic peak, appearance of the most recent peak, change in the peak form, onset temperature/melting point, relative peak area, or enthalpy [37].

8.2.6 Zeta potential

Zeta potential was assessed using a Horiba SZ 100Z particle size instrument with the zeta potential measurement mode. The lead to a zeta potential of 25 mV confirms the advance's stability. (Sahu D, Pratap R, Rajput S, Patel L, Dewangan P. An updated review on formulation, characterization, and evaluation of herbal and synthetic liposome Vol. 9, International Journal of Creative Research Thoughts. 2021. Available from: www.ijcrt.org). For example, samples were separated into water and placed under 15 minutes of sonication. Before testing, the samples were diluted with water (1:10). Meconazole's zeta potential in the phytosomes zeta potential was calculated using the zeta potential measuring mode on a Horiba SZ 100Z particle size analyzer. The compound's stability is indicated by the resulting zeta potential of 25 mV [36].

9. Novel targeted drug delivery systems

Novel targeted drug delivery systems are a type of medication delivery strategy that differs from traditional drug delivery methods. In the case of herbosomes, it is important to note that the effectiveness of herbal therapy depends on delivering the right amount of therapeutically active components. The negative impact of specific plant components can be minimized with this approach. Traditional herbal remedies were not commonly used in modern formulations due to their fast effects, lack of scientific explanation, and difficulties in processing, such as standardization, extraction, identification of specific components, and blending with other excipients. However, current phytopharmaceutical research has addressed scientific requirements such as pharmacokinetics, mechanism of action, site of action, precise dose forms, additional binding agents, and more. This has led to the incorporation of herbal remedies into novel targeted drug delivery systems, which can be broadly classified [24].

Vesicular delivery systems:

a. Liposomes

b. Ethosomes

c. Transferosomes

Particulate delivery systems:

a. Microsphere

b. Nanoparticle

c. Micro pellets

Biphasic delivery systems:

a. Micro/Nanoemulsion

9.1 Vesicular delivery systems

- Vesicular drug delivery systems are highly organized assemblies composed of one or more circumferential bilayers created due to amphiphilic building blocks self-assembling in the presence of water. They are essential for the targeted administration of medicines because of their capacity to localize drug activity at the site or organ of action, minimizing its concentration at various locations in the body [37].

9.1.1 Liposomes

- Liposomes are colloidal, concentric bilayered vesicles in which the aqueous compartment is surrounded by a bilayer membrane consisting primarily of natural or synthesized lipids. Phospholipids are critical liposomal drug delivery system components, while cholesterol is a fluidity buffer. Liposomes have become popular medication carriers for targeted drug delivery [38].

9.1.2 Ethosomes

- Ethosomes are lipid, soft, pliable vesicles comprised of phospholipid, ethanol, and water that act as a permeability modifier. They have the impact of enhanced cell membrane lipid fluidity induced by Ethosomes' ethanol, which results in increased skin permeability, while this is focused on the deep skin layer [39].

9.1.3 Transfersomes

- Transfersomes are organisms that transport bodies. It is a highly deformable, stress-sensitive complex vesicle with an aqueous core surrounded by a tough bilayer of lipids. These synthetic vesicles are made up of one natural amphiphilic lipid and a bilayer softener, which is a biocompatible surfactant. Amphiphilic surfactants allow transferosomes to reversibly adjust their membrane composition to pass through tiny skin pores (**Table 1**) [40].

9.2 Particulate delivery systems

The most modern treatments include medications made up of micro-nanosized particles (particulate DDS) that can diffuse into the circulation and be carried into arteries, veins, and capillaries while crossing barriers, preventing big particles and organisms from exiting the system. The cardiovascular system uses two mass transport mechanisms to transmit drug particles: advection and diffusion. As a consequence of advection, the medication particles are translated while in suspension of the blood, which flows at varying speeds in different parts of the cardiovascular system. As a result of diffusion, drug particles diffuse in the circulation from a high-concentration zone to a low-concentration region *via* Brownian motion. This is explained by particle diffusion rules, namely the diffusion–advection equation.

9.2.1 Microsphere

Microspheres are tiny, spherical particles with a 1–1000 nm size range. These particles comprise a polymer matrix that uniformly contains medicine and are released using first-order kinetics. Microspheres can be manufactured from natural or synthetic polymers. Due to their high surface-to-volume ratio, microspheres and micro pellets are commonly used for sustained drug delivery. For this purpose, gastroretentive floating microspheres of silymarin are particularly effective.

9.2.2 Nanoparticle

Nanoparticles are submicron-sized particles with a diameter of around 200 nm composed of biodegradable and nonbiodegradable polymers. They enhance component solubility, better absorb integrated medication, and reduce dosage and dose-related adverse effects. They are chiefly used for controlled release and medication targeting particle tissue and organs.

Vascular system	Description	Applications
Aquasomes	Aquasomes have water-like properties with a diameter from 30 to 500 nm. They are nanoparticulate carrier systems with a three-layered self-assembled structure. The particle core is composed of nanocrystalline calcium phosphate coated with a polyhydroxy oligomeric film.	Specific targeting, molecular shielding, carrier for delivering vaccine, hemoglobin, drugs, dyes, and enzymes.
Archaesomes	Archaeosomes, which possess potent adjuvant activity, were obtained from archaebacteria that are capable of producing methane. The vesicles are made up of glycerolipids that belong to the archive and exhibit strong adjuvant activity.	It is used in delivering cancer antigens in combination with checkpoint inhibitor immunotherapies. Poor adjuvant activity.
Colloidosomes	A new type of microcapsules called colloidosomes have been developed. These microcapsules have shells that are made up of coagulated or fused colloid particles located at the interface of emulsion droplets. Colloidosomes are hollow shells that have controllable permeability and elasticity.	Use in drug targeting.
Cryptosomes	The topmost stratum of phosphatidylcholine is a preferred polyoxyethylene derivative originating from phosphatidyl ethanolamine.	Use in drug targeting and ligand-mediated drug delivery.
Carbohydrase	Multidimensional structures are created using carbohydrate-based lipids that can be zwitterionic, cationic, or anionic in nature in this new formulation.	Use in drug targeting.
Cubosomes	The bi-continuous cubic phases are made up of two hydrophilic regions that are separate and continuous. These regions are not intersecting, and they are divided by a lipid layer.	Use in drug targeting.
Escheriosomes	Lipid vesicles made from polar lipids extracted from Escherichia coli.	Use in drug targeting.
Genomes	A functional gene transfer can be facilitated through the use of a synthetic macromolecular complex.	Cell-specific gene transfer.
Layersome	The layersomes consist of several layers and are coated with biocompatible polyelectrolytes to reinforce their structure.	Oral administration and incorporation in biomaterials
Pharmacosomes	Pharmacosomes consist of drugs and lipids that form an amphiphilic structure. The drugs are conjugated to lipids with the help of hydrogen bonds. Pharmacosomes can exist in the form of ultrafine vesicular, micellar, or hexagonal aggregates.	Improving the solubility and bioavailability of various drugs while reducing their gastrointestinal toxicity can be achieved through the delivery of hydrophilic and lipophilic drugs.
Transfersomes	Ultra-deformable and self-optimized aggregates called transfersomes are utilized for transdermal application. These aggregates contain lipids and membrane softeners that are biocompatible.	Use in drug targeting.

Table 1.
Vesicular systems and their applications.

9.2.3 Micro pellets

- Micro pellets are tiny solid particles ranging from 1 to 1000 nm. The medicine contained within these micro pellets can be dissolved or scattered in polymeric solutions using a method known as spray drying. This quick-drying approach is a one-step process and can be easily scaled up, making it ideal for use with heat-sensitive pharmaceuticals. Researchers have discovered that micro pellets made from alginate-based andrographolide derived from Andrographis paniculate can release medication away from the upper gastrointestinal tract. This can help prevent GIT irritation and related issues such as nausea, loss of appetite, and vomiting [41].

9.3 Biphasic delivery systems

Biphasic vesicles are a novel lipid-based delivery technology that combines the benefits of liposomes and emulsions. Concentric phospholipid bilayers enclose aqueous, oil, and micellar compartments in these vesicles. Structural investigations demonstrate a specific scattering characteristic distinguishing biphasic vesicles from simple liposome-emulsion mixes. These cysts have an average diameter from 1 to 10 m, with submicron emulsion droplets at 300 nm and micellar compartments at 50 nm. A phospholipid phase (soya phosphatidylcholine, cholesterol, monolauroyl lysine, and propylene glycol) and a submicron emulsion phase (vegetable oil, surfactant, fatty alcohol, glycerol ester, and wax) comprise the composition. Biphasic vesicles can be customized for drug delivery, including permeability enhancers for transdermal or more profound tissue drug administration.

9.3.1 Micro/nanoemulsion

The o/w type emulsions are micro and nanoemulsions, with sizes ranging from a few nanometers to a few microns. It is a surfactant-stabilized thermodynamically stable dispersion of two immiscible liquids. High-pressure homogenization and microfluidization procedures are used to prepare them. Many herbal medicines and phytoconstituents are mixed into microemulsions for various uses [41].

10. Current strategy of herbal drug formulation

Charles K Armes established phyto technologies, advanced aromatherapy, and herbal medicine. The company produces concentrated liquid phytopharmaceutical extractions from plants and incorporates phytochemical components into body care products. Herbo technologies markets its products directly to consumers and natural practitioners through the Internet. The company also sells some of its products, such as the hair coloring line and the nasal spray, through drug stores and other mass outlets. Furthermore, customers can purchase products online from health food stores and other outlets.

11. Benefits of herbal formulations

a. Some substances can have a higher bioavailability.

b. The delivery of substances to various biological tissues is pharmacologically ensured.

c. Nutrient safety is not compromised.

d. A reduced dosage of the main ingredient can be used due to increased absorption.

e. The drug loading efficiency is predetermined and high because of drug and lipid conjugation, forming cysts.

f. There is no issue with drug entrapment.

g. Herbosomes are superior to liposomes in skin care products.

h. The unique structure of herbosomes has advantages in cosmetic applications.

i. Herbosomes can cross cell membranes and enter cells more efficiently.

12. Future aspects

Herbosomes offer several features that make them appealing as medication carriers for topically administered medicines. They differ in size and surface features, and they can operate as sustained release depots, releasing encapsulated medicines with half lifetimes ranging from 0.6 to 11 days. Furthermore, because of their collagen surface features, a new generation of liposomes known as "collagen-modified Herbosomes" can modulate the herbosomes' and herbosomes' cell contact. Topically applied ribosomal formulations, particularly those made from lipid mixes comparable to the stratum corneum's composition, might be an effective delivery strategy for treating skin problems. In the future, herbosomes will be created for medication delivery with little toxicity and maximum efficacy.

Author details

Aneri Joshi[1], Vaibhavi Patel[2], Achal J. Yeola[2] and Pranav Y. Dave[2]*

1 School of Pharmacy, National Forensic Sciences University, Gujarat, India

2 School of Engineering and Technology, National Forensic Sciences University, Gujarat, India

*Address all correspondence to: pranav.y.dave@nfsu.ac.in

References

[1] Nagar G. Phytosomes: A novel drug delivery for herbal extracts. International Journal of Pharmaceutical Sciences and Research. 2019;**4**(3):949-959

[2] Saurabh KV, Kesari A. Herbosome a novel carrier for herbal drug delivery. International Journal of Current Pharmaceutical Research. 2011;**3**(3):36-41

[3] Barnes PM, Powell G, McFann N. Complementary and alternative medicine use among adults. United States Advanced Data. 2004;**27**(343):1-19

[4] Kumar VS. Herbosome, novel carrier for herbal drug delivery. Current Pharmaceutical Research. 2007;**3**(3):24-27

[5] Mukherjee PK, While A. Integrated approaches towards drug development from Ayurveda and other Indian system of medicine. Journal of Ethnopharmacology. 2006;**103**:25-35

[6] Singh A, Singh AP, Verma N. Phytosome: A revolution in herbal drug delivery system. Asian Journal of Chemistry. 2011;**23**(12):5189

[7] Chaudhury I, Deb P, Das S. A review on formulation and characterization of ribosome complex. International Journal of Current Pharmaceutical Research. 2019;**11**(4)

[8] Howard AC, Nicholas PG. Pharmaceutical Dosage Forms and Drug Delivery System. New Delhi, first Indian reprint 2010: Wolters Kluwer(India) Pvt. ltd. pp. 294-296

[9] Bombardelli E, Mustich G. Bilobalide Phospholipid Complex, its Uses, and its Formulation. New York: U.S. Patent; 1991

[10] Patel J, Patel R, Khambholja K, Patel N. An overview of phytosomes as an advanced herbal drug delivery system. Asian Journal Pharmaceutical Science. 2009;**4**:363-371

[11] La Grange L, Wang M, Watkins R, Ortiz D, Sanchez ME, Konst J, et al. Protective effects of the flavonoid mixture, silymarin, on fetal rat brain and liver. Journal of Ethnopharmacology. 1999;**65**(1):53-61

[12] Kalita B, Das MK. Resveratrol-phospholipid complexes (pyrosomes) with improved physicochemical properties favorable for drug delivery via the skin. World Journal of Pharmaceutical Research. 2015;**4**(5):1497-1517

[13] Singh RP, Chavan R. Phytosome: Recent advance research for novel drug delivery system. Asian Journal of Pharmaceutical Research and Development. 2014;**2**(3):15-29

[14] Upase AU, Bhusnure OG, Gholve SB, Giram PS, Wattamwar PB. A review on phytosome loaded with novel herbal drug and their formulation, standardization, and applications. Journal of Drug Delivery and Therapeutics. 2019;**9**(3-s):765-769

[15] Sriya KC, Sai D, Sankar PR. Phytosomes: A novel approach to enhancing the bioavailability of herbal phytochemicals. International Journal of Pharmaceutical Sciences Review and Research. 2020;**6**:21-26

[16] Li J, Wang X, Zhang T, Wang C, Huang Z, Luo X, et al. A review on phospholipids and their main applications in drug delivery systems. Asian Journal of Pharmaceutical Sciences. 2015;**10**(2):81-98

[17] Mozafari MR, Mortazavi SM. Nanoliposomes: From Fundamentals to Recent Developments. Oxford, UK: Trafford Publishing Ltd; 2005. ISBN 1-4120-5545-8

[18] More MS, Shende MA, Kolhe DB, Jaiswal NM. Herbosomes: Herbo-phospholipid complex is an approach for absorption enhancement. International Journal of Bio-Pharma Research. 2012;**3**(8):946-955

[19] Kidd PM. Bioavailability and activity of phytosome complexes from botanical polyphenols: The silymarin, curcumin, green tea, and grape seed extracts. Alternative Medicine Review. 2009;**14**:226-246

[20] Nimbekar T, Wanjari B, Bais Y. Herbosomes- herbal medicinal system for managing periodontal disease. International Journal of Biomedical and Advance Research. 2012;**3**(6):468-472

[21] Allen TM, Cullis PR. Liposomal drug delivery systems: From concept to clinical applications. Advanced Drug Delivery Reviews. 2013;**65**(1):36-48

[22] Anwana U, Adesuwa Eghianruwa Q. Herbosomes in the Delivery of Phytotherapeutics and Nutraceuticals: Concepts, Applications and Future Perspective. Available from: https://www.researchgate.net/publication/299456386

[23] Dewan N, Chowdhary G, Pandit S, Ahmed P, Dasgupta D. Review on-Herbosomes, a new arena for drug delivery. Journal of Pharmacognosy and Phytochemistry. 2016;**5**(4)

[24] Akki R, Navya Sri K, Govardhani KL, Gayatri Ramya M. Phytosomes: A Novel Drug Delivery for Herbal Extracts. 2019. Available from: www.rjlbpcs.com

[25] Saraf S, Kaur C. Phytoconstituents as photoprotective novel cosmetic formulations. Pharmacognosy Reviews. 2010;**4**:1-11

[26] Sriya KC, Sai D, Sankar PR. Phytosomes: A novel approach for herbal phytochemicals to enhance bioavailability. International Journal of Pharmaceutical Sciences Review and Research. 2020;**6**:21-26

[27] Saha S, Sarma A, Saikia P, Chakrabarty T. Phytosome: A brief overview. Scholars Academic Journal of Pharmacy. 2013;**2**(1):12-20

[28] Singh A, Kumar K, Gupta A, Singh S. Phytosomes: A newer approach towards drug delivery system. World Journal of Pharmaceutical Sciences. 2019;**7**(10):39-43

[29] Tedesco D, Steidler S, Galletti S, Tameni M, Sonzogni O, Ravarotto L. Efficacy of the silymarin-phospholipid complex in reducing the toxicity of aflatoxin B1 in broiler chicks. Poultry Science. 2004;**83**:1839-1843

[30] Hikino H, Kiso Y, Wagner H, Fiebig M. Antihepatotoxic actions of flavonolignans from silybummarianum fruits. Planta Medica. 1984;**50**:248-250

[31] Valenzuela A, Aspillaga M, Guerra R. Selectivity of silymarin on the increase of glutathione containing in different tissues of rat. Planta Medica. 1989;**55**:42

[32] Sahu D, Pratap R, Rajput S, Patel L, Dewangan P. An updated review on formulation, characterization, and evaluation of herbal and synthetic liposome. International Journal of Creative Research Thoughts. 2021;**9**

[33] Maffei Facino R, Carini M, Aldini G, Bombardelli E, Morazzoni P, Morelli R.

Free radical scavenging action and anti-enzyme activities of procyanidines from Vitis vinifera. Arzneimittel-Forschung. 1994;**44**(5):592-601

[34] Bachhav YG, Patravale VB. Formulation of meloxicam gel for topical application; in vitro and in vivo evaluation. Acta Pharmaceutica. 2010;**60**:153-163

[35] Ittadwar PA, Puranik PK. Novel umbelliferone phytosomes: Development and optimization using experimental design approach and evaluation of photoprotective and anti-oxidant activity. International Journal of Pharmacy and Pharmaceutical Sciences. 2017;**9**(1):1-11

[36] Sundari PP, Prathima S, Madhava RB. Miconazole-loaded novel phytosomal topical gels. World Journal of Pharmacy and Pharmaceutical Sciences. 2015;**4**(10):2305-2320

[37] Jain S, Jain V, Mahajan SC. Lipid-based vesicular drug delivery systems. Advances in Pharmaceutics. 2014;**2014**:1-12

[38] Shashi K, Satinder K, Bharat P. A complete review of liposomes. International Research Journal of Pharmacy. 2012;**3**(7):10-16

[39] Tiwari A. Development and Characterization of Herbosomes Complex. 2020. Available from: www.iajpr.com.

[40] Prajapati ST, Patel CG, Patel CN. Transfersomes: A vesicular carrier system for transdermal drug delivery. Asian Journal of Biochemical and Pharmaceutical Research. 2011;**2**(1):507-524

[41] Shukla A, Pandey V, Shukla R, Bhatnagar P, Jain S. Herbosomes: A current concept of herbal drug technology an overview. Journal of Medical Pharmaceutical and Allied Sciences. 2012;**1**:39-56

Chapter 5

Phytosome: A Novel Drug Delivery Approach in Herbal Medicine

Sakineh Shabanpour

Abstract

Phytomedicine is known widely in novel drug delivery systems due to its herbal properties. Extracting the effective substance of plants and targeting the drug to the desired site is a challenging task. Many biologically active constituents are water soluble, which reduce their absorption and thus their bioavailability. Phytosome technology has solved this problem. Phytosomes, due to amphiphilic properties, can effectively absorb from a hydrophilic environment to a lipophilic environment such as a cell membrane and finally reach the blood circulation system. The increase in bioavailability also reduces the side effects of the drug. Due to the easy preparation of the bilayer vesicles and their potency, phytosomes have been comprehensively employed and confirmed by the scientific literature. In this chapter, phytosome technology, its structural components, its physicochemical properties, formulation techniques, approaches as well as advantages and disadvantages are discussed.

Keywords: drug delivery system, phytosome, bioavailability, phytoconstituent, phospholipid, herbal

1. Introduction

In drug therapy, it is significant to provide therapeutic levels of the drug to the site of action and keep them up during the treatment [1]. The capability of the dosage form to convey the medicament to its site of action is critical to the efficacy of any drug, whether it comes from an animal, plant, or a synthetic base. However, a wide range of pharmacokinetic difficulties appear due to one or more biological barriers throughout the body. Moreover, systemic bioavailability can also be reduced due to factors preventing drug flux. For example, the destruction of medicine before crossing the biomembrane or ejection of the drug from the body after uptake by efflux transport systems. Therefore, it is obvious that several parameters are needed to evaluate before designing the drug carriers [2].

Preparations of plants or parts of them have been extensively used in medicine from the past up to now. The use of phytomedicine is well-documented in the world. In the past hundred years, pharmacological and chemical studies have been conducted on a considerable number of plant extracts to recognize their chemical composition and confirm any medicinal effects. Although there were implications of partial loss in the active properties of the purified components of a given plant in case of separation and purification. Phytosome is a patented technology developed by a leading traditional medicine manufacturer. It incorporates standardized plant extracts or water soluble phytoconsituents into phospholipids to produce lipid compatible molecular complexes. Phytosomes vastly enhance phospholipids absorption and bioavailability [3].

2. Phytosome technology

Phytosomes or herbosomes are an advanced novel form of phytoconstituents which are better absorbed orally, topically, and transdermally. Phytosome is a phospholipid complexation invented in 1989 by Indena, an Italian nutraceutical and pharmaceutical company [4]. The term phytosome is made of two terms, 'Phyto' which indicates plant, and 'some' which is cell-like, in which the chemical constituents shield within the phospholipid bilayer [2].

Phytosomes are a product of the stoichiometric quantity of the phospholipid (phosphatidylcholine) and the polyphenolic constituents (like simple flavonoids) reacting inside a non-polar solvent. Phosphatidylcholine is a bifunctional compound, The lipophilic part of it is phosphotidyl. The other part is hydrophilic which is the choline. The latter is the head responsible for binding to the compound molecules. The lipid soluble phosphatidyl portion comprising the body and a tail envelopes the choline bound material. As a result, the phytoconstituents produce a lipid compatible molecular complex with phospholipids, also called phyto-phospholipid complex [3]. **Figure 1** describes the structure of phosphatidylcholine.

In phytosomal complexes, standardized extracts of plant or hydrophilic phytoconstituents are incorporated into phospholipid molecules to form a lipid compatible vesicular complex. As a novel formulation, phytosomes demonstrate excellent benefits as compared to the conventional formulations of herbal extracts and bioactive components. Phytosome technology primarily increases the bioavailability, lipid solubility, and gastrointestinal solubility of the bioactive compounds. For example, vasicine is utilized for the treatment of bronchitis and asthma and is a potential bronchodilator. Due to low solubility, its absorption in GIT is decreased leading to low bioavailability of vasicine. By employing the phytosome technology, its solubility and absorption were increased which led to better bioavailability of vasicine. Other benefits include incremented ability to cross cell membranes, stability, sustained delivery, and prevention from toxicity and chemical or physical degradation. Research have proven the higher efficacy of the phytosomes, in aspects of both reduced dosage and pharmacological potential. Phytosomes exhibit better transdermal drug distribution and have an extensive scope in cosmeticology. Phytosomes of various plants such as *Hedyotis corymbosa*, *Terminalia Arjuna*, *Nicotiana tabacum* var. *Virginia*, *Punica granatum* L., *Geophila repens*, *Vaccinium macrocarpon*, *Intsia bijuga*, *Aloe*

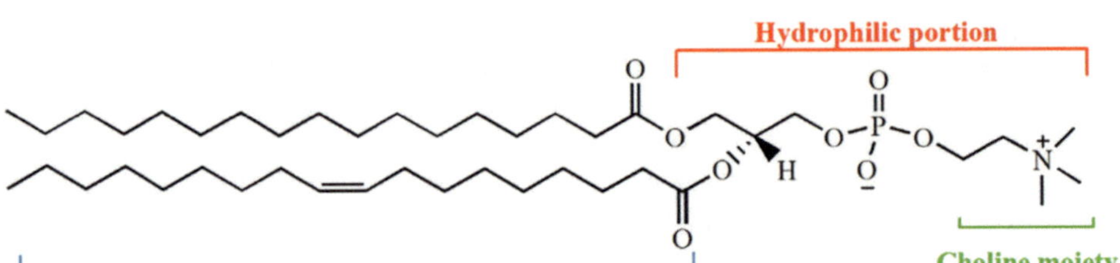

Figure 1.
Structure of phosphatidylcholine.

vera, *Trigonella foenum-graecum*, *Moringa oleifera*, *Centella asiatica* L., *Ginkgo biloba*, *Bombax ceiba*, *Diospyros kaki* L., *Annona muricata* L., *Cinnamon*, *Vitis vinifera* L., *Abutilon indicum* and *Piper longum*, *Aegle marmelos* have been reported with enhanced bioavailability and pharmacological properties. In nutshell, phyto-phospholipid technology carry out as a boon for the badly absorbed phytochemicals and herbal extract [4].

Phospholipids have outstanding properties of amphiphilicity and excellent biocompatibility. These considerable characteristics make phospholipids the most appropriate to be utilized as a crucial pharmaceutical agent and have several applications in drug delivery systems. Phospholipids are basically lipids consisting of a polar part, phosphorus, and non-polar components in their molecular structures. Phospholipids are compounds in which the hydrophilic portion and the hydrophobic acyl chains are bonded to the alcohol group. There is a vast variety of phospholipids due to variations in the polar head portion, alcohols, and aliphatic chains [4].

3. Physicochemical properties of phytosomes

Mixing polyphenols or polyphenol extracts with phospholipids in a hydrophobic solvent is the usual preparation method at the beginning of its synthesis. Later, it was found that hydro-alcoholic solvents have been used to make the phytosome. Since it has an amphiphilic nature, it helps improve the biopharmaceutical aspects of phytomedicines. In the presence of water, phytosomes assume the shape of the micelle. Thus, its systemic availability is increased as related to the traditional herbal extracts, framing a liposome-like structure.

Basal differences exist well among both phytosomes and liposomes. In liposomes, the active moiety is dissolved in the central portion so that no interaction occurs between the nearby lipid and the polar ingredient. Conversely, the inner layer of the lipid membrane in a phytosome can act as a critical part. Since the complex is made inside where the hydrophilic functional group of lipophilic moiety interacts by hydrogen bonds with the hydrophilic head of a phospholipid (i.e., phosphate and ammonium group), building an exclusive arrangement. It helps significantly in the permeability of biomembranes with improved systemic availability too [2].

4. Differences between phytosome and liposome

Based on some observations of high absorption and proper bioavailability, it can be implied that phytosomes have excellent therapeutic efficacy over liposomes. Phytosomes and liposomes are compared in **Table 1** along with their structure in **Figure 2** [5].

Sr. no	Properties	Phytosome	Liposome
1	Bonding	Associated with few molecules (mainly with phospholipid and polyphenol extract)	Number of molecules and even they are not connected well
2	Oral drug delivery	Best for oral delivery	Connected well poor oral bioavailability
3	Phospholipid ratio	Preferably 1:1, 1:2 ratio is preferred for its preparation	

Table 1.
Comparison between phytosome and liposome.

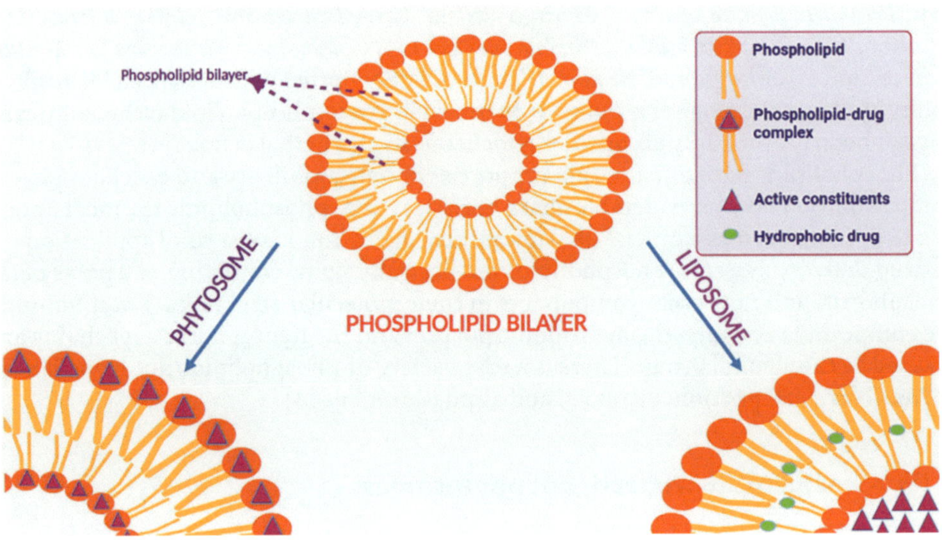

Figure 2.
Comparison between phytosome and liposome.

5. Methods of formulation of phytosomes

Phytosomes are fabricated by the treatment of plant extract into phospholipids mostly phosphatidylcholine. Several techniques have been proposed for the formulation of phytosomes. They include the solvent evaporation method, thin layer hydration technique, antisolvent precipitation technique, co-solvent lyophilization method, and salting-out technique. These techniques are given in **Figure 3** [4].

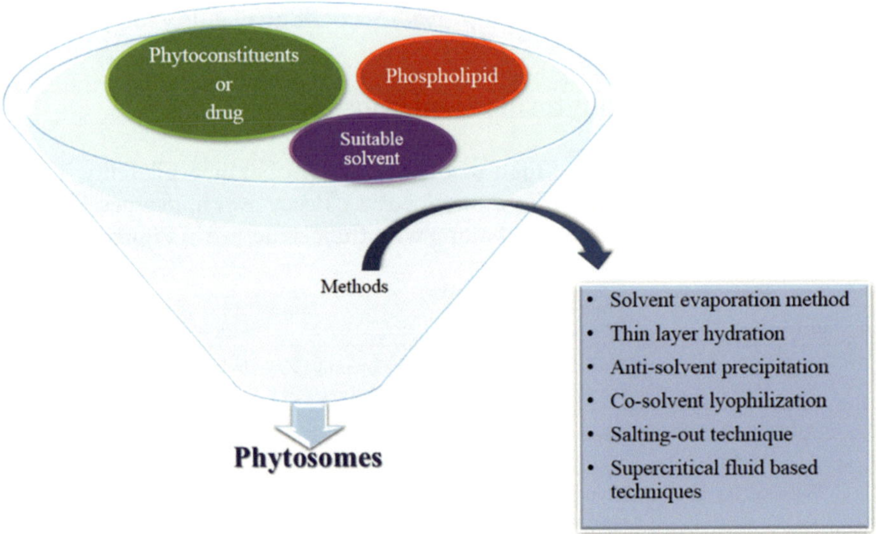

Figure 3.
Fabrication of phytosome.

6. Advantages of phytosome technology

- Phytosomes demonstrate an excellent feature such as better absorption, which leads to better bioavailability than simple plant extracts. An improved absorption leads to a lower dosage of phytoconstituents required for a biological effect.

- Phytosomes are cell-like in which all the important constituents of plant extract are prevented from degradation by gut bacteria and digestive secretions. The formation of phytosomal complexes can also prevent phytochemicals from degradation.

- Phytosomes solubility in an aqueous medium is decreased. It ensures the formulation of stable creams or emulsions.

- Phytosomes exhibit better drug entrapment efficiency and stability because of chemical bonds between the bioactive compounds and phospholipid molecules. It ensures proper drug delivery to the target tissues.

- Enhanced absorption of bioactive phytochemicals across the skin makes phyto-phospholipid complexes being widely employed in cosmetics for their higher lipid profile and better skin penetration.

- Phytosomes have a higher rate of drug complexation. Furthermore, the fabrication of phytosomes is not a complicated process. The methods of phytosomes preparation are simple easily reproducible, but non-conventional.

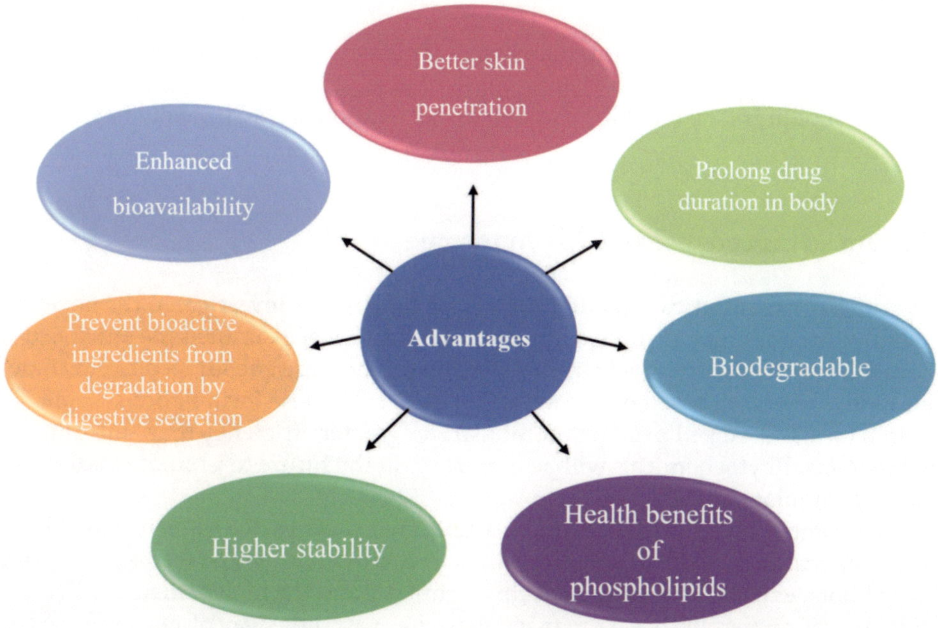

Figure 4.
Advantages of phytosome technology.

- Phytosomal complexation prolongs the duration of the drug. In addition, frequent administration of Naringenin is required due to its shorter half-time and rapid removal from the body. Phospholipid complexes of Naringenin were fabricated with a motive to enhance its duration in the blood circulatory system. In another study, the half-life of andrographolide-phospholipid complexes was incremented 3.34 times than that of pure andrographolide.

- As the phytosomal complexes are biodegradable, drug entrapment is not an issue.

The advantages of phytosome technology are shown case by case in **Figure 4**.

7. Disadvantages

- Despite of exhibiting a wide range of benefits as a drug delivery system, phytosomal products are not prevalent in the market.

- A major drawback of phytosome is the leaching of phytochemicals off the 'some' which decreases the desired concentration of drug which indicates their unstable nature.

- It exhibits a short half-life.

- Hydrolysis, leakage, fusion, and oxidation are undergone by phospholipid molecules.

- Its cost of production is high and allergic reactions to the phytosomal components may also be observed sometimes.

- Their larger size, may cause some issues while targeting the tissues.

- Phospholipids (soy lecithin) can cause proliferation on MCF-7 cell lines of breast cancer.

8. Recent advanced research in phytosome

Various pharmaceutical manufacturers and researchers investigated the novelty and biological activities of phytosome formulations. They examined the enhanced bioavailability of polar phytochemicals. The researchers are encouraged to continue their field of research based on the overall evidence for these formulations. Clinical research on standardized products demonstrates greater efficiency than unformulated extracts. Phytochemicals will be important in the future to promote awareness of these technologies.

Some plant extracts are getting more attention nowadays due to their potent biological applications, such as quercetin, silymarin, curcumin, grape seed extract, and ginkgo biloba extract. The efficacy of this technique and the high demand of herbal medicines for numerous disease management, has paved the way of newer research. Various phytosomal formulations utilizing medicinal plants and phytochemicals have been reported since the development of the phytosome technology [4].

Remarkably, quercetin has been described to exert a specific antiviral effect. In the latest viral pandemic, the phytosome form of quercetin could be a possible candidate as an anti-COVID-19 [6].

A view of literature on a few of the latest reported phytosomal formulations is given in **Table 2**.

Sr. no	Phytosomal formulations	Method employed for fabrication	Biological applications	References
1	Quercetin loaded nano-phytosome	Thin layer hydration method	Anti-leishmania and antimalarial effects	[7]
2	Bergamot essential oil with spironolactone containing phytosomes	Thin film hydration technique	Treatment of acne vulgaris	[8]
3	*Nicotiana tabacum* var. *Virginia* leaves extract loaded phytosomes	Solvent displacement method	Antioxidant and anti-inflammatory activities	[9]
4	*Hedyotis corymbosa* L. extract loaded phytosomes	Phospholipid encapsulation	Enhanced delivery of extract for the efficient relief from neuropathic pain	[10]
5	Phytosomes containing carotenoids of *Nyctanthes arbor-tristis* and *Tagetes patula*	Lipid film hydration technique	Protect skin aging induced due to D-galactose	[11]
6	Phytosomes of Parthenolide	Solvent evaporation method	Parthenolide containing phytosomes attenuate the renal dysfunction and also structural damage by decreasing inflammation, oxidative stress, and apoptosis in kidney.	[12]
7	Genistein phytosome	Solvent evaporation method	Breast cancer treatment	[13]
8	Scorpion venom-standardized quercetin loaded phytosomal complexes	Antisolvent precipitation	Anticancer activity against MCF-7 Cells in breast cancer management	[14]
9	Silybin loaded phytosome	Solvent evaporation method	Neuro-protective activity and attenuates cerebral ischemia-reperfusion injury	[15]
10	Polyphenols from *Moringa oleifera* leaf loaded phytosome	Nano-precipitation method	Treatment against cell lines of breast cancer	[16]
11	*Geophila repens* phytosome loaded intranasal gel formulation	Co-solvency method	Efficient treatment of Alzheimer's disease	[17]
12	Phytosome of *Punica granatum* L. peel extract	Thin film hydration method	Anti-infective, antimicrobial, antioxidative, antidiarrheal, hepato-protection, antiatherogenicity, and anti-inflammation therapy	[18]

Sr. no	Phytosomal formulations	Method employed for fabrication	Biological applications	References
13	Novel diammonium glycyrrhizinate containing phytosome	Solvent evaporation technique	Induce nasal immune responses	[19]
14	*Intsia bijuga* heartwood extract loaded phytosome	Solvent evaporation technique	Serve as an antioxidant, tyrosinase inhibitor, and sun protector	[20]
15	Phytosomes of *Aloe vera* extract	Phospholipid encapsulation	Anticancer activity	[21]
16	Leucoselect phytosome containing grape seed procyanidin extract	Phospholipid complexation	Antineoplastic and anti-inflammatory activity	[22]
17	Phytosome loading allicin-rich extract	Solvent evaporation technique	Extensive pharmacological activities, including antihypertensive, antioxidant, cardioprotective, antimicrobial, antidiabetic, nephroprotective, anticarcinogenic and a cytochrome activity.	[23]
18	*Centella asiatica* L. phytosomes	Phytosome complexation	Antioxidant and anti-inflammatory activity; promoting Bdnf expression leading to improvement in cognitive action	[24]
19	*Trigonella foenum-graecum* phytosomes	Thin film hydration technique	Anti-inflammatory and antiarthritic activity	[25]
20	Naringenin-loaded dipalmitoylphosphatidylcholine phytosomes	Solvent evaporation and a freeze-drying method	Utilized in the inhaled treatment of mild lung damage	[26]
21	Icariin containing phytosomes	Antisolvent precipitation	Incremented cytotoxicity against ovarian cancer cells	[14]
22	Thymoquinone loaded phytosomes	Refluxing in combination with antisolvent precipitation	Anticancer effects on human cells of lung cancer	[27]
23	Selenium-deposited tripterine phytosomes	In situ reduction technique or melting-hydration	Boost the antiarthritic effectiveness a synergistic sensitization	[28]
24	Cocoa pod husk containing phytosomes	Thin-layer method	Antioxidant and tyrosinase inhibitory effects	[29]
25	Chrysin-loaded phytosomes	Solvent evaporation method	Enhanced solubility and improved glucose uptake in C2-C12 muscle cells.	[30]
26	*Diospyros kaki* L. extract containing phytosomes	Phytosomal complexation	Helpful in reducing oxidative degradation caused due to the reactive oxygen species	[31]

Sr. no	Phytosomal formulations	Method employed for fabrication	Biological applications	References
27	Diosgenin derivative loaded phytosomes	Thin-film rehydration method	Anticancer action against lung cancer cells	[32]
28	Phytosomes loading aqueous extract of *Annona muricata* L.	Phytosome complexation	In vivo depression treatment	[33]
29	Curcumin loaded phytosomes	Solvent evaporation method	Helpful in the treatment of human diseases, including cancer, retinopathy, diabetic microangiopathy osteoarthritis, and inflammatory diseases	[34]

Table 2.
Recent advances of phytosome technology.

9. Conclusion

Phytosome is an emerging technique that has shown its potential in drug delivery. Phytoconstituents are water soluble bioactive compounds surrounded by phospholipid. Due to lipid solubility in the outer layer, phytosome technology yields more absorption. Therefore, compared to other drug delivery techniques, it provides high bioavailability. Phytosome's formulation method is replicable, simple, and non-conventional. Nowadays, phytosome is used as an antioxidant, antibiotic, antidiabetic, as liver and heart protector, as treatment of cancer, and its impact on the nervous system research findings. A number of data seem to suggest phytosome as a potential technology candidate for the treatment of viral pandemics. It appears that phytosome technology is promising in the treatment of emerging diseases in the future.

Acknowledgements

The author appreciates the assistance of Dr. Ab. Bagheri, H.R. Rahbari and Milad Karami.

Author details

Sakineh Shabanpour
Independent Researcher, Tehran, Iran

*Address all correspondence to: s.shabanpour90@gmail.com

References

[1] Shabanpour S, Shariati FP, Khatibani AB. Potential alendronate sodium drug carrier by preparation and characterization of sodium alginate cross-linked montmorillonite. Brazilian Journal of Pharmaceutical Sciences. 2022;**58**:e20243

[2] Hari Priya VM, Kumaran A. Recent trends in phytosome nanocarriers for improved bioavailability and uptake of herbal drugs. Pharmaceutical Sciences. 2023;**29**(3):298-319

[3] Jain N, Gupta BP, Thakur N, Jain R, Banweer J, Jain DK, et al. Phytosome: A novel drug delivery system for herbal medicine. International Journal of Pharmaceutical Sciences and Drug Research. 2010;**2**(4):224-228

[4] Mehmood H. Phytosome as a novel carrier for delivery of phytochemicals: A comprehensive review. Middle East Journal of Applied Science & Technology. 2023;**06**(04):21-51

[5] Khanzode MB, Kajale AD, Channawar MA, Gawande SR. Review on phytosomes: A novel drug delivery system. GSC Biological and Pharmaceutical Sciences. 2020;**13**(1):203-211

[6] Di Pierro F, Khan A, Bertuccioli A, Maffioli P, Derosa G, Khan S, et al. Quercetin Phytosome® as a potential candidate for managing COVID-19. Minerva Gastroenterology [Internet]. May 2021;**67**(2):190-195. [cited 2024 Apr 2]

[7] Hanif H, Abdollahi V, Javani Jouni F, Nikoukar M, Rahimi Esboei B, Shams E, et al. Quercetin nano phytosome: As a novel anti-leishmania and anti-malarial natural product. Journal of Parasitic Diseases. 2023;**47**(2):257-264

[8] Albash R, Badawi NM, Hamed MIA, Ragaie MH, Mohammed SS, Elbesh RM, et al. Exploring the synergistic effect of bergamot essential oil with spironolactone loaded nano-phytosomes for treatment of acne vulgaris: In vitro optimization, in silico studies, and clinical evaluation. Pharmaceuticals. 2023;**16**(1):128

[9] Chittasupho C, Chaobankrang K, Sarawungkad A, Samee W, Singh S, Hemsuwimon K, et al. Antioxidant, anti-inflammatory and attenuating intracellular reactive oxygen species activities of *Nicotiana tabacum* var. *Virginia* leaf extract phytosomes and shape memory gel formulation. Gels. 2023;**9**(2):78

[10] Kumar M. Hepatoprotective study of curcumin-soya lecithin complex. Scientia Pharmaceutica. 2008;**76**(4):761-774

[11] Naik AA, Gadgoli CH, Naik AB. Formulation containing phytosomes of carotenoids from nyctanthes arbor-tristis and tagetes patula protect D-galactose induced skin aging in mice. Clinical Complementary Medicine and Pharmacology. 2023;**3**(1):100070

[12] Albalawi RS, Binmahfouz LS, Hareeri RH, Shaik RA, Bagher AM. Parthenolide phytosomes attenuated gentamicin-induced nephrotoxicity in rats via activation of Sirt-1, Nrf2, OH-1, and NQO1 axis. Molecules. 2023;**28**(6):2741

[13] Komeil IA, Abdallah OY, El-Refaie WM. Surface modified genistein phytosome for breast cancer treatment: In-vitro appraisal, pharmacokinetics, and in-vivo antitumor efficacy. European Journal of Pharmaceutical Sciences. 2022;**179**:106297

[14] Alhakamy NA,Fahmy U, Badr-Eldin S, Ahmed O, Asfour H, Aldawsari H, et al. Retracted: Optimized icariin phytosomes exhibit enhanced cytotoxicity and apoptosis-inducing activities in ovarian cancer cells. Pharmaceutics. 2020;**12**(4):346

[15] Pasala PK, Uppara RK, Rudrapal M, Zothantluanga JH, AbdK U. Silybin phytosome attenuates cerebral ischemia-reperfusion injury in rats by suppressing oxidative stress and reducing inflammatory response: In vivo and in silico approaches. Journal of Biochemical and Molecular Toxicology. 2022;**36**(7):e23073

[16] Wanjiru J, Gathirwa J, Sauli E, Swai HS. Formulation, optimization, and evaluation of *Moringa oleifera* leaf polyphenol-loaded phytosome delivery system against breast cancer cell lines. Molecules. 2022;**27**(14):4430

[17] Rajamma SS, Krishnaswami V, Prabu SL, Kandasamy R. Geophila repens phytosome-loaded intranasal gel with improved nasal permeation for the effective treatment of Alzheimer's disease. Journal of Drug Delivery Science and Technology. 2022;**69**:103087

[18] Kazemi D, Nejad Ebrahimi S, Mohsenian KR. Fabrication and optimization of physicochemical properties of nano-phytosome from *Punica granatum* L. peel enriched polyphenol extract. Journal of Medicinal Plants. 2022;**21**(83):60-71

[19] Chen X, Fan X, Li F. Development and evaluation of a novel diammonium glycyrrhizinate phytosome for nasal vaccination. Pharmaceutics. 2022;**14**(10):2000

[20] Sari RK, Prayogo YH, Sari RAL, Asidah N, Rafi M, Wientarsih I, et al. Intsia bijuga heartwood extract and its phytosome as tyrosinase inhibitor, antioxidant, and sun protector. Forests. 2021;**12**(12):1792

[21] Murugesan MP, Venkata Ratnam M, Mengitsu Y, Kandasamy K. Evaluation of anti-cancer activity of phytosomes formulated from aloe vera extract. Materials Today Proceedings. 2021;**42**: 631-636

[22] Mao JT, Xue B, Fan S, Neis P, Qualls C, Massie L, et al. Leucoselect phytosome modulates serum eicosapentaenoic acid, docosahexaenoic acid, and prostaglandin E3 in a phase I lung cancer chemoprevention study. Cancer Prevention Research (Philadelphia, Pa.). 2021;**14**(6):619-626

[23] Nining N, Srifiana Y, Fadlianty EM. Preparation and characterization of enteric-coated delayed-release microsphere of phytosome loading allicin-rich extract. International Journal of Applied Pharmaceutics. 10 Mar 2021;**13**:71-75

[24] Sbrini G, Brivio P, Fumagalli M, Giavarini F, Caruso D, Racagni G, et al. *Centella asiatica* L. phytosome improves cognitive performance by promoting bdnf expression in rat prefrontal cortex. Nutrients. 2020;**12**(2):355

[25] Sharma N, Singh S, Laller N, Arora S. Application of central composite design for statistical optimization of *Trigonella foenum-graecum* phytosome-based cream. Research Journal of Pharmacy and Technology. 2020;**13**(4):1627

[26] Yu Z, Liu X, Chen H, Zhu L. Naringenin-loaded dipalmitoyl-phosphatidylcholine phytosome dry powders for inhaled treatment of acute lung injury. Journal of Aerosol Medicine and Pulmonary Drug Delivery. 2020;**33**(4):194-204

[27] Alhakamy N, Badr-Eldin S, Fahmy U, Alruwaili N, Awan Z, Caruso G, et al. Retracted: Thymoquinone-loaded soy-phospholipid-based phytosomes exhibit anticancer potential against human lung cancer cells. Pharmaceutics. 2020;**12**(8):761

[28] Zhu S, Luo C, Feng W, Li Y, Zhu M, Sun S, et al. Selenium-deposited tripterine phytosomes ameliorate the antiarthritic efficacy of the phytomedicine via a synergistic sensitization. International Journal of Pharmaceutics. 2020;**578**:119104

[29] Pariani SE, Aprilia S, Aryani R, Purwanti L. Antioxidant and tyrosinase inhibitory activity of face serum containing cocoa pod husk phytosome (*Theobroma cacao L.*). Journal of Applied Pharmaceutical Science. Oct 2019;**9**(10): 110-115

[30] Kim SM, Jung JI, Chai C, Imm JY. Characteristics and glucose uptake promoting effect of chrysin-loaded phytosomes prepared with different phospholipid matrices. Nutrients. 2019;**11**(10):2549

[31] Direito R, Reis C, Roque L, Gonçalves M, Sanches-Silva A, Gaspar MM, et al. Phytosomes with persimmon (*Diospyros kaki* L.) extract: Preparation and preliminary demonstration of in vivo tolerability. Pharmaceutics. 2019;**11**(6):296

[32] Xu L, Xu D, Li Z, Gao Y, Chen H. Synthesis and potent cytotoxic activity of a novel diosgenin derivative and its phytosomes against lung cancer cells. Beilstein Journal of Nanotechnology. 2019;**10**:1933-1942

[33] Mancini S, Nardo L, Gregori M, Ribeiro I, Mantegazza F, Delerue-Matos C, et al. Functionalized liposomes and phytosomes loading *Annona muricata* L. aqueous extract: Potential nanoshuttles for brain-delivery of phenolic compounds. Phytomedicine. 2018;**42**:233-244

[34] Mirzaei H, Shakeri A, Rashidi B, Jalili A, Banikazemi Z, Sahebkar A. Phytosomal curcumin: A review of pharmacokinetic, experimental and clinical studies. Biomedicine & Pharmacotherapy. 2017;**85**:102-112

Section 3

Colloidal Drug Delivery System

Chapter 6

Unlocking the Synergy: Exploring the Solubility Permeability Interplay in Microemulsion-Based Skin Drug Delivery

Neha Verma, Sonam Rai, Nishant Gaur and Nitin Kumar

Abstract

In recent years, the pharmaceutical industry has witnessed a growing demand for drug delivery systems that are both effective and targeted. This surge in demand has sparked considerable interest in microemulsions as carriers for delivering drugs to the skin. This chapter aims to delve into the intricate relationship between solubility and permeability within microemulsion-based delivery systems, with the objective of unraveling the synergistic effects that govern their efficacy. This review investigates the physicochemical properties of microemulsions and their role in enhancing drug solubility and skin permeability. By examining current literature and experimental data, we aim to demonstrate how microemulsions can improve drug delivery, particularly in cases where conventional formulations struggle with poor solubility and limited skin permeation. The outcomes of this review chapter are poised to hold significant promise for the pharmaceutical industry by offering strategies for optimizing drug delivery systems. These findings improve our understanding of microemulsion-based drug delivery and guide the design of more effective formulations, advancing transdermal drug delivery. By highlighting key research findings and identifying areas for future investigation, this chapter aims to open new avenues for improving therapeutic outcomes and patient care in the field of dermatology and beyond.

Keywords: microemulsion, solubility, permeability, surfactant, targeted drug delivery

1. Introduction

The transdermal mode of administration presents numerous benefits over traditional routes, specifically injectable or oral methods, in the treatment of diverse diseases and applications in cosmetics. The skin functions as a reservoir, facilitating the sustained delivery of the absorbed drug over extended periods. This mechanism reduces local irritation and toxicity by providing multiple absorption sites and allows for the avoidance of systemic side effects. While the transdermal route offers several benefits, its suitability for drug delivery is limited due to the practical constraints associated with effectively delivering only a select number of drugs through this method.

The skin's stratum corneum functions as a robust barrier, creating challenges for the penetration of most drugs and making it difficult for them to cross through the skin. Fortunately, there are non-invasive methods available that can effectively enhance the permeation of drugs through this obstacle. Utilizing nanocarriers to expand the spectrum of drugs available for transdermal delivery has emerged as a promising and valuable alternative. Nanocarriers offer the potential to deliver both lipophilic and hydrophilic drugs along the stratum corneum, providing the option for systemic or local effects in the treatment of various diseases [1]. In transdermal administration, the primary aim of the dosage form is to maximize the permeation through the skin and facilitate absorption into the systemic circulation. This administration route, the oldest to employ the microemulsion technique, has historical significance. A beneficial approach to enhance percutaneous flux involves elevating the concentration of the drug or utilizing a suitable vehicle that can improve transdermal delivery [2].

The term "microemulsion" was initially coined by Hoar and Schulman in the early 1940s. The formation of a transparent single-phase solution was accomplished by titrating a milky emulsion with hexanol. Microemulsions represent clear, isotropic, thermodynamically stable colloidal dispersions composed of water, oil, and a surfactant, frequently augmented by the inclusion of a cosurfactant. These simulations demonstrate elevated stability, extremely low interfacial tension, a substantial interface area, diminished viscosity, and straightforward preparation [3]. The ME system distinguishes itself from other colloidal alternatives like liposomes, noisomes, and nanoparticles by its unique capacity to spontaneously form and sustain thermodynamic stability without the need for external energy. Additionally, the ME system exhibits improved solubilizing efficiency of drugs, which can consequently enhance drug permeability through skin and bioavailability [4]. The preparation of microemulsions involves blending water, oil, and surfactant/cosurfactant in various ratios, considering the specific type of microemulsion, whether it be oil/water or water/oil [5]. These systems can be categorized into two fundamental types: water-in-oil (w/o) and oil-in-water (o/w). Microemulsions are transparent systems of surfactant, cosurfactant, oil, and an aqueous phase [6]. Amphiphiles, which comprise a mixture of surfactant and co-surfactant, reduce the interfacial tension between oil and water through interfacial adsorption. This procedure reduces the positive free energy change linked with the formation of dispersion at the surface [5]. The primary distinction between emulsions and microemulsions lies in the size and configuration of the dispersed droplets within the continuous phase, indicative of variations in the thermodynamic stability of these two systems. Emulsions exhibit kinetic stability but lack thermodynamic stability; with time or storage, droplets coalesce, leading to the separation of the two phases. Conversely, microemulsions are thermodynamically stable, and their components do not segregate into distinct phases over time [7].

2. Characterization of microemulsions

Characterizing microemulsions poses a challenge given their intricate nature, diverse structures, and the multitude of components involved in these systems. Additionally, each technique employed for characterization comes with its limitations. Yet, obtaining this knowledge is crucial for the effective commercial utilization of microemulsions. Studies on phase behavior become indispensable in understanding surfactant systems, and this is achieved through the analysis of phase diagrams. These diagrams offer insights into the boundaries of various phases concerning composition variables and temperatures. Most importantly, they allow inferences about the structural organization of the microemulsions [8]. The field of microemulsion science extensively depends on characterization techniques, serving both the fundamental clarification of phase and nanostructural behavior and the identification of distinctive properties that render them suitable for the mentioned applications. The practical use of these systems frequently requires the incorporation of additional elements like drugs, polymers, and nanoparticles, thereby increasing the intricacy of the systems. Microemulsion characterization demands the integration of multiple complementary techniques. Recent progress in electron microscopy allows for the examination of the nanoscale morphology of diverse microemulsion structures. Scattering techniques, complementing imaging methods by offering nanostructural information under ambient conditions, have been widely employed for characterizing different types of microemulsions. This involves both model-independent data and model-dependent analyzes [9]. Various scattering techniques, including static light scattering, dynamic light scattering (DLS), small-angle neutron scattering (SANS), and small-angle X-ray scattering (SAXS) offer a detailed understanding of the microstructure [10, 11]. Characterizing a microemulsion necessitates performing measurements encompassing refractive index, pH, viscosity, phase separation, turbidity, density, and droplet size [12].

3. Co-surfactant and surfactant role in microemulsion system

Microemulsions are the preparations that come under the novel &and fruitful formulation because they give their action for a long period and also make them stable, enhancing the solubilization property of the drug with the easiest form of preparation and delivery. In microemulsions, key components such as surfactants and co-surfactants possess the ability to facilitate the formulation of mild, clinically acceptable, and stable microemulsions when utilized at their optimal concentrations. Microemulsions are of two types, The first one is the o/w type where water is dispersed medium/continuous phase and oil is the dispersion phase and the second one is the w/o type where oil is the continuous phase and water is dispersion phase. Microemulsion formulation stability and solubility can be improved with surfactant and co-surfactant. This phenomenon, which involves the incorporation of the solute by amounts of surfactant molecules, is considered solubilization (**Figure 1**).

4. Surfactant

The term “Surfactant” was initially coined by Antara Product in the year 1950. Surfactants can solubilize both organic and inorganic drugs. Surfactants after reaching their Critical Micellar Concentration (CMC) produce micelles/reverse micelles which indeed work as nano-sized supra-molecules in solubilization, emulsification of drugs. This wonderful quality of surfactants is most useful in the bio-medical and bio-chemical fields to improve the production, purification, and delivery of drugs. In recent years various strategies have been used to tackle this challenge and the use of various kinds of surfactants to increase the solubility of drugs is one of them. Surfactants can act as wetting agents which decreases the surface tension and allows the liquid to spread easily. Apart from that, surfactants can also be used as solubilizers and emulsifiers in other formulations [13, 14].

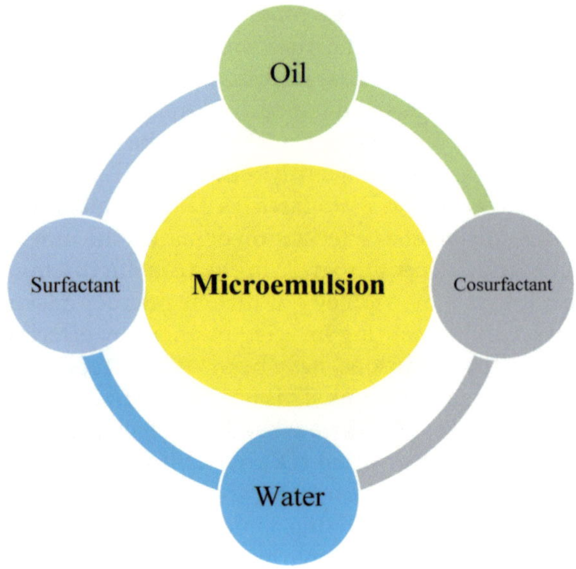

Figure 1.
Components of microemulsion [12].

5. Classifications of surfactants

Surfactants can be divided into four different classes which are based on their charge of the water-soluble segment of the surfactant and have their specific uses in bio-medicinal and pharmaceutical fields. These four classes are shown as follows (**Table 1**) [16].

- *Cationic (positive charge)*: Its exceptional disinfectant and bactericidal properties make it a preferred choice for treating burns and wounds.
- *Anionic (negative charge)*: It finds application in preoperative skin cleansers and medicated shampoos, showcasing bacteriostatic capabilities.
- *Nonionic (no charge)*: It works as nanocarriers like niosomes, liposomes, and polymersomes.
- *Amphoteric (containing a positive and a negative)*: It plays an excellent role in dermatological properties.

The latest developments in pharmaceutical science research and development have sparked significant interest among researchers in a unique type of surface-active agent called microbial surfactants, which are formed by microorganisms. These biosurfactants are regarded as a boon in the biomedical field, especially when synthetic surfactants may not be as advantageous and could potentially cause adverse effects on the skin or other areas. Microbial surfactants (biosurfactants) have some essential features like a less pollutant in nature, biodegradable, less toxic, and easy to recycle. This kind of quality makes them superior to synthetic surfactants. Biosurfactants or microbial surfactants increase steadily better for the hydrophobic drugs i.e. increase solubility (**Table 2**).

S. No.	Classes	Examples
1.	Surfactants with negative charge	Na dodecyl sulfate
		Na dodecyl benzene sulfonate
		Na stearate
2.	Surfactants with positive charge	Lauryl amine hydrochloride
		Trimethyl dodecylammonium chloride
		Cetyl Triammonium bromide
3.	Surfactants with no-charge	Polyoxyethylene alcohol
		Alkylphenolethoxylate
		Propylene oxide-modified polymethylsiloxane (PO = propyleneoxy, EO = ethyleneoxy)
4.	Surfactants with both charges	Lauramidopropyl betaine
		Dodecyl betaine
		Cocoamido-2-hydroxypropyl sulfo betaine

Table 1.
Exploring surfactants: Categorizing varieties with illustrative examples [15].

S. No.	Types	Characterizations	Examples	Uses
1.	Bioemulsifiers (High molecular weight)	Based on emulsification	Lipoproteins	Industrial
			Lipopolysaccharides	Food industry
			Heteropolysaccharides	Cosmetic industry
			Proteins	Biomedicine
				Pharmaceutical industry
				Clean products industry
2.	Biosurfactants (Low molecular weight)	Based on concentration	*Glycolipids e.g.* Sophorolipids, rhamnolipids, mannosylerythritol lipids, succinoyl trehalose lipids	Environmental
			Lipopeptides e.g. Fengycin, surfactin	

Table 2.
Microbial surface-active agents [17].

6. Properties of surfactants

1. *Wetting* - Three types of phenomena are adhesion, spreading, and immersion.

2. *Emulsification* - Surfactants play a crucial role in formulating a stable emulsion comprising two or more liquids that are typically immiscible, such as oil and water. The emulsification phenomenon has worked on different mechanisms like interfacial tension, Interfacial double layer, and Electrical double layer.

3. *Detergency* - Detergents are surfactants used for the removal of dirt by wetting dirt particles and removing the insoluble dirt as a deflocculated particle.

4. *Solubilization* - Surfactants form aggregates called micelles; their role is crucial in the solubilization of immiscible liquids. The micelles formation in polar and non-polar solvents relies on the concentration of surfactant present in the specific solvent. Inpolar and non-polar solvents micelles are formed but it is based on the quantity or concentration of that particular surfactant that is used.

5. *Micellization* - Process of preparing clear solution.

7. Principle for use of surfactants

In microemulsions which are the ternary system, the surfactant has a structure in which the head works as hydrophilic, and the tail performs as a hydrophobic nature. Surfactant molecules can create a monolayer at the interface of two liquids that do not mix, like water and oil. In this arrangement, the hydrophobic tails of the surfactant molecules are immersed in the oil phase, while the hydrophilic heads align with the water phase [18]. In binary systems such as oil/surfactant or water/surfactant, diverse self-assembled structures can emerge. These structures encompass various forms, including cylindrical micelles and (inverted) spherical, as well as bi-continuous microemulsions and lamellar phases, often characterized by a predominant presence of oil/liquid phases. Transcutaneous permeation is impacted by three main factors: the drug's presence in the carrier, its release from the carrier, and its penetration into the skin [19]. These elements impact either the thermodynamic activity propelling the drug into the skin or the drug's permeability within the skin, particularly in the stratum corneum [20].

8. Role of surfactants in microemulsions

Surfactants are available in the formulation of microemulsion with a requirement of large amounts along with co-surfactant in microemulsion, if needed. This large amount of surfactant plays a significant role in producing lower droplet sizes of dispersed phases in microemulsions, concentration of the surfactant is a crucial element in any kind of preparation. It means, that the surfactants (synthetic ones and biological), usually upgrade polypeptide stabilization at below Critical Micelle Concentration (CMC), while the concentrations are higher than the CMC, there is a different or opposite effect, they upgrade aggregation, and decrease the function of proteins in biological system [21]. Oil and surfactant ratio may affect the significant change in the formation of droplets, drug permeability, and solubilization which have a great extent influence the safety and therapeutic effects of microemulsion [22]. Surfactant's contribution to interfacial film formation, and solubilization is more important for stabilizing the dispersed phase in microemulsion. The general truth behind its nanoscale stabilization is the preparation of a monomolecular layer around dispersed phase/internal phase droplets which results in the formation of various microstructures [23, 24]. Three phenomenological constants, namely tension, bending rigidity, and spontaneous curvature, characterize the film of the surfactant or surface-active agent. The films created by surface-active agents contribute to the static

S. No.	Surfactant	Type of surfactant	HLB value	Properties
1.	Tween 80	Non-ionic	15	Emulsifier and detergent
2.	Tween 40	Non-ionic	15.6	Emulsifier and detergent, micellar
3.	Triton X-100	Non-ionic	13.51	Emulsifier
4.	Lecithin	Amphoteric	8	Emulsifier, detergency, solubilizer
5.	Brij-58	Non-ionic	15.73	Emulsifier, detergency, solubilizer
5.	Cremophor El	Non-ionic	13.5	Emulsifier, micellar, solubilizer
7.	PEG 400	Amphoteric	14	Emulsifier, wetting
8.	Benzethonium	Cationic	15	Micellar, emulsifier
9.	Sodium dodecyl sulfate	Ionic	15.40	Detergent, wetting
10.	Sodium stearate	Ionic	8.3	Detergent, wetting

Table 3.
Various surfactants used in microemulsion and their HLB values are as follows [25].

and dynamic characteristics of microemulsions. These encompass phase behavior and stability, structural attributes, and the capacity for solubilization (**Table 3**) [26, 27].

9. Advantages of surfactants in microemulsion

1. It is useful to increase the absorption rate.
2. Surfactants can eliminate absorption variability.
3. It is useful in the solubilization process of hydrophobic drugs.
4. Useful to increase bioavailability.
5. Less amount of energy requirement
6. In-liquid dosage forms enhance patient adherence [28].

10. Role of co-surfactant in microemulsions

Generally, co-surfactants are short-chain amines or alcohols. Co-surfactants have the property that the various drugs solubility increased by decreasing the interfacial tensions between water and oil, whenever used co-surfactant it is important to adjust them at lower concentrations with surfactants. When using any co-surfactant, the co-surfactant must be non-irritant to the skin. However desirable concentrations of co-surfactant should have the capability to produce more availability of drug across skin. Co-surfactants have different classes, but ionic or nonionic type co-surfactants help in the stabilization of a system via the establishment of dynamic micelles formation and further decrease the interfacial tension of immiscible liquids [29]. Co-surfactants are commonly employed alongside surfactants in the formulation of microemulsions. They decrease the interfacial tension between immiscible liquids, like water and oil, to a temporarily negative value. At this juncture, fine droplets form due to the

S.No.	Co-surfactant	Classified	Preferred surfactant	Solubility
1.	Ethanol	Short chain alcohol	Ethoxylates	70%
2.	Glycerol	Alkane diols and triols	Trisiloxane surfactants	40%
3.	Sodium deoxycholate	Bile salts	Tween 20, Tween 60	40%
4.	Caprylic acid	Organic acids and salts	Polyglyceryl fatty acid esters	80%
5.	Sodium caprylate	Organic acids and salts	n-octanoate	62.40%
6.	Potassium sorbate	Organic acids and salts	Poly alcohol	58.20%
7.	Propylene glycol	Alkane diols and triols	Ethoxylates	100%
8.	2-Pyrrolidone	Pyrrolidone derivative	Alkyl sulfates	100%
9.	Butylene glycol	Alkane diols and triols	Guanine crystals	40%
10.	Isopropanol	Short chain alcohol	Ethoxylates	70%

Table 4.
Classification of co-surfactants with preferred surfactants [18, 30, 31].

expansion of the interphase, and a significant amount of surfactant/co-surfactant is absorbed onto the surface until the bulk condition is substantial enough to restore a positive interfacial tension. Short to medium chain-length alcohols, serving as co-surfactants, ensure the flexibility of the interfacial film, allowing it to easily deform around droplets (**Table 4**) [32].

11. Insights into pseudo ternary phase diagram

The formulation of microemulsions involves the amalgamation of oil and water phases, supported by surfactant molecules, and complemented by cosurfactants. This combination ensures their thermodynamic stability, isotropy, and transparency, creating dispersions with these desirable characteristics [33]. Even though there are many more formulation components; with the help of a ternary phase diagram, it is easy to suppose the microstructure of microemulsion which carries oil/surfactant/co-surfactant/water type systems [34].

In microemulsion systems, the diagrams that illustrate the composition and behavior of the system are known as "pseudoternary phase diagrams." The diagrams adopt the shape of equilateral triangles, with the vertices commonly representing a binary combination of two elements, like water/drug, surfactant/cosurfactant, or oil/drug. This is particularly applicable when the formulation comprises more than three components. The creation of ternary phase diagrams is a time-intensive process; however, it stands as a crucial and indispensable step in the development of micro-emulsion formulations. These diagrams serve the purpose of identifying the region where microemulsion exists and examining how varying surfactant/co-surfactant weight ratios impact the extent of a stable microemulsion area. A straightforward and favored approach for constructing the ternary phase diagram involves arranging and graphing experimental data in terms of percentages of oil, water, and surfactant [35]. The development and formulation of microemulsion-based formulations necessitate diverse techniques for analyzing microstructure and formation conditions. These methods encompass the examination of ternary phase diagrams, hydration effects, particle size, and other relevant factors [36].

12. Approaches to skin permeation

The skin consists of two main layers: the underlying active layer known as the dermis, and the outermost layer referred to as the epidermis. The dermis houses essential components such as hair muscles, nerve receptors, sebaceous glands, and blood vessels. Below the dermis lies a layer of fat. Despite its heterogeneity with various cell types, the stratum corneum is the key layer regulating drug penetration. Although it measures only 15–20 μm in thickness, the stratum corneum serves as a highly effective barrier. Drug permeation through the skin occurs via appendageal, intercellular, and transcellular routes, involving hair follicles or eccrine glands (sweat) [37]. The permeability of transdermal drugs is primarily determined by three crucial factors: the mobility of the drug within its carrier, its release from the carrier, and its penetration through the skin [38]. Consequently, researchers face the challenge of developing formulations that enhance drug permeability while preserving the integrity of the skin barrier function. Potential strategies to improve drug penetration involve directly influencing the skin and adjusting the formulation to alter partition, diffusion, or solubility (**Figure 2**) [39, 40].

13. Microemulsion utilizations in dermal and transdermal delivery

The utilization of microemulsion carriers for delivering drugs to the skin is increasingly favored due to their remarkable capacity to dissolve a diverse array of both lipophilic and hydrophilic substances. Extensive research has been conducted on microemulsion systems, especially in their potential applications within the pharmaceutical industry. Enhanced dermal drug delivery has been noted in these systems compared to traditional topical formulations like emulsions and gels. The effectiveness of delivering drugs through the skin using microemulsions depends not only on the vehicle components but also substantially on the composition and internal structure of the phase. This structure plays a crucial role in potentially slowing down drug diffusion within vehicles [41]. Microemulsion works by lowering the interfacial tension on the skin surface and effectively solubilizing the drug. In certain formulations, a permeation enhancer, which could be a surfactant or lipid, is employed. By disrupting or dissolving the lipid bilayer structure of the stratum corneum, this enhancer reduces the barrier function of the skin's outermost layer. This, in turn, establishes a pore or pathway for facilitating the transfer of the drug across the skin.

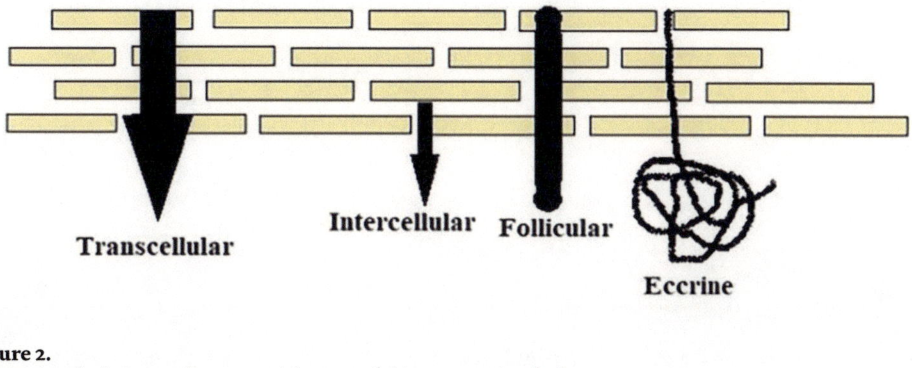

Figure 2.
Illustration depicting various potential routes of skin penetration [37].

Although there has been extensive research and promising results regarding the use of microemulsions in skin drug delivery systems, there is a scarcity of studies dedicated to examining the mechanisms responsible for the enhanced transdermal drug delivery enabled by microemulsions. **Figure 3** delineates the intricate mechanism through which microemulsion components play a pivotal role in augmenting drug permeation. The figure serves as a valuable guide for understanding the intricate details of the microemulsion-mediated mechanisms that contribute to heightened drug permeation, offering insights into how these components synergistically work to optimize transdermal drug delivery.

El Maghraby reported seven potential mechanisms, based on speculative considerations, that define the enhanced transdermal delivery [42–44]. These mechanisms are outlined as follows:

1. The initial hypothesis proposes that the substantial microemulsion drug-loading capacity may act as a mechanism, creating a heightened concentration gradient and thereby bolstering the driving force across the skin.

2. An alternative potential mechanism suggests that the enhanced penetration characteristics of microemulsion components contribute to improved delivery through the skin. This concept finds support in the recognized penetration-enhancing effects commonly associated with oils, surfactants, and cosurfactants.

3. Another possible scenario relies on the penetration of microemulsion components into the skin in their monomeric form, leading to increased drug solubility within the skin. The increased solubility of the drug elevates its partitioning into the skin, leading to elevated drug concentrations in the upper layers of the skin. As a result, this generates an enhanced propelling force for transdermal drug delivery.

4. The fourth mechanism investigates the potential for the drug to transfer directly to the stratum corneum from the microemulsion droplet. This idea is based on the drug's presence within the microstructure of the microemulsion,

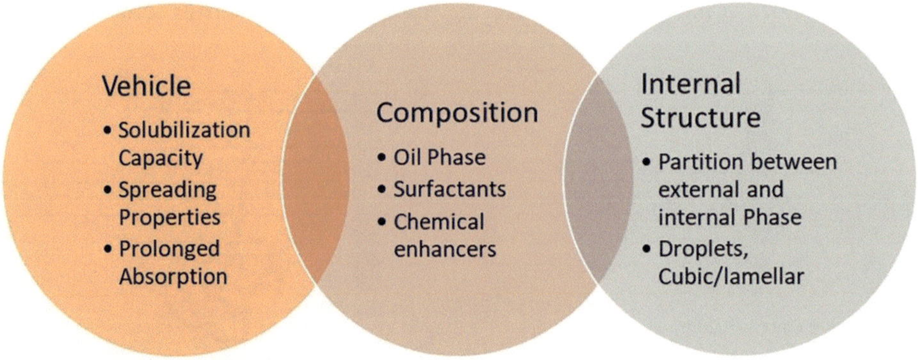

Figure 3.
Elucidating the mechanism through which the components of a microemulsion can actively participate in augmenting drug permeation.

distinguished by its small droplet sizes, creating a substantial surface area that facilitates effective drug transfer to the skin.

5. Another potential mechanism involves leveraging an extremely low interfacial tension, promoting enhanced contact, and spreading between the microemulsion and the surface of the skin. This promotes the penetration of the vehicle into even the microscopic gaps and wrinkles in the skin, thereby facilitating the transfer of the drug from the vehicle to the skin.

6. The sixth mechanism depends on the possibility of an in-situ supersaturation process occurring, which enhances the thermodynamic activity and amplifies the driving force for drug transfer through the skin. Achieving supersaturation involves rapidly introducing a nonsolvent into the drug solution, leading to a state where the concentration of the drug surpasses its equilibrium solubility.

7. The final potential mechanism involves enhanced permeation into and through the follicle. Support for this concept is evident in the observed twofold rise in trans follicular penetration of the drug after the application of liposomes or microemulsions, in contrast to conventional multiple coarse emulsions.

14. Recent developments in microemulsion-based approaches

In recent years, microemulsion has emerged as a versatile and effective tool in various drug delivery systems, demonstrating significant advancements in diverse therapeutic applications. Among these applications is the delivery of drugs from the nose to the brain, targeting neurological and psychiatric conditions [45], as well as insulin-based oral delivery for diabetes treatment [46]. Furthermore, microemulsion has been successfully employed in topical delivery systems, such as the administration of ivermectin for the treatment of parasite infestations [47].

In the realm of cancer treatment, microemulsion has exhibited noteworthy potential, particularly in Paclitaxel Delivery. Poly [2-methacryloyloxyethyl phosphorylcholine (MPC)-co-n-butyl methacrylate (BMA)-co-p-nitrophenyl-oxycarbonyl polyethylene glycol-methacrylate (ME-ONP)] (PMBN) has been identified as a promising way for the effective treatment of cancer [48]. Ocular drug delivery has also benefited from microemulsion technology, with a focus on enhancing the solubility and permeability of sparfloxacin and improving its residence time in the Cul de sac [49].

Microemulsion-based formulations have contributed to advancements in dermatological applications, including the creation of efinaconazole formulations for the specific treatment of onychomycosis via the transungual route [50]. Intranasal drug delivery has been explored for glioblastoma treatment, with microemulsions facilitating the intranasal delivery of mebendazole [51]. A notable frontier in drug delivery system innovation involves the development of a curcumin-loaded turmeric oil microemulsion designed for brain targeting. This formulation not only offers a novel approach for drug delivery but also holds promise in probing protective effects for the treatment of neurodegenerative disorders [52]. The recent advancements made in the utilization of microemulsion-based approaches underscore their potential to revolutionize drug delivery systems. These diverse applications, ranging from neurological conditions to cancer and beyond, highlight the significant impact of microemulsion technology in advancing therapeutic interventions. This comprehensive overview serves as a valuable contribution to the current literature on drug delivery systems. Microemulsion systems are recognized as advanced drug delivery platforms capable of facilitating extended or regulated drug release through diverse administration routes, such as transdermal, intravenous, nasal, oral, topical, and ophthalmic, among others. Employing microemulsions for drug delivery represents a viable approach to enhance pharmacological target specificity, increase therapeutic effectiveness, and reduce potential toxicity. The notable existence of diverse polarity domains within microemulsion systems emphasizes their substantial potential as carriers for drug delivery across a broad spectrum of pharmaceuticals [53].

15. Future directions

Innovations in pharmaceuticals, such as Novel Drug Delivery Systems, provide healthcare professionals with a diverse array of tools to address diseases with unprecedented levels of effectiveness, safety, and precision. From a clinical perspective, Novel Drug Delivery Systems not only alleviate the fluctuating pattern of drug levels in the bloodstream but also enable precise drug targeting to their intended site of action, consequently minimizing side effects associated with dosage. Uncovering novel drugs and optimizing their optimal Drug Delivery Systems (DDS) stands as a primary challenge in the medical field, significantly influencing the effectiveness and outcomes of various diseases and treatments. The fundamental attributes of an ideal Drug Delivery System (DDS) encompass drug loading capacity and subsequent release, crucial factors contributing to heightened drug bioavailability, the capability to reach specific targets, and controlled, timely release. Hence, a variety of drug delivery vectors, including polymeric, cellular carriers, macromolecular, and particulate, have been developed to serve diverse functions in the transportation of drugs. Microspheres, micelles, liposomes, and nanoparticles represent various colloidal forms of Drug Delivery Systems (DDS). Microemulsions, emerging as innovative Drug Delivery Systems (DDS), consist of essential components such as water, oil, and surfactants. A critical aspect in formulating these systems optimally lies in addressing the safety and biocompatibility of the materials employed. Microemulsions were formulated using microbial surfactants and natural oils. Microemulsions present a diverse array of applications, including but not limited to targeted drug delivery, controlled drug administration, sustained drug release, taste masking, improvement of bioavailability, and enzyme immobilization. Due to the instability of hydrophilic drugs when orally administered in the gastrointestinal tract (GIT), there is a necessity to investigate innovative methods incorporating biocompatible elements for active targeting in clinical trial practices.

Author details

Neha Verma, Sonam Rai, Nishant Gaur* and Nitin Kumar
Saraswathi College of Pharmacy, Hapur, India

*Address all correspondence to: nkgaur29@gmail.com

References

[1] Yu YQ, Yang X, Wu XF, Fan YB. Enhancing permeation of drug molecules across the skin via delivery in nanocarriers: Novel strategies for effective transdermal applications. Frontiers in Bioengineering and Biotechnology. 2021;**9**:646554

[2] Jadhav KR, Shaikh IM, Ambade KW, Kadam VJ. Applications of microemulsion based drug delivery system. Current Drug Delivery. 2006;**3**(3):267-273

[3] Moghimipour E, Salimi A, Leis F. Preparation and evaluation of tretinoin microemulsion based on pseudo-ternary phase diagram. Advanced Pharmaceutical Bulletin. 2012;**2**(2):141

[4] Vicentini FT, Vaz MM, Fonseca YM, Bentley MV, Fonseca MJ. Characterization and stability study of a water-in-oil microemulsion incorporating quercetin. Drug Development and Industrial Pharmacy. 2011;**37**(1):47-55

[5] Suhail N, Alzahrani AK, Basha WJ, Kizilbash N, Zaidi A, Ambreen J, et al. Microemulsions: Unique properties, pharmacological applications, and targeted drug delivery. Frontiers in Nanotechnology. 2021;**3**:754889

[6] Shinde U, Pokharkar S, Modani S. Design and evaluation of microemulsion gel system of nadifloxacin. Indian Journal of Pharmaceutical Sciences. 2012;**74**(3):237

[7] Singh V, Bushettii SS, Raju SA, Ahmad R, Singh M, Bisht A. Microemulsions as promising delivery systems: A review. Indian Journal of Pharmaceutical Education and Research. 2011;**45**(4):392-401

[8] Jha SK, Dey S, Karki S. Microemulsions-potential carrier for improved drug delivery. Asian Journal of Biomedical and Pharmaceutical Sciences. 2011;**1**(1):5-9

[9] Acharya DP, Hartley PG. Progress in microemulsion characterization. Current Opinion in Colloid & Interface Science. 2012;**17**(5):274-280

[10] Lawrence MJ, Rees GD. Microemulsion-based media as novel drug delivery systems. Advanced Drug Delivery Reviews. 2012;**64**:175-193

[11] Paul S, Panda AK. Combined phase behavior, dynamic light scattering, viscosity and spectroscopic investigations of a pyridinium-based ionic liquid-in-oil microemulsion. RSC Advances. 2014;**4**(61):32383-32390

[12] Sujatha B, Himabindu E, Bttu S, Abbulu K. Microemulsions - A review. Journal of Pharmaceutical Sciences and Research. 2020;**12**(6):750-753

[13] Aguirre-Ramírez M, Silva-Jiménez H, Banat IM, Díaz De Rienzo MA. Surfactants: Physicochemical interactions with biological macromolecules. Biotechnology Letters. 2021;**43**:523-535

[14] Sadaghiani AS. Conductometry technique to study the surfactants in pharmaceutical formulations. Journal of Advanced Chemical and Pharmaceutical Materials (JACPM). 2020;**3**(3):266-268

[15] Sekhon BS. Surfactants: Pharmaceutical and medicinal aspects. Journal of Pharmaceutical Technology, Research and Management. 2013;**1**(1):43-68

[16] Eras-Muñoz E, Farré A, Sánchez A, Font X, Gea T. Microbial biosurfactants: A review of recent environmental applications. Bioengineered. 2022;**13**(5):12365-12391

[17] Wei Z, Wang JJ, Gaston LA, Li J, Fultz LM, DeLaune RD, et al. Remediation of crude oil-contaminated coastal marsh soil: Integrated effect of biochar, rhamnolipid biosurfactant, and nitrogen application. Journal of Hazardous Materials. 2020;**396**:122595

[18] Ande NS, Sonone BK, Bakal LR, Ajmire VP, Sawarkar SH. Role of surfactant and co-surfactant in microemulsion: A review. Research Journal of Pharmacy and Technology. 2022;**15**(10):4829-4834

[19] Morris SA, Anantha-padmanabhan KP, Kasting GB. Anionic surfactant–induced changes in skin permeability. Journal of Pharmaceutical Sciences. 2019;**108**(11):3640-3648

[20] Ohadi M, Shahravan A, Dehghannoudeh N, Eslaminejad T, Banat IM, Dehghannoudeh G. Potential use of microbial surfactant in microemulsion drug delivery system: A systematic review. Drug Design, Development and Therapy. 2020;**14**:541-550

[21] Malik NA. Surfactant–amino acid and surfactant–surfactant interactions in aqueous medium: A review. Applied Biochemistry and Biotechnology. 2015;**176**:2077-2106

[22] Sarheed O, Dibi M, Ramesh KV. Studies on the effect of oil and surfactant on the formation of alginate-based O/W lidocaine nanocarriers using nanoemulsion template. Pharmaceutics. 2020;**12**(12):1223

[23] Yuan JS, Yip A, Nguyen N, Chu J, Wen XY, Acosta EJ. Effect of surfactant concentration on transdermal lidocaine delivery with linker microemulsions. International Journal of Pharmaceutics. 2010;**392**(1-2):274-284

[24] Molle B, De Geyer A, Guillermo A, Farago B. Steric interactions in cellular structures formed in a water/oil/surfactant/cosurfactant mixture. Physical Review Letters. 2003;**90**(6):068305

[25] Matsaridou I, Barmpalexis P, Salis A, Nikolakakis I. The influence of surfactant HLB and oil/surfactant ratio on the formation and properties of self-emulsifying pellets and microemulsion reconstitution. AAPS PharmSciTech. 2012;**13**:1319-1330

[26] Sandhu RK, Kaur A, Kaur P, Rajput JK, Khullar P, Bakshi MS. Solubilization of surfactant stabilized gold nanoparticles in oil–in–water and water–in–oil microemulsions. Journal of Molecular Liquids. 2021;**336**:116305

[27] Ahmed N, Kermanshahi B, Ghazani SM, Tait K, Tcheng M, Roma A, et al. Avocado-derived polyols for use as novel co-surfactants in low energy self-emulsifying microemulsions. Scientific Reports. 2020;**10**(1):5566

[28] Bhura MR, Shahiwala A. Poorly water-soluble drugs and formulation strategy to improve oral bioavailability. In: Novel Drug Delivery Technologies: Innovative Strategies for Drug Re-Positioning. 2019. pp. 11-28

[29] Duangjit S, Chairat W, Opanasopit P, Rojanarata T, Panomsuk S, Ngawhirunpat T. Development, characterization and skin interaction of capsaicin-loaded microemulsion-based nonionic surfactant. Biological and Pharmaceutical Bulletin. 2016;**39**(4):601-610

[30] Azeem A, Rizwan M, Ahmad FJ, Khar RK, Iqbal Z, Talegaonkar S. Components screening and influence of surfactant and cosurfactant on nanoemulsion formation. Current Nanoscience. 2009;**5**(2):220-226

[31] Elnikova L. 3D lattice model for the phase transition in a water/oil/surfactant/cosurfactant mixture. Solid State Phenomena. 2006;**115**:315-318

[32] Abd Sisak MA, Daik R, Ramli S. Study on the effect of oil phase and co-surfactant on microemulsion systems. Malaysian Journal of Analytical Sciences. 2017;**21**:1409-1416

[33] Zhang H, Cui Y, Zhu S, Feng F, Zheng X. Characterization and antimicrobial activity of a pharmaceutical microemulsion. International Journal of Pharmaceutics. 2010;**395**(1-2):154-160

[34] Burguera JL, Burguera M. Analytical applications of emulsions and microemulsions. Talanta. 2012;**96**:11-20

[35] Berkman MS, Güleç K. Pseudo ternary phase diagrams: A practical approach for the area and centroid calculation of stable microemulsion regions. İstanbul Journal of Pharmacy. 2021;**51**(1):42-49

[36] Hickey S, Hagan SA, Kudryashov E, Buckin V. Analysis of phase diagram and microstructural transitions in an ethyl oleate/water/Tween 80/Span 20 microemulsion system using high-resolution ultrasonic spectroscopy. International Journal of Pharmaceutics. 2010;**388**(1-2):213-222

[37] Kogan A, Garti N. Microemulsions as transdermal drug delivery vehicles. Advances in Colloid and Interface Science. 2006;**123**:369-385

[38] Peltola S, Saarinen-Savolainen P, Kiesvaara J, Suhonen TM, Urtti A. Microemulsions for topical delivery of estradiol. International Journal of Pharmaceutics. 2003;**254**(2):99-107

[39] Hadgraft J. Skin, the final frontier. International Journal of Pharmaceutics. 2001;**224**(1-2):1-8

[40] Williams AC, Barry BW. Penetration enhancers. Advanced Drug Delivery Reviews. 2012;**64**:128-137

[41] Santos P, Watkinson AC, Hadgraft J, Lane ME. Application of microemulsions in dermal and transdermal drug delivery. Skin Pharmacology and Physiology. 2008;**21**(5):246-259

[42] Kreilgaard M. Influence of microemulsions on cutaneous drug delivery. Advanced Drug Delivery Reviews. 2002;**54**:S77-S98

[43] El Maghraby GM. Transdermal delivery of hydrocortisone from eucalyptus oil microemulsion: Effects of cosurfactants. International Journal of Pharmaceutics. 2008;**355**(1-2):285-292

[44] El Maghraby GM. Microemulsions as transdermal drug delivery systems. Current Nanoscience. 2012;**8**(4):504-511

[45] Froelich A, Osmałek T, Jadach B, Puri V, Michniak-Kohn B. Microemulsion-based media in nose-to-brain drug delivery. Pharmaceutics. 2021;**13**(2):201

[46] Momoh MA, Franklin KC, Agbo CP, Ugwu CE, Adedokun MO, Anthony OC, et al. Microemulsion-based approach for oral delivery of insulin: Formulation design and characterization. Heliyon. 2020;**6**(3):e03650

[47] Das S, Lee SH, Chia VD, Chow PS, Macbeath C, Liu Y, et al.

Development of microemulsion based topical ivermectin formulations: Pre-formulation and formulation studies. Colloids and Surfaces B: Biointerfaces. 2020;**189**:110823

[48] Gharbavi M, Sharafi A, Motamed Fath P, Oruji S, Pakzad H, KheiriManjili H. Formulation and biocompatibility of microemulsion-based PMBN as an efficient system for paclitaxel delivery. Journal of Applied Biotechnology Reports. 2021;**8**(1):51-62

[49] Dhaval M, Devani J, Parmar R, Soniwala MM, Chavda J. Formulation and optimization of microemulsion based sparfloxacin in-situ gel for ocular delivery: In vitro and ex vivo characterization. Journal of Drug Delivery Science and Technology. 2020;**55**:101373

[50] Agrawal V, Patel R, Patel M, Thanki K, Mishra S. Design and evaluation of microemulsion-based efinaconazole formulations for targeted treatment of onychomycosis through transungual route: Ex vivo and nail clipping studies. Colloids and Surfaces B: Biointerfaces. 2021;**201**:111652

[51] Mena-Hernández J, Jung-Cook H, Llaguno-Munive M, García-López P, Ganem-Rondero A, López-Ramírez S, et al. Preparation and evaluation of mebendazole microemulsion for intranasal delivery: An alternative approach for glioblastoma treatment. AAPS PharmSciTech. 2020;**21**:1-2

[52] More S, Pawar A. Brain targeted curcumin loaded turmeric oil microemulsion protects against trimethyltin induced neurodegeneration in adult zebrafish: A pharmacokinetic and pharmacodynamic insight. Pharmaceutical Research. 2023;**40**(3):675-687

[53] Yadav KS, Soni G, Choudhary D, Khanduri A, Bhandari A, Joshi G. Microemulsions for enhancing drug delivery of hydrophilic drugs: Exploring various routes of administration. Medicine in Drug Discovery. 2023;**20**:100162

Chapter 7

Solid Lipid Nanoparticles: A Promising Drug Delivery System and Their Potential for Peptide and Protein Therapeutics

Soheil Mehrdadi

Abstract

The discovery of peptide and protein therapeutics such as insulin and adrenocorticotrophic hormone in the twentieth century was a breakthrough in drug discovery. However, peptide and protein therapeutics due to their characteristics are predisposed to denaturation and degradation and their delivery and formulation have been a persistent challenge for the biotech and pharmaceutical industry. Their bioavailability is very low mainly due to low gastrointestinal solubility and permeability resulting from low membrane penetration, high molecular weight, proteolytic chemical and enzymatic degradation which altogether urge a compatible drug delivery system. Numerous drug delivery systems with modifiable properties have been synthesized. Solid Lipid Nanoparticles (SLNs) protect the encapsulated peptide and protein therapeutics against first-pass effect and proteolytic degradation, thus enhance drug stability, dissolution rate, absorption and bioavailability. The physicochemical properties of SLNs such as small size, high surface area and surface modification improve their mucosal adhesion, tissue-targeted distribution, controlled drug release and half-life. Besides, SLNs can be encapsulated by both hydrophilic and lipophilic drugs which also offer simplicity of preparation, large-scale manufacturing, biodegradability, biocompatibility, low toxicity, low adverse effects and various drug release profile.

Keywords: solid lipid nanoparticles, drug delivery, drug discovery, peptide and protein therapeutics, nanomedicine

1. Introduction

With the breakthrough of novel techniques in pharmaceutical biotechnologies, molecular pharmacology, and medicinal chemistry in recent decades, new approaches have spawned in both drug discovery and drug delivery – as two sides of a coin – to improve the therapeutic efficiency of some of the already-existing drugs and/or introduce new molecular entities (NMEs) into the market. The past decades have witnessed a booming market for protein and peptide drugs (PPDs), owing to their

IntechOpen

superior efficiency and biocompatibility compared to their chemical counterparts, "small molecular drugs".

With the introduction of more advanced biomedical analytical methods, and novel genetic and molecular engineering methods in recent decades peptides and proteins, among all endogenous biomolecules of the body, have been the focus of studies and research sector leading to the recognition of various peptides and proteins as NMEs, large-scale protein production and a better-defined role of peptides and proteins as regulatory components of numerous diseases [1], which eventually rendered them as Active Pharmaceutical Ingredients (API) of a new category and generation of medicinal products – e.g. biopharmaceuticals – for the treatment of diseases [2] and recently as a vaccine [3] turning them into the fastest growing sector in pharmaceutical and biotechnology industry [4].

Peptides and proteins have various physiological functions such as hormones, enzyme substrates, enzyme inhibitors, antibiotics, biological regulators, structural components, cellular signaling factors, growth factors, ion channel ligands, neurotransmitters, and catalyzers, and any disorder/dysfunction in their structure or function leads to serious diseases and pathological conditions such as diabetes [5], dwarfism [6], cystic fibrosis [7], thalassemia [8], or impaired blood clotting [9], among many others [10, 11].

PPDs, due to their intrinsic biological characteristics – poor in-vivo stability, poor membrane penetration, low tissue distribution, and low bioavailability [12, 13]– lack the necessary physicochemical requirements and fail to penetrate through biological barriers, implying the importance of proper nanoparticle systems to maintain their biological integrity with the maximum therapeutic concentration and minimum adverse effect [14].

This chapter discusses PPDs, their historical development, pharmaceutical characteristics, studies for their therapeutic application, formulation challenges, and the importance of systematic preformulation studies for their translation into the clinical setting by solid lipid nanoparticles (SLNs) as a promising system for their delivery. There are numerous studies in the literature on the various methodologies of the synthesis of SLNs [15, 16].

2. The journey of "drug discovery" toward peptide/protein therapeutics

In recent decades, the old paradigm of drug discovery – identification of endogenous active compounds/natural products, followed by chemical modifications to optimize their characteristics in in-vivo models – has switched to the modern paradigm, which relies mainly on target-based drug discovery (**Figure 1**), i.e. in-vitro screening to identify compounds – also known as "leads" – that bind to and inhibit/activate a biological target and then optimize their pharmacological properties, such as target selectivity, pharmacokinetics, and safety, by changing the chemical structure [17].

Hence, receptors as "drug targets" have been the focus of pipeline studies and research for introducing novel drug candidates [18]. The vast majority of drugs exert their effects by interacting with their receptors, which are macromolecules yielding a biological response upon interaction with a drug molecule, followed by a chain of physicochemical events leading to a particular pharmacological response. However, some drugs act extracellularly without involving a drug–receptor interaction at non-cellular constituents of the body (e.g. neutralization of gastric acid by antacid drugs)

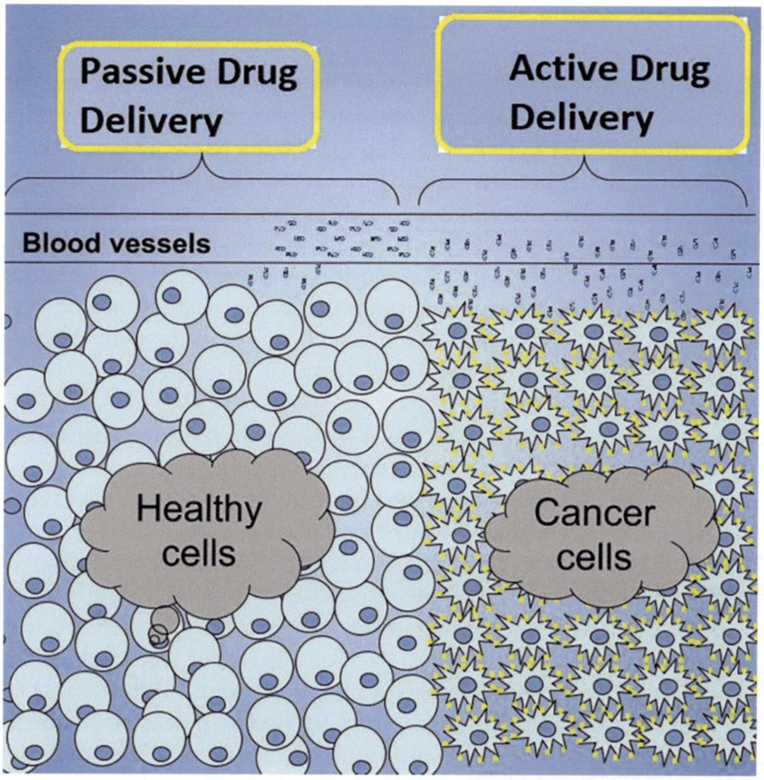

Figure 1.
Passive (non-targeted) versus active (targeted) drug delivery; cancer cells overexpressing a specific receptor can be identified and targeted with surface-modified nanoparticles.

by acting through macromolecular components, while the biological effects result from non-specific effects of the chemical properties of the drugs (e.g. alcohol acting by destroying the integrity of the cell through disrupting the cellular constituents) [15].

There are basically four classes of receptor molecules – lipoproteins (or glycoproteins), proteins, nucleic acids, and lipids – where proteins and recently peptides have been the main protagonists for drug discovery [19].

The classical strategy in drug discovery revolved around four concepts: improvement of existing drugs, systematic screening, exploitation of biological information, and rational approaches. However, with the advent of genomics in the 1990s, the classical strategies were doubted and questioned, mainly owing to their limited research and development (R&D) productivity in the pharmaceutical sector to introduce potential drug candidates into the market [20]. With the great progress in the development of new tools to identify targets (e.g. RNA interference), optimize their structure (e.g. X-ray crystallography and computational modeling and screening), and compounds that interact with these targets novel preclinical strategies to identify potential drug candidates were brought up namely as target-based screening, phenotypic screening, modification of natural substances and biologic-based approaches, where the first and second accounted mostly for the innovative medicines and their respective molecular mechanism of action with focusing on target-centric approach and limited use of phenotypic screening in studying receptor-drug interactions in diseases' pathogenesis.

3. Peptides and proteins as an emerged category of drugs

The isolation of insulin as the first peptide in 1921, brought up the potential of peptides and proteins as therapeutic agents. The first application of peptides and proteins as therapeutic drugs in a clinical setting dates back to the 1920s in the endocrinology and hematology fields with insulin and factor VIII, respectively [21]. Over the upcoming decades, with the technologies used for protein purification and synthesis, structure elucidation, and sequencing, enormous studies have been made on the other natural human hormones such as insulin, oxytocin, vasopressin, and gonadotropin-releasing hormone (GnRH) [12] to explore their efficacy as drug candidates, which led to the approval of the first-ever peptide drug product in the early 1980s and the approval of more than 80 peptide drugs and a total of 33 non-insulin peptide drugs onward [22].

Since then, with the exploitation of novel methods in pharmaceutical biotechnologies [23], peptide and protein synthesis and delivery have become a major source of R&D in the pipeline of pharmaceutical and biotechnology enterprises, with over 240 approved PPDs by the FDA and a variety of potential drug candidates in clinical trials [24, 25]. According to 2018 and 2019 PhRMA reports [26] there were respectively 4751 and 5422 novel biotechnological medicines of various therapeutic categories such as insulin, human growth hormone, monoclonal antibodies, interferons, erythropoietin, biopharmaceuticals, biologics, vaccines, therapeutic blood products (such as IVIG), gene therapy and cell therapy (for instance, stem cell therapies) for more than 100 diseases in human clinical trials or under review by the Food and Drug Administration (FDA) [26] including autoimmune disorders, blood disorders, cancer, cardiovascular disease, diabetes-related conditions, GI disorders, ocular conditions, genetic disorders, infectious diseases, musculoskeletal disorders, neurologic disorders, respiratory disorders, skins diseases, transplantation, antiparasitic diseases, AIDS/HIV, etc. [27–31].

Most of the studies and research conducted on peptides and proteins have been mostly focused on insulin and different delivery routes for insulin. Nevertheless, the high demands urged the pharmaceutical market to shift from human insulin to animal-derived bovine and porcine insulin products until the introduction of recombinant insulin [32, 33], which paved the way for other synthetic peptides' synthesis, namely synthetic oxytocin [34], synthetic vasopressin [35], and recombinant human insulin [36, 37] alongside natural peptides.

Peptides and proteins have also been used as targeting moieties and surface ligands (e.g. antibodies) on DDSs to promote drug uptake by cancer cells via receptor-mediated endocytosis [38] and the passage through physiological barriers like the blood-brain barrier (BBB) [15]. This strategy has been successfully used in cancer studies for the design and formulation of chemotherapeutic-loaded DDSs (**Figure 2**) [39].

The aforementioned technologies have eliminated the classical methods of peptide and protein extraction and purification from human and animal cells and tissues and resulted in the production of PPDs in commercial quantities. Besides, they can easily be synthesized with chemical synthesis methods (e.g. Merrifield's solid-phase peptide synthesis method), in which the amino acid sequence of the peptide of interest can be precisely synthesized at the molecular level [40].

The Nordic Council on Medicines in 1976 presented the ATC system as a "drug substances" classification system, which was adopted and recommended by the World Health Organization (WHO) in 1981 as a classification for all global drug

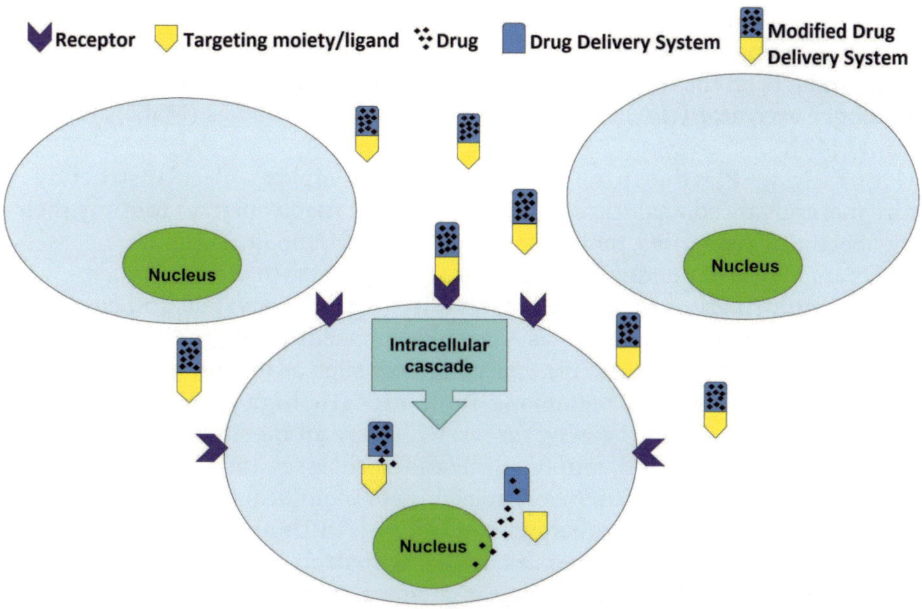

Figure 2.
Schematic depiction of cancer cell targeting by nanoparticles modified with receptor- specific surface targeting moieties/ligands.

utilization studies. However, contemporary emerging trends along with the renewed R&D strategies prompted a new category of biotechnology-driven drugs with potential therapeutic efficiency and lower costs of formulation and marketing. Biotechnology-driven products use genetically modified living organisms to produce protein or peptidyl products, while other pharmaceutical drugs and small molecule drugs (SMDs) (also known as micromolecules) have a low molecular weight of ≤1000 daltons and size of 1 nm that usually derive from chemical synthesis and could regulate a biological process as a drug, which comprises the majority of medicinal products in the market.

4. Advantages and drawbacks of peptide and protein therapeutics

PPDs, in contrast to the SMDs, offer higher potency, selectivity, and specificity for their extracellular targets (as more than 90% of the PPDs have extracellular targets) [25], have biodegradability of non- to low-toxicity metabolites, therapeutic efficiency at low doses, low drug–drug interactions, lower immunogenicity, and allergic reactions, which in turn facilitates the regulatory procedures for their market approval [41]. The large size and flexible backbone of peptide drugs also render them potent inhibitors of PPIs [42]. Other benefits of peptides and proteins as drugs include biocompatibility, cost-benefit, modifiable in-vivo bioactivity, specific targeting, chemical diversity, higher in-vivo activity, stability, and lower expenses favoring them over other categories of drugs for regulatory approval (higher than 20%) which is twice the rate of small molecules [43].

PPDs overcome issues of source availability and safety (transmission of blood-borne pathogens or prion diseases), function as an alternative to direct extraction methods from inappropriate or hazardous sources (e.g. human urine, vipers), and, with their engineering methods, offer clinical advantages over the equivalent natural products on the market (e.g. faster or slower-acting insulins, modified tissue plasminogen activator (tPA), humanized monoclonal antibodies (Mabs), fusion proteins) [44].

Nevertheless, PPDs due to their larger and more complex molecular structure require more advanced analytical methods (e.g. mass spectrometry) to study their physicochemical properties, molecular structure, and biological activity.

PPDs are highly dependent on the production process to maintain their molecular conformation and biological activity (e.g. non-covalent and covalent forces) of peptides and proteins – as Active Pharmaceutical Ingredients (API) – hence, they are sensitive to environmental factors such as temperature, oxidation, light, non-aqueous solvents, metal ions, ionic strength, high pressure, detergents, adsorption, agitation, and shearing forces, which are all inevitably part of the manufacturing, sterilization, and lyophilization processes and eventually might damage the developing peptide/protein leading to biological inactivation, aggregation, immunogenicity and precipitation [45, 46]. PPDs are also vulnerable to numerous physicochemical properties including hydrolysis, oxidation, racemization, β-elimination, disulfide exchange as chemical instability and denaturation, adsorption to surfaces, non-covalent self-aggregation, and precipitation as physical instability. Stringent conditions should also be maintained for their proper storage to avoid degradation.

Antigenicity and immunogenicity of biotech drugs emerging from the application of specific solvents have been voiced as an issue and challenge that remains to be addressed [47].

5. The demand for peptide and protein drug delivery systems

Only recently peptides and proteins have been considered as therapeutic agents while they had never been considered as potential therapeutic agents [43] mostly due to their protease degradation, metabolic instability, short half-life, challenges of the delivery route, low penetration through biological barriers (e.g. blood-brain barrier [15], GI tract [16]), manufacturing complications and high expenses, which in long-term administration render them unfavorable in terms of processing costs and patient compliance especially with regard to parenteral administration as the majority of peptides (10%) have a very low oral bioavailability.

As "drug discovery" of peptide and protein therapeutics has been increasingly addressing an ever-growing range of medical conditions, the pharmaceutical industry is today more in demand of "drug delivery" technologies for their efficient penetration and distribution across biological barriers. Undesired physicochemical features of PPD remain a serious challenge for formulation scientists in the pharmaceutical and biotechnology sectors and enterprises.

Numerous criteria are involved in introducing parenteral and non-parenteral drug delivery systems for PPDs, namely as bioavailability, therapeutic dose and respective release profile (e.g. controlled, sustained release), clinical demand of the market, general or local delivery, disease pathogenesis, the desired delivery route, duration of treatment, patient convenience and compliance, systemic toxicity, synthesis conditions, and process costs. The classical drug delivery of PPDs was based on the parenteral route of liquid formulations which was the invasive and undesired route in terms of patient compliance eventually leading to further investigations on novel DDSs for non-parenteral and non-invasive delivery routes such as oral, nasal, and pulmonary routes for systemic administration and dermal and ocular for topical administrations.

Hence, in recent decades a variety of nanoparticle systems have been introduced and formulated that can provide the desired release profile, improve bioavailability and biodistribution, and when surface-modified are able to passively or actively deliver the therapeutic agent (**Figure 1**).

The oral delivery with the most consistent formulation and delivery challenges has been the most investigated route and to address low oral bioavailability novel strategies have been introduced in the course of years namely as chemical modification (lipidization, cationization, PEGylation, prodrug formation, peptide cyclization, and unnatural amino acids substitution), addition of effective agents (absorption enhancers, modulation of pH, proteolytic enzyme inhibitor, mucolytic agents, cell-penetrating peptides), medical devices (biodegradable microneedle-based delivery system, ingestible self-orienting system, intestinal mucoadhesive patches), formulation technology with combinational strategies (Transient Permeation Enhancer® (TPE®), Gastrointestinal Permeation Enhancement Technology (GIPET®), peptelligence technology, ThioMatrix™ technology, transferrin-based recombinant fusion protein technology, Oral sCT (Ostora™) technology, Oramed and Orasome technology, Q-Sphera™ technology, Nano Inclusion technology, Oleotec™, and Soctec™ gastro-retentive technology) [48].

6. Solid lipid nanoparticles

Solid lipid nanoparticles (SLNs) belong to lipid-based drug delivery systems and, since the 1990s, have been under investigation as a substitute to address some of the issues of the other DDSs (**Figure 3**) [49]. SLNs offer biocompatibility, higher penetration capacity, lipophilicity with no need for surface modification, lower toxicity, simple fabrication, stability, low costs, and industrial-scale production. However, they have a low drug-loading capacity justifying partly the reason behind the small number of SLN-marketed products (**Table 1**) [23].

SLNs are formulated only with solid lipids which although limit their encapsulation capacity but gives them more controlled drug release due to limited drug mobility

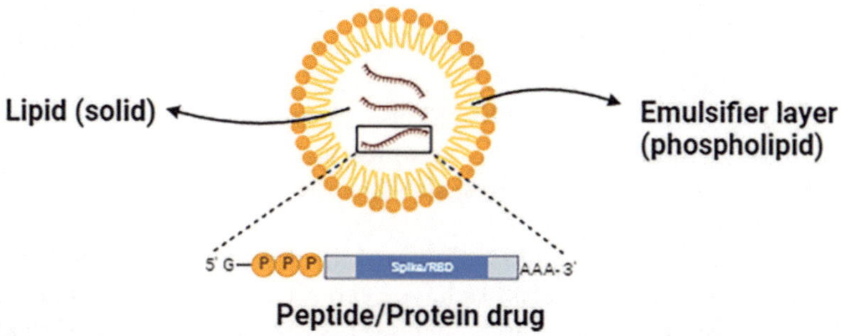

Figure 3.
Solid lipid nanoparticles (SLNs) and their constituents.

Advantages	• Encapsulation capacity for both hydrophilic and lipophilic drugs; • Potential encapsulation with a wide range of therapeutic molecules, such as oligonucleotides, peptides, genes, and superparamagnetic iron oxide particles; • Protection of the loaded therapeutic molecule from RES clearance; • Poor water solubility favoring the encapsulated substance for controlled and sustained release; • Long-term stability and lower toxicity making them applicable for long-term administration; • Biocompatibility, easily sterilized, and no need for organic solvents use which might influence the toxicity of the final product; • Large-scale industrial production capacity; • Modifiable targeting features for tissue-targeted drug delivery
Disadvantages	• Encapsulated therapeutic particles export, • Gelation predisposition, • Low encapsulation efficiency

Table 1.
Advantages and disadvantages of SLNs.

and have been formulated as oral pellets and retard capsules (e.g. Mucosolvan®), as microparticles by spray drying and oral nano pellets. There have been plenty of studies regarding their characteristics and properties [50].

Based on the desired release profile, there are three types of SLNs where the therapeutic molecules can be incorporated in the core, matrix, or attached on the surface (in the case of a high surface/volume ratio) [51]. The latter results in a longer half-life, systemic circulation, and increased mean residence time (**Figure 4**, **Table 2**) [52].

SLNs are composed of different lipids and surfactants/co-surfactants for solidness at various temperatures and low melting points. The choice of lipids, surfactants, and the composition of SLNs (the solid core: 0.1–30% w/w, surfactants: 0.5–5% w/v) determines release profile, drug encapsulation, stability over time, surface charge, polydispersity index, size, and physicochemical features.

Crystallization process during synthesis leads to low encapsulation efficiency of SLNs limiting the internal space of the lipid core for therapeutic substance encapsulation [53]. The highly ordered crystalline structure of the lipids in an SLN has been recently studied with a detailed description of the internal and external structure of SLN [51].

Since their introduction in the 1990s, SLNs have been used as DDSs in various therapeutic fields including anticancer therapies, antimicrobials, central nervous system (CNS) diseases and/or disorders, site-specific treatments, and various conditions/diseases.

Numerous drugs with large and small lipophilic molecules, high polarity, hydrophilic, and hydrophobic characteristics have been efficiently encapsulated into SLNs proving the versatility of these nanoparticles. SLNs can also be surface-modified with peptide/protein-based targeting moieties and surface ligands (e.g. antibodies) for active targeted drug delivery toward receptor-overexpressing cancer cells (**Figure 2**) [38].

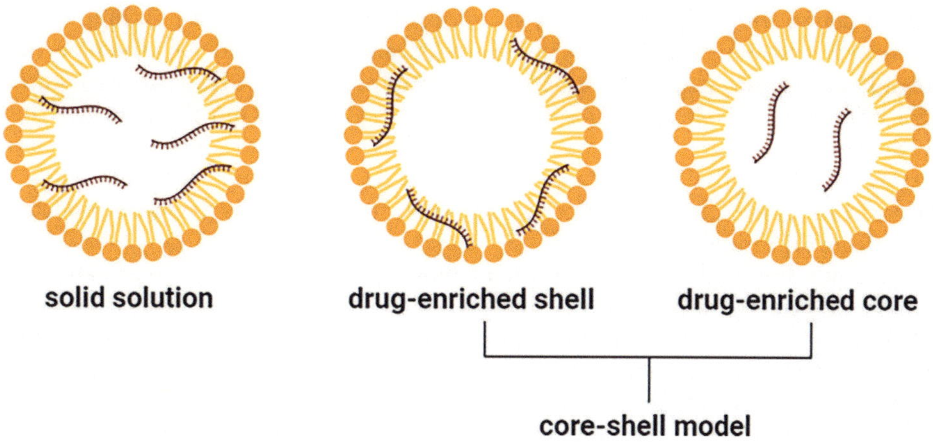

Figure 4.
Different modes of drug encapsulation in solid lipid nanoparticles.

Model	Drug loading site	Drug release pattern
Homogenous matrix of solid solution	Homogeneous drug dispersion in the lipid matrix of the particles	Diffusion from the solid lipid matrix and/or by degradation of lipid matrix in the GI tract
Drug-enriched shell	Drug concentration on the outer shell of the nanoparticles	Burst release is modified by varying the formulation conditions: production temperature (preferably cold homogenization) and surfactant concentration
Drug-enriched core	Drug concentration in the core of the nanoparticles	Prolonged drug release

Table 2.
Models of drug incorporation for the lipid nanoparticles.

7. Biological barriers and peptide and protein drug delivery by SLNs

7.1 Parenteral route

Although an invasive route, parenteral drug delivery has been the most common route of PPD administration as it avoids the challenges of other routes, especially the oral route [54]. The intravenous (I.V.) route basically uses two separate bodily systems – the blood system and lymphatic system – for the drug's general distribution and in-site deposition with defined pharmacodynamics properties. The uptake of nanoparticles by the reticuloendothelial system (RES) and their transfer to the spleen and kidney have been a challenge, hence the application of polyethylene (PEGs) and "stealth technology" to prolong nanoparticles blood circulation time [55–57]. Peptide and protein drug delivery through the lymphatic system has also been voiced as an undesired route by some studies as the delayed time of distribution might result in peptide and protein enzymatic degradation [58, 59]. The transcellular pathway of nanoparticles leads to their uptake by M cells and transport to the lymph [60].

Furthermore, extensive preformulation studies are required for in-vivo assays of PPD parenteral delivery as they have larger molecular sizes than their chemical drug counterparts which is critical in the design of an effective delivery method for their vascular penetration. The anatomical structure of endothelium (i.e. continuous, fenestrated, and sinusoidal) varies in different organs hence rendering them permeable only to peptides and proteins of a specific molecular size [61]; particles >7 μm in size accumulate in the lung capillaries, while particles of 0.1-7 μm clear through the RES (lowering half-life of peptides); while particles <0.1 μm are collected in the bone marrow [62]. Nevertheless, the large molecular size of PPDs imparts them a good steric and electronic complementarity between ligands, which is the most important prerequisite for binding.

The other drawbacks of the I.V. route include unfavorable patient compliance, variable clearance (few minutes to few days), high risks of vascular extravasation and undesired general distribution, repeated injections for the required therapeutic efficacy leading to local tissue necrosis/phlebitis [63, 64], which altogether might result in severe adverse effects. Besides, I.V. preparations are required to be sterile in order to avoid septicemia, thromboembolism, and thrombophlebitis [62].

The subcutaneous (S.C.) and intramuscular (I.M.) routes have been also investigated for PPDs with the former for vaccines. Based on studies [64], the S.C. route offers a 100% bioavailability for PPDs resulting from different factors such as molecular weight, site of injection, local injection site activity, and pathological conditions. Following S.C. administration, PPDs are absorbed based on their molecular weight; high molecular weight drugs (<16,000 Da) either through the endothelial cells of vessels to capillaries or the local lymphatic system to the thoracic duct and general blood circulation, while small molecular weight ones through the local capillaries [64].

7.2 Non-parenteral routes

Non-parenteral delivery of peptide and protein drugs has been investigated extensively as a non-invasive route to address the issues associated with the parenteral route, patient compliance above all. Oral delivery has been the focus of the majority of studies while there have also been numerous studies investigating nasal, pulmonary, transdermal, and ophthalmic routes for PPDs [65–73]. Mucosae which have been neglected for drug delivery seem to be a promising approach for drug absorption, especially efficient for biomolecules of large size and molecular weight [65, 74]. The advantages of mucosal surfaces for drug delivery over skin and GI tract can be named as fewer biological barriers to pass for systemic diffusion, rapid absorption, and evading hepatic first-pass effect. However, one practical challenge of mucosae is related to the preparations that are formulated for long-term and local treatment.

Oral drug delivery, despite being a desired route in terms of patient compliance and convenience, faces numerous challenges in formulating DDSs to maintain the biological and chemical integrity of PPDs while distributing through barriers.

The first and foremost challenge of oral delivery is the low oral bioavailability (1%) [75] and subsequent short half-life (<1%) resulting mainly from enzymatic degradation and poor intestinal penetration of PPDs which is claimed to have been increased to 30–50% by pharmaceutical enterprises [76, 77]. Enzymatic degradation results from the susceptibility of PPDs to stomach's salt-laden pepsin, pancreatic proteases (trypsin, chymotrypsin, elastase, and carboxypeptidase A and B), intestinal brush-border peptidases (endo-, amino- and carboxypeptidases) [65] and intracellular enzymes (cytosolic and lysosomal peptidases) [78] which eventually lead to physical instability [79], aggregation, adsorption, denaturation, enzymatic degradation, poor intestinal penetration, short plasma half-life, and immunogenicity [80, 81]. Poor intestinal penetration and the subsequent low blood absorption and diffusion result from large molecular size, hydrophilicity, charge, and relatively high molecular weight (>500 Da) of PPDs.

PPDs due to their larger molecular size require specific epithelial transporters for their general blood distribution [82]. Their large molecular size allows for specific drug-target interaction with binding pockets that are not normally available to small molecular drugs. These targets are part of intracellular protein-protein interaction networks, which have been recognized in numerous diseases. PPDs in order to interact with such targets must penetrate cells; however, most of them are known to have extracellular targets [83] and are parenterally administered; hence, cellular penetration is not their ordinary route as it is for mucosal surfaces. Currently, the main obstacle to the oral administration of these novel categories of drugs for their maximum therapeutic effects could be addressed as the penetration through intestinal and target cellular membranes. The GI tract is covered with different types of cells (enterocytes, M cells, goblet cells, and paneth cells) and their respective target cells, which allow for broad surface modification of DDSs for passive or active targeting.

The mucous layer covering the epithelium of the GI tract is another barrier that is 400–450 μm thick in some parts of the GI tract and 100–200 μm in the duodenum and jejunum. Mucus is composed of different bodily secretions, including mucins and glycoproteins of high molecular weight, which, owing to the presence of the sialic and sulphonic acid functional groups, possesses negative charges, enabling it to interact with positively-charged peptides and functional groups, which in turn lowers their diffusion rate and absorption.

Moreover, the epithelial cell monolayer membrane of the GI tract, tight junctions, and efflux proteins such as P-glycoprotein aggravate the condition of low oral bioavailability and permeability [84, 85]. PPDs surviving physical and GI enzymatic degradation when absorbed in the general circulation are still subject to liver's first-pass effect enzymatic metabolism, enzymatic degradation by plasma, and clearance via the kidneys.

Nevertheless, the oral route is non-invasive, painless, easy to self-administrate, has minimum risk of cross-contamination, high patient convenience/compliance, outpatient feasibility, and cost-benefit (no need for sterile manufacturing) [86]. Besides, the oral route does not face the drawbacks of I.V. route: drug extravasation from blood, catheter-related infectious complications, and thrombosis, and is expensive and invasive, especially for chronic conditions.

In recent years, the nasal route has been studied extensively for PPD delivery as an alternative to other routes as it evades the first-pass effect and GI enzymatic degradation, especially as a "shortcut" for CNS diseases/disorders by by-passing BBB and distributing through the olfactory nerve (cranial nerve I) and trigeminal nerve (cranial nerve V) [15, 87]. The nasal route has been promising owing to porous epithelial layers, large surface area, microvilli, and highly vascularized mucose, which collectively favor quick general circulation and distribution of drugs [88, 89].

The governing factors for PPD penetration in intranasal tissue are molecular weight, lipophilicity, and dissociation rate, hence the low penetration of PPDs [90]. The nasal mucosa, due to its vast lymphoid tissue, is considered a desirable site for vaccine delivery than other delivery routes as both local and systemic immune systems can be stimulated [90], especially against respiratory infections, with the nasal mucosa as the first site of contact with the causative pathogens/antigens. One study on respiratory syncytial virus (RSV) proved higher immunization with nasal vaccine delivery than intramuscular or oral vaccination [91].

Pulmonary drug delivery has been increasingly under investigation in recent years as it can be exploited to address both local (e.g. asthma, chronic obstructive pulmonary disease (COPD), cystic fibrosis, pulmonary arterial hypertension, tuberculosis, lung cancer, etc.), and systemic diseases/conditions (e.g. cancer, diabetes, acute pain, immune deficiencies, autoimmune diseases, infections, etc.) [92].

The major challenges of the pulmonary route are first the highly-evolved defensive system of the respiratory tract with its mucociliary clearance for exhaling exogenous materials or depositing and deactivating them [93], and second the use of inhaler devices such as pressurized metered dose inhalers (pMDIs) and dry powder inhaler (DPIs) for the efficient therapeutic regimen [94], which partly justify the slow progress of studies and innovations of the pharmaceutical and biotech industry in this sector.

Lungs with alveolar epithelium, vast vasculature system, and large surface area are desirable sites as they allow for high and rapid absorption of poorly water-soluble drugs with low oral bioavailability [95–97]. Since the extra- and intra-cellular enzyme activity of lung cells is low, drug degradation is low which provides a higher extension of absorption even for drugs with low absorption rates [98]. However, based on studies peptide/protein adsorption through the pulmonary route is quick leading to quick peak serum levels (which is undesirable when the slow-release profile is required) [99, 100] rendering the pulmonary route a desirable route only when low doses of PPDs are required causing no adverse effects at high peak serum levels.

Dermal and transdermal delivery have also been studied as an area of great interest for topical dermal treatment and other general conditions [71]. Although the stratum corneum, the outermost layer of skin, is the major barrier responsible for low skin penetration, it also functions as a defensive barrier against exogenous particles such as microorganisms [101] and drug delivery systems. However, due to the high amount of lipid in the stratum corneum, lipid-based nanoparticles have demonstrated great biocompatibility and biodegradability for drug delivery [102], as quickly bind to the surface of the skin and facilitate lipid exchange between the stratum corneum's outer layers [103, 104]. Lipid-based nanoparticles protect the encapsulated drug from bodily chemical degradation, modulate the release profile of interest, and allow for an occlusive effect by an adhesive lipid film formation [105].

Ocular drug delivery has also been under investigation for topical ophthalmic treatment. However, eyes due to their unique anatomical structure (e.g. blood-retina barrier, corneal epithelium) and physiological mechanisms (e.g. the short drug residence time) pose a serious challenge for the local delivery of antibiotics, plasmids, anti-inflammatory, and immunosuppressive agents [106]. Based on studies, the anionic nature of the ocular mucosae can contribute to the development and adhesion of positively charged DDSs on the cornea by increasing drug residence time [106, 107].

8. Protein and peptide drug delivery

Due to the hydrophilic properties of SLNs dispersed phase technologies have been employed for their synthesis. The encapsulation of proteins in the lipophilic matrix of the solid lipid core results in the partition of the aqueous phase during formulation hence surfactants (e.g. emulsion and stabilizers) are used [108]. In one study [109] lyophilic ion coupling improved and facilitated encapsulation of leuprolide and insulin within SLNs where stoichiometry of the ion pair was employed for the former molecule. Various peptides and proteins with different properties have been used for cancer studies implying the multifunctionality of SLNs for both hydrophilic and hydrophobic drugs [110].

The first investigation on peptide drug encapsulation in SLNs was done to incorporate LHRH and thymopentin [111], followed by other studies on insulin with an encapsulation efficiency of about 80% [112]. In another study [113], positively and negatively charged lipid nanoparticles were encapsulated by protein antigens (HBsAg) for intranasal immunization against hepatitis B. So far, different strategies have been employed to increase the bioavailability of peptide and protein therapeutics including:

- Co-administration of enzyme inhibitors such as aprotinin (natural inhibitor of trypsin) [113], ethylenediaminetetraacetic acid (EDTA) [114], sodium glycocholate, camostat mesylate [113, 115], or bacitracin [116]);

- Absorption enhancers such as low molecular weight surfactants, bile salts, calcium ion chelators, or cyclodextrins [117, 118];

- Altering the gastrointestinal retention time using mucoadhesive polymers such as chitosans [119];

- And peptide/protein conjugation to a suitable nanosystem [120].

Among numerous DDSs, SLNs seem a very promising system and their properties mentioned in this chapter offer the four abovementioned opportunities for drug delivery of peptide and protein drugs.

9. Future perspectives and conclusion

After the introduction of insulin as the first peptide drug in the 1920s the progress of marketing peptide and protein drugs has been very limited hence numerous approaches were introduced. The information presented in this chapter provided concepts regarding SLNs and their promising characteristics as a DDS for peptide and protein drug delivery. However, further studies are still required for their translation into clinical settings as there are currently no SLNs for peptide and protein drug delivery in clinical evaluation stages and trials, hence more time is expected for their marketing in the pharmaceutical sector. Proof that they are still in their initial stages of research can be seen in the literature, of which most are in-vitro and in-vivo and limited to research. The majority of SLN reports are based on experimental drugs and are not transferable to clinical trials. However, the studies have demonstrated positive results for their application as they are biocompatible and can be encapsulated by a variety of drugs and also can improve the efficacy and pharmacokinetic profile of the encapsulated drugs. Their limiting factors for their marketing still remain to be addressed namely large-scale manufacturing processes, sterilization, tailoring strategies, and stability issues. The hydrophobic constituents of SLNs render them a favorable scaffold for the encapsulation of hydrophobic and lipophilic drugs where the pharmaceutical market and trends are increasing for the latter.

Author details

Soheil Mehrdadi
Department of Pharmaceutical and Pharmacological Sciences, University of Padova, Padua, Italy

*Address all correspondence to: soheilmehrdadi@gmail.com

References

[1] Adessi C, Soto C. Strategies to improve stability and bioavailability of peptide drugs. Frontiers in Medicinal Chemistry - Online. 2004;**1**(1):513-528. DOI: 10.2174/9781608052042104010105 13

[2] Hussain N. Recent advances in the understanding of uptake of microparticulates across the gastrointestinal lymphatics. Advanced Drug Delivery Reviews. 2001;**50**(1-2):107-142. DOI: 10.1016/s0169-409x(01)00152-1

[3] Wang F, Kream RM, Stefano GB. An evidence based perspective on mRNA-SARS-CoV-2 vaccine development. Medical Science Monitor. 2020;**26**:e924700. DOI: 10.12659/MSM.924700

[4] Park K, Kwon IC, Park K. Oral protein delivery: Current status and future prospect. Reactive and Functional Polymers. 2011;**71**(3):280-287. DOI: 10.1016/j.reactfunctpolym.2010.10.002

[5] Vajo Z, Fawcett J, Duckworth WC. Recombinant DNA technology in the treatment of diabetes: Insulin analogs. Endocrine Reviews [Internet]. 2001;**22**(5):706-717. DOI: 10.1210/edrv.22.5.0442

[6] Takeda A, Cooper K, Bird A, Baxter L, Frampton GK, Gospodarevskaya E, et al. Recombinant human growth hormone for the treatment of growth disorders in children: A systematic review and economic evaluation. Health Technology Assessment. Sep 2010;**14**(42):1-209, iii-iv. DOI: 10.3310/hta14420

[7] Cutting GR. Modifier genetics: Cystic fibrosis. Annual Review of Genomics and Human Genetics. 2005;**6**(1):237-260. DOI: 10.1146/annurev.genom.6.080604.162254

[8] Weatherall DJ. Phenotype—Genotype relationships in monogenic disease: Lessons from the thalassaemias. Nature Reviews Genetics. 2001;**2**(4):245-255. DOI: 10.1038/35066048

[9] Powell JS. Lasting power of new clotting proteins. Hematology. 2014;**5**(1):355-363. DOI: 10.1182/asheducation-2014.1.355

[10] Hirschhorn JN, Lohmueller K, Byrne E, Hirschhorn K. A comprehensive review of genetic association studies. Genetics in Medicine. 2002;**4**(2):45-61. DOI: 10.1097/00125817-200203000-00002

[11] Savic S, McDermott MF. New monogenic diseases span the immunological disease continuum. Nature Reviews Rheumatology. 2014;**11**(2):67-68. DOI: 10.1038/nrrheum.2014.215

[12] Craik DJ, Fairlie DP, Liras S, Price D. The future of peptide-based drugs. Chemical Biology & Drug Design. 2013;**81**:136-147. DOI: 10.1111/cbdd.12055

[13] Fosgerau K, Hoffmann T. Peptide therapeutics: Current status and future directions. Drug Discovery Today. 2015;**20**:122-128. DOI: 10.1016/j.drudis.2014.10.003

[14] Uekama K, Hirayama F, Irie T. Cyclodextrin drug carrier systems. Chemical Reviews. 1998;**98**:2045-2076. DOI: 10.1021/cr970025p

[15] Mehrdadi S. Drug delivery of solid lipid nanoparticles (SLNs) and nanostructured lipid carriers (NLCs) to target brain Tumors. Advanced Pharmaceutical Bulletin. 2023;**13**(3):512-520. DOI: 10.34172/apb.2023.062

[16] Mehrdadi S. Lipid-based nanoparticles as oral drug delivery systems: Overcoming poor gastrointestinal absorption and enhancing bioavailability of peptide and protein therapeutics. Advanced Pharmaceutical Bulletin. 2024;**14**(1):48-66. DOI: 10.34172/apb.2024.016

[17] Swinney DC, Anthony J. How were new medicines discovered? Nature Reviews. Drug Discovery. 2011;**10**(7):507-519. DOI: 10.1038/nrd3480

[18] Harvey AL, Edrada-Ebel R, Quinn RJ. The re-emergence of natural products for drug discovery in the genomics era. Nature Reviews. Drug Discovery. 2015;**14**(2):111-129. DOI: 10.1038/nrd4510

[19] Teague SJ. Implications of protein flexibility for drug discovery. Nature Reviews. Drug Discovery. 2003;**2**(7):527-541. DOI: 10.1038/nrd1129

[20] Mohs RC, Greig NH. Drug discovery and development: Role of basic biological research. Alzheimer's & Dementia: Translational Research & Clinical Interventions. 2017;**3**(4):651-657. DOI: 10.1016/j.trci.2017.10.005

[21] Van der Walle C. Peptide and Protein Delivery. London: Academic Press; 2011

[22] Scioli Montoto S, Muraca G, Ruiz ME. Solid lipid nanoparticles for drug delivery: Pharmacological and biopharmaceutical aspects. Frontiers in Molecular Biosciences. 2020;**7**:587997. DOI: 10.3389/fmolb.2020.587997

[23] Morrison C, Lähteenmäki R. Public biotech in 2015 - the numbers. Nature Biotechnology. 2016;**34**(7):709-715. DOI: 10.1038/nbt.3630

[24] Henninot A, Collins JC, Nuss JM. The current state of peptide drug discovery: Back to the future? Journal of Medicinal Chemistry. 2018;**61**:1382-1414. DOI: 10.1021/acs.jmedchem.7b00318

[25] Lau JL, Dunn MK. Therapeutic peptides: Historical perspectives, current development trends, and future directions. Bioorganic & Medicinal Chemistry. 2018;**26**:2700-2707. DOI: 10.1016/j.bmc.2017.06.052

[26] Report: Biotechnology Medicines in Development. The Pharmaceutical Research and Manufacturers of America (PhRMA). Washington DC: Pharmaceutical Research and Manufacturers Association; 2019. Available from: https://phrma.org/en/resource-center/Topics/Access-to-Medicines/PhRMA-Welcomes-2019-Special-301-Report

[27] Fisher E, Pavlenko K, Vlasov A, Ramenskaya G. Peptide-based therapeutics for oncology. Pharmaceutical Medicine. 2019;**33**:9-20. DOI: 10.1007/s40290-018-0261-7

[28] Iyengar S, Ossipov MH, Johnson KW. The role of calcitonin gene-related peptide in peripheral and central pain mechanisms including migraine. Pain. 2017;**158**:543-559. DOI: 10.1097/j.pain.0000000000000831

[29] Sloan LA. Review of glucagon-like peptide-1 receptor agonists for the treatment of type 2 diabetes mellitus in patients with chronic kidney disease and their renal effects. Journal of Diabetes. 2019;**11**:938-948. DOI: 10.1111/1753-0407.12969

[30] Peterson SC, Barry AR. Effect of glucagon-like peptide-1 receptor agonists on all-cause mortality and cardiovascular outcomes: A meta-analysis. Current Diabetes Reviews. 2018;**14**:273-279. DOI: 10.2174/1573399813666170414101450

[31] Torres MDT, Sothiselvam S, Lu TK, de la Fuente-Nunez C. Peptide design principles for antimicrobial applications. Journal of Molecular Biology. 2019;**431**:3547-3567. DOI: 10.1016/j.jmb.2018.12.015

[32] Mathieu C, Gillard P, Benhalima K. Insulin analogues in type 1 diabetes mellitus: Getting better all the time. Nature Reviews. Endocrinology. 2017;**13**:385-399. DOI: 10.1038/nrendo.2017.39

[33] Zaykov AN, Mayer JP, DiMarchi RD. Pursuit of a perfect insulin. Nature Reviews. Drug Discovery. 2016;**15**:425-439. DOI: 10.1038/nrd.2015.36

[34] Sawyer WH, Manning M. Synthetic analogs of oxytocin and the vasopressins. Annual Review of Pharmacology and Toxicology. 1973;**13**:1-17. DOI: 10.1146/annurev.pa.13.040173.000253

[35] Spiegelman AR. Synthetic vasopressin and diabetes insipidus. Journal of the American Medical Association. 1964;**187**:1035. DOI: 10.1001/jama.1964.03060260063027

[36] Keen H et al. Human insulin produced by recombinant DNA technology: Safety and hypoglycaemic potency in healthy men. Lancet. 1980;**2**:398-401. DOI: 10.1016/s0140-6736(80)90443-2

[37] Johnson IS. Human insulin from recombinant DNA technology. Science. 1983;**219**:632-637. DOI: 10.1126/science.6337396

[38] Shi J, Kantoff PW, Wooster R, Farokhzad OC. Cancer nanomedicine: Progress, challenges and opportunities. Nature Reviews. Cancer. 2017;**17**:20-37. DOI: 10.1038/nrc.2016.108

[39] Rajpoot K, Jain SK. Oral delivery of pH-responsive alginate microbeads incorporating folic acid-grafted solid lipid nanoparticles exhibits enhanced targeting effect against colorectal cancer: A dual-targeted approach. International Journal of Biological Macromolecules. 2020;**151**:830-844. DOI: 10.1016/j.ijbiomac.2020.02.132

[40] Rubert Pérez CM, Stephanopoulos N, Sur S, Lee SS, Newcomb C, Stupp SI. The powerful functions of peptide-based bioactive matrices for regenerative medicine. Annals of Biomedical Engineering. 2014;**43**(3):501-514. DOI: 10.1007/s10439-014-1166-6

[41] Lax R. The future of peptide development in the pharmaceutical industry. In: PharManufacturing: The International Peptide Review. 2010. Available from: https://www.semanticscholar.org/paper/The-Future-of-Peptide-Development-in-the-Industry-Lax/91e7e891ef217610b8f1d04a6d920a20c74e4091 [Accessed: March 25, 2013]

[42] Petta I, Lievens S, Libert C, Tavernier J, De Bosscher K. Modulation of protein-protein interactions for the development of novel therapeutics. Molecular Therapy. 2016;**24**(4):707-718. DOI: 10.1038/mt.2015.214

[43] Lax RT. The future of peptide development in the pharmaceutical industry. In: Pharmanufacturing: The International Peptide Review. London: World Business Journals, Pharmaceutical Division; 2010

[44] Longstaff C, Whitton CM, Stebbings R, Gray E. How do we assure the quality of biological medicines? Drug Discovery Today. 2009;**14**(1-2):50-55. DOI: 10.1016/j.drudis.2008.09.010

[45] Frokjaer S, Otzen DE. Protein drug stability: A formulation challenge. Nature Reviews Drug Discovery.

2005;**4**(4):298-306. DOI: 10.1038/nrd1695

[46] Wang W. Protein aggregation and its inhibition in biopharmaceutics. International Journal of Pharmaceutics. 2005;**289**(1-2):1-30. DOI: 10.1016/j.ijpharm.2004.11.014

[47] Davda J, Declerck P, Hu-Lieskovan S, et al. Immunogenicity of immunomodulatory, antibody-based, oncology therapeutics. Journal for Immuno Therapy of Cancer. 2019;**7**:105. DOI: 10.1186/s40425-019-0586-0

[48] Chen G, Kang W, Li W, Chen S, Gao Y. Oral delivery of protein and peptide drugs: From non-specific formulation approaches to intestinal cell targeting strategies. Theranostics. 2022;**12**(3):1419-1439. DOI: 10.7150/thno.61747

[49] Müller RH, Radtke M, Wissing SA. Solid lipid nanoparticles (SLN) and nanostructured lipid carriers (NLC) in cosmetic and dermatological preparations. Advanced Drug Delivery Reviews. 2002;**54**:S131-S155. DOI: 10.1016/S0169-409X(02)00118-7

[50] Eldem T, Speiser P, Hincal A. Optimization of spray-dried and congealed lipid micropellets and characterization of their surface morphology by scanning electron microscopy. Pharmaceutical Research. 1991;**8**:47-54. DOI: 10.1023/a:1015874121860

[51] Pink DL, Loruthai O, Ziolek RM, Wasutrasawat P, Terry AE, Lawrence MJ, et al. On the structure of solid lipid nanoparticles. Small. 2019;**15**(45):e1903156. DOI: 10.1002/smll.201903156

[52] Li SD, Huang L. Pharmacokinetics and biodistribution of nanoparticles. Molecular Pharmaceutics. 2008;**5**(4):496-504. DOI: 10.1021/mp800049w

[53] Mehnert W, Mäder K. Solid lipid nanoparticles: Production, characterization and applications. Advanced Drug Delivery Reviews. 2001;**47**:165-196. DOI: 10.1016/s0169-409x(01)00105-3

[54] Donnelly M, Hodge S. Overview of selected novel drugs approved in 2018. Annual Review of Changes in Healthcare. Vol. 3. 2019. Available from: https://www.semanticscholar.org/paper/Overview-of-Selected-Novel-Drugs-Approved-in-2018-Hodge/5f18f8343eb42c16c55c6ba2319d45e42cd5bbf7

[55] Yoo J-W, Doshi N, Mitragotri S. Adaptive micro and nanoparticles: Temporal control over carrier properties to facilitate drug delivery. Advanced Drug Delivery Reviews. 2011;**63**(14-15):1247-1256. DOI: 10.1016/j.addr.2011.05.004

[56] Moghimi SM, Hunter AC, Murray JC. Long-circulating and target-specific nanoparticles: Theory to practice. Pharmacological Reviews. 2001;**53**(2):283-318

[57] Cavadas M, González-Fernández Á, Franco R. Pathogen-mimetic stealth nanocarriers for drug delivery: A future possibility. Nanomedicine: Nanotechnology, Biology and Medicine. 2011;**7**(6):730-743. DOI: 10.1016/j.nano.2011.04.006

[58] Crommelin DJA, Storm G, Verrijk R, et al. Shifting paradigms: Biopharmaceuticals versus low molecular weight drugs. International Journal of Pharmaceutics. 2003;**266**:3-16. DOI: 10.1016/s0378-5173(03)00376-4

[59] Saltzman M. Drug Delivery: Engineering Principles for Drug Therapy. New York: Oxford University Press; 2001. DOI: 10.1093/oso/9780195085891.003.0005

[60] Mrsny RJ. Perspective: Oral drug delivery research in Europe. Journal of Controlled Release. 2012;**161**:247-253

[61] Sarin H. Physiologic upper limits of pore size of different blood capillary types and another perspective on the dual pore theory of microvascular permeability. Journal of Angiogenesis Research. 2010;**2**:14. DOI: 10.1186/2040-2384-2-14

[62] Banerjee PS, Hosny EA, Robinson JR. Parenteral delivery of peptide and protein drug. In: Lee VHL, editor. Peptide and Protein Drug Delivery. New York: Marcel Dekker; 1991. pp. 487-543

[63] Tauzin B. Report: Biotechnology Medicines in Development. Washington DC: Pharmaceutical Research and Manufacturers Association; 2006

[64] Crommelin D, van Winden E, Mekking A. Delivery of pharmaceutical proteins. In: Aulton ME, editor. Pharmaceutics: The Science of Dosage Forms Design. Edinburgh: Churchill Livingstone; 2001. pp. 544-553

[65] Pettit DK, Gombotz WR. The development of site-specific drug-delivery systems for protein and peptide biopharmaceuticals. Trends in Biotechnology. 1998;**16**(8):343-349. DOI: 10.1016/s0167-7799(98)01186-x

[66] Ugwoke MI, Agu RU, Verbeke N, et al. Nasal mucoadhesive drug delivery: Background, applications, trends and future perspectives. Advanced Drug Delivery Reviews. 2005;**57**:1640-1665. DOI: 10.1016/j.addr.2005.07.009

[67] Myles ME, Neumann DM, Hill JM. Recent progress in ocular drug delivery for posterior segment disease: Emphasis on transscleral iontophoresis. Advanced Drug Delivery Reviews. 2005;**57**:2063-2079. DOI: 10.1016/j.addr.2005.08.006

[68] Smart JD. Buccal drug delivery. Expert Opinion on Drug Delivery. 2005;**2**:507-517. DOI: 10.1517/17425247.2.3.507

[69] Mackay M, Phillips J, Hastewell J. Peptide drug delivery: Colonic and rectal absorption. Advanced Drug Delivery Reviews. 1997;**28**:253-273. DOI: 10.1016/S0169-409X(97)00076-8

[70] Hussain A, Ahsan F. The vagina as a route for systemic drug delivery. Journal of Controlled Release. 2005;**103**:301-313. DOI: 10.1016/j.jconrel.2004.11.034

[71] Schuetz YB, Naik A, Guy RH, et al. Emerging strategies for the transdermal delivery of peptide and protein drugs. Expert Opinion on Drug Delivery. 2005;**2**:533-548. DOI: 10.1517/17425247.2.3.533

[72] Agu RU, Ugwoke MI, Armand M, et al. The lung as a route for systemic delivery of therapeutic proteins and peptides. Respiratory Research. 2001;**2**:198-209. DOI: 10.1186/rr58

[73] Bosquillon C, Préat V, Vanbever R. Pulmonary delivery of growth hormone using dry powders and visualization of its local fate in rats. Journal of Controlled Release. 2004;**96**:233-244. DOI: 10.1016/j.jconrel.2004.01.027

[74] Ghilzai NMK, Desai A. Facing the challenges of transmucosal absorption—Buccal, nasal and rectal routes. In: Pharma Tech 2004. London: Business Briefing World Market Series; 2004. pp. 104-106

[75] Mahato RI, Narang AS, Thoma L, Miller DD. Emerging trends in oral delivery of peptide and protein drugs. Critical Reviews in Therapeutic Drug Carrier Systems. 2003;**20**(2-3):153-214

[76] Lee HJ. Protein drug oral delivery: The recent progress. Archives of Pharmacal Research. 2002;**25**(5):572-584. DOI: 10.1007/BF02976925

[77] Vincent HL, Satish DK, George MG, et al. Oral route of protein and peptide drug delivery. In: Vincent HL, editor. Peptide and Protein Drug Delivery. New York: Marcel Dekker; 1991. pp. 691-738

[78] Langguth P, Bohner V, Heizmann J, Merkle HP, Wolffram S, Amidon GL, et al. The challenge of proteolytic enzymes in intestinal peptide delivery. Journal of Controlled Release. 1997;**46**:39-57

[79] Ikesue K, Kopečkovà P, Kopeček J. Degradation of proteins by Guinea pig intestinal enzymes. International Journal of Pharmaceutics. 1993;**95**(1-3):171-179. DOI: 10.1016/0378-5173(93)90404-4

[80] Saffran M, Kumar G, Savariar C, Burnham J, Williams F, Neckers D. A new approach to the oral administration of insulin and other peptide drugs. Science. 1986;**233**(4768):1081-1084. DOI: 10.1126/science.3526553

[81] Fix JA. Oral controlled release technology for peptides: Status and future prospects. Pharmaceutical Research. 1996;**13**(12):1760-1764. DOI: 10.1023/a:1016008419367

[82] Yun Y, Cho YW, Park K. Nanoparticles for oral delivery: Targeted nanoparticles with peptidic ligands for oral protein delivery. Advanced Drug Delivery Reviews. 2013;**65**(6):822-832. DOI: 10.1016/j.addr.2012.10.007

[83] Tsomaia N. Peptide therapeutics: Targeting the undruggable space. European Journal of Medicinal Chemistry. 2015;**94**:459-470. DOI: 10.1016/j.ejmech.2015.01.014

[84] Ensign LM, Cone R, Hanes J. Oral drug delivery with polymeric nanoparticles: The gastrointestinal mucus barriers. Advanced Drug Delivery Reviews. 2012;**64**:557-570. DOI: 10.1016/j.addr.2011.12.009

[85] Murakami T, Takano M. Intestinal efflux transporters and drug absorption. Expert Opinion on Drug Metabolism & Toxicology. 2008;**4**:923-939. DOI: 10.1517/17425255.4.7.923

[86] Choonara BF, Choonara YE, Kumar P, et al. A review of advanced oral drug delivery technologies facilitating the protection and absorption of protein and peptide molecules. Biotechnology Advances. 2014;**32**:1269-1282. DOI: 10.1016/j.biotechadv.2014.07.006

[87] Mehrdadi S. Acute bacterial meningitis: Diagnosis, treatment and prevention. Journal of Archives in Military Medicine. 2018;**6**(4):e84749. DOI: 10.5812/jamm.84749

[88] Durga P et al. Pulmonary nanomedicine. In: Nasal and Pulmonary Delivery of Macromolecules to Treat Respiratory and Nonrespiratory Diseases. Singapore: Pan Stanford Publishing; 2012. pp. 45-102

[89] Alam MI, Beg S, Samad A, Baboota S, Kohli K, Ali J, et al. Strategy for effective brain drug delivery. European Journal of Pharmaceutical Sciences. 2010;**40**(5):385-403. DOI: 10.1016/j.ejps.2010.05.003

[90] Illum L. Nasal drug delivery–Possibilities, problems and solutions. Journal of Controlled Release. 2003;**87**(1-3):187-198. DOI: 10.1016/s0168-3659(02)00363-2

[91] Yu JR, Kim S, Lee JB, Chang J. Single intranasal immunization with recombinant adenovirus-based vaccine induces protective immunity against respiratory syncytial virus infection. Journal of Virology. 2008;**82**(5):2350-2357. DOI: 10.1128/JVI.02372-07

[92] Kohlhäufl M. The lung and basic considerations for lung delivery. In:

Bechtold-Peters K, Luessen H, editors. Pulmonary Drug Delivery. Aulendorf: Editio Cantor Verlag für Medizin und Naturwissenschaften GmbH; 2007. pp. 15-44

[93] Labiris NR, Dolovich MB. Pulmonary drug delivery. Part I: Physiological factors affecting therapeutic effectiveness of aerosolized medications. British Journal of Clinical Pharmacology. 2003;**56**(6):588-599. DOI: 10.1046/j.1365-2125.2003.01892.x

[94] Newman S. Improving inhaler technique, adherence to therapy and the precision of dosing: Major challenges for pulmonary drug delivery. Expert Opinion on Drug Delivery. 2014;**11**(3):365-378. DOI: 10.1517/17425247.2014.873402

[95] Heinemann L, Pfützner A, Heise T. Alternative routes of administration as an approach to improve insulin therapy: Update on dermal, oral, nasal and pulmonary insulin delivery. Current Pharmaceutical Design. 2001;7(14):1327-1351. DOI: 10.2174/1381612013397384

[96] Yang W, Peters JI, Williams RO 3rd. Inhaled nanoparticles–A current review. International Journal of Pharmaceutics. 2008;**356**(1-2):239-247. DOI: 10.1016/j.ijpharm.2008.02.011

[97] Gehr P, Bachofen M, Weibel ER. The normal human lung: Ultrastructure and morphometric estimation of diffusion capacity. Respiration Physiology. 1978;**32**(2):121-140. DOI: 10.1016/0034-5687(78)90104-4

[98] Bur M, Henning A, Hein S, Schneider M, Lehr CM. Inhalative nanomedicine–Opportunities and challenges. Inhalation Toxicology. 2009;**21**(1):137-143. DOI: 10.1080/08958370902962283

[99] Patton JS. Pulmonary delivery of drugs for bone disorders. Advanced Drug Delivery Reviews. 2000;**42**(3):239-248. DOI: 10.1016/s0169-409x(00)00064-8

[100] Cryan SA, Sivadas N, Garcia-Contreras L. In vivo animal models for drug delivery across the lung mucosal barrier. Advanced Drug Delivery Reviews. 2007;**59**(11):1133-1151. DOI: 10.1016/j.addr.2007.08.023

[101] Neubert RH. Potentials of new nanocarriers for dermal and transdermal drug delivery. European Journal of Pharmaceutics and Biopharmaceutics. 2011;**77**(1):1-2. DOI: 10.1016/j.ejpb.2010.11.003

[102] Souto EB, Doktorovova S, Boonme P. Lipid-based colloidal systems (nanoparticles, microemulsions) for drug delivery to the skin: Materials and end-product formulations. Journal of Drug Delivery Science and Technology. 2011b;**21**(1):43-54. DOI: 10.1016/S1773-2247(11)50005-X

[103] Zur Mühlen A, Schwarz C, Mehnert W. Solid lipid nanoparticles (SLN) for controlled drug delivery–Drug release and release mechanism. European Journal of Pharmaceutics and Biopharmaceutics. 1998;**45**(2):149-155. DOI: 10.1016/s0939-6411(97)00150-1

[104] Schäfer-Korting M, Mehnert W, Korting HC. Lipid nanoparticles for improved topical application of drugs for skin diseases. Advanced Drug Delivery Reviews. 2007;**59**(6):427-443. DOI: 10.1016/j. addr.2007.04.006

[105] Battaglia L, Gallarate M. Lipid nanoparticles: State of the art, new preparation methods and challenges in drug delivery. Expert Opinion on Drug Delivery. 2012;**9**(5):497-508. DOI: 10.1517/17425247.2012.673278

[106] Araújo J, Gonzalez E, Egea MA, Garcia ML, Souto EB. Nanomedicines for

ocular NSAIDs: Safety on drug delivery. Nanomedicine. 2009;**5**(4):394-401. DOI: 10.1016/j.nano.2009.02.003

[107] Başaran E, Demirel M, Sirmagül B, Yazan Y. Cyclosporine-A incorporated cationic solid lipid nanoparticles for ocular delivery. Journal of Microencapsulation. 2010;**27**(1):37-47. DOI: 10.3109/02652040902846883

[108] Almeida AJ, Souto E. Solid lipid nanoparticles as a drug delivery system for peptides and proteins. Advanced Drug Delivery Reviews. 2007;**59**(6):478-490. DOI: 10.1016/j.addr.2007.04.007

[109] Gallarate M, Battaglia L, Peira E, Trotta M. Peptide-loaded solid lipid nanoparticles prepared through coacervation technique. International Journal of Chemical Engineering. 2011;**2011**:6. Article ID 132435. DOI: 10.1155/2011/132435

[110] Bayón-Cordero L, Alkorta I, Arana L. Application of solid lipid nanoparticles to improve the efficiency of anticancer drugs. Nanomaterials (Basel). 2019;**9**(3):474. DOI: 10.3390/nano9030474

[111] Morel S, Ugazio E, Cavalli R, Gasco MR. Thymopentin in solid lipid nanoparticles. International Journal of Pharmaceutics. 1996;**132**:259-261

[112] Trotta M, Cavalli R, Carlotti ME, Battaglia L, Debernardi F. Solid lipid micro-particles carrying insulin formed by solvent-in-water emulsion-diffusion technique. International Journal of Pharmaceutics. 2005;**288**(2):281-288. DOI: 10.1016/j.ijpharm.2004.10.014

[113] Yamamoto A, Taniguchi T, Rikyuu K, Tsuji T, Fujita T, Murakami M, et al. Effects of various protease inhibitors on the intestinal absorption and degradation of insulin in rats. Pharmaceutical Research. 1994;**11**(10):1496-1500. DOI: 10.1023/a:1018968611962

[114] Bernkop-Schnürch A, Krajicek ME. Mucoadhesive polymers as platforms for peroral peptide delivery and absorption: Synthesis and evaluation of different chitosan-EDTA conjugates. Journal of Controlled Release. 1998;**50**(1-3):215-223. DOI: 10.1016/s0168-3659(97)00136-3

[115] Tozaki H, Emi Y, Horisaka E, Fujita T, Yamamoto A, Muranishi S. Degradation of insulin and calcitonin and their protection by various protease inhibitors in rat caecal contents: Implications in peptide delivery to the colon. The Journal of Pharmacy and Pharmacology. 1997;**49**(2):164-168. DOI: 10.1111/j.2042-7158.1997.tb06773.x

[116] Kramer TH, Toth G, Haaseth RC, Matsunaga TO, Davis P, Hruby VJ, et al. Influence of peptidase inhibitors on the apparent agonist potency of delta selective opioid peptides in vitro. Life Sciences. 1991;**48**(9):881-886. DOI: 10.1016/0024-3205(91)90034-9

[117] Kanwar JR, Long BM, Kanwar RK. The use of cyclodextrins nanoparticles for oral delivery. Current Medicinal Chemistry. 2011;**18**(14):2079-2085. DOI: 10.2174/092986711795656243

[118] Shaji J, Patole V. Protein and peptide drug delivery: Oral approaches. Indian Journal of Pharmaceutical Sciences. 2008;**70**(3):269-277. DOI: 10.4103/0250-474X.42967

[119] Khutoryanskiy VV. Advances in mucoadhesion and mucoadhesive polymers. Macromolecular Bioscience. 2011;**11**(6):748-764. DOI: 10.1002/mabi.201000388

[120] Griffin BT, O'Driscoll CM. Opportunities and challenges for oral delivery of hydrophobic versus hydrophilic peptide and protein-like drugs using lipid-based technologies. Therapeutic Delivery. 2011;**2**(12):1633-1653. DOI: 10.4155/tde.11.128

Section 4

Nano-Based Drug Delivery System

Chapter 8

The Application of Nanotechnology in the Pharmaceutical Treatment of Common Diseases

Morteza Rabiei and Seyedeh Sabereh Samavati

Abstract

The use of chemical drugs to treat disease always imposes certain limitations, including, but not limited to, drug side effects, loss of a significant portion of the dose, inappropriate method of administration to the patient, and the development of resistance to the prescribed dose. Recently, nanotechnology has been utilized to develop drug delivery systems to overcome these limitations through the improvement of methods for controlled release. Limited drug absorption by nervous, bone, and cartilage tissues has led to modification of the delivery methods to increase the accumulation of drugs in these specific tissues. Topical administration of drugs in skin diseases prevents drug waste typically occurring in systemic administration, and topical use has gained more patient acceptance and eliminated common side effects. The controlled release of diabetes drugs since explosive release or depletion of the drug exposes diabetes patients to serious health risks. Nanotechnology and its controlled drug release technologies have facilitated the sustained plasma concentration of diabetes medications. Given the worldwide prevalence of diseases of the nervous, musculoskeletal, and respiratory systems as well as skin diseases and diabetes, effective treatments are highly sought after as they bring many advantages for both the healthcare systems and more importantly the patient.

Keywords: nanotechnology, drug delivery, controlled release, brain, bone, cartilage, diabetes, musculoskeletal, respiratory system, skin diseases

1. Introduction

In recent years, nanoscience has emerged as an important tool in the treatment of diseases. Therapeutic approaches have benefited from the application of nanotechnology including drug delivery, wound dressings, tissue engineering, gene delivery, photothermal therapy, vaccination, and treatment of infectious diseases. Among these techniques, the most tremendous studies have been done on focused and controlled drug delivery, in regards to cancer therapy. The severe side effects associated with chemotherapy have probably provided the most powerful incentive for the pursuit of research on effective targeted drug delivery of therapeutic agents to tumor tissue [1]. Notwithstanding the comprehensive studies undertaken within the drug delivery area for the remedy of cancer, other serious human diseases are confronted with similar demanding situations. The advent of nanotechnology into the field of drug delivery is paving the way for the more effective treatment of a myriad of diseases. Neurological diseases with a low treatment success rate such as Alzheimer, Parkinson disease (PD), and multiple sclerosis (MS) [2], and musculoskeletal diseases such as osteoarthritis, Rheumatoid Arthritis, and osteoporosis, known as the diseases of the present century, all present the challenge of drug delivery [3]. Biological barriers, such as the presence of the blood–brain barrier (BBB) and the absence of blood vessels in cartilage tissue have rendered drug delivery to the relevant organs difficult [4, 5]. Nanotechnology has provided a variety of means to target and effectively deliver drugs for treatment of brain diseases by increasing drug retention within the brain or by circumventing the BBB via intranasal delivery [4]. With the aid of nanotechnology targeted drug delivery for the treatment of musculoskeletal diseases has enabled increased retention of drugs [5]. Nanotechnology has also been applied in the field of tissue engineering for cartilage and bone repair allowing for targeted delivery of growth factors to cells [6]. Control of drug concentration, a critical requirement for treatment of diabetes, another disease with low treatment success rate, has become possible by utilizing nanoparticles (NPs) responsive to glucose concentration and NPs enabling controlled drug release [7]. By allowing modification of the methods of delivery and usage of drugs application of nanotechnology in the field of drug delivery has led to an improvement in the quality of medical treatments. Delivery of nanodrugs via skin particularly using skin patches has enabled released control of the drug without side effects, thereby gaining widespread acceptance by patients [8]. In addition, utilization of nanomaterials to build skin patches has improved their quality and performance [9]. The method of drug delivery for the treatment of respiratory diseases has been notably facilitated by nanotechnology. NPs are capable of deep penetration into the respiratory system, and by designing NPs as aerosols local delivery to the respiratory tissues can be accomplished [10]. In this article, drug delivery to brain, bone, cartilage, skin, and the respiratory system as well as drug delivery for treatment of diabetes is discussed, and the unresolved challenges, solutions, and the progress made to date in this area is discussed.

2. Drug delivery to brain

Systemic and nonsurgical techniques for treatment of neurological diseases present a major challenge in medicine which is associated with the condensation and coherence of the brain tissue. The coherence structure of the brain is due to the presence of continuous layer of capillary endothelial cells known BBB. The BBB is highly selective and prevents most substances from entering the brain tissue, so permitting only metabolic substance and nutrients to pass through. Although this property has caused challenges in the treatment of neurological diseases, it has opened up a wide research area in the field of drug delivery [11]. **Figure 1** schematically illustrates the BBB.

The limitations related to brain drug delivery include both the specific properties of the drug to be delivered and characteristics of the BBB. The unidirectional action of epithelial cells in BBB prevents substances from entering to the brain. The barrier characteristic of this layer is associated with adherence junctions and tight junctions between the epithelial cells, which block intercellular passage of substances [13]. The molecules introducing the brain also confront transfer limitations. Both hydrophilic

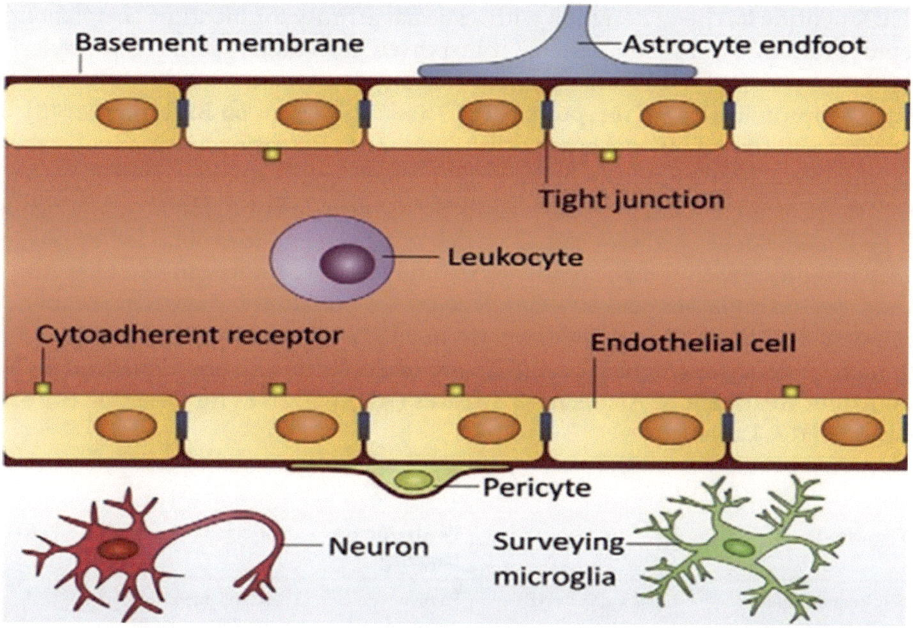

Figure 1.
Schematic illustration of BBB, capillary endothelial cell, astrocytes, pericytes, basement membrane, and tight junction [12].

and charged molecules are unable of passing the BBB [13]. Depending on their concentration gradient only certain solutes and ions may pass via the barrier. The drug molecules less than 50 nm with molecular weight less than 400–500 Da can pass through the BBB. Larger molecules can gain entry via receptors and transporters [14].

In last years, with the entrance of nanotechnology in drug delivery, huge research has been taking place in the brain drug delivery. Nanoparticles (NPs) provide properties such as lipophilicity, modifiable electrical surface charge, and small size and are suitable for drug delivery to the brain. Furthermore, targeting the NPs toward the endothelial of brain can intercellularly convey the drug to brain. NPs protect drug molecules and improve their solubility as well [15]. The highly applicable NPs in brain drug include liposomes, nanostructured lipid carriers (NLCs), solid lipid nanoparticles (SLNs), micelles, and polymeric NPs. Also, the intranasal drug delivery using mucoadhesive using polymeric NPs can bypass the brain pathway [16]. Photothermal therapy for neurological disease treatment also was used. For instance, graphene or gold NPs which have high thermal conductivity when exposed to near-infrared (NIR) beams, oscillate, produce thermal energy, and kill the brain tumors [17].

The high selectivity of the BBB has directed most investigations on brain drug delivery using active approaches. Presence of specific transporters and receptors on the brain cells surface can be utilized for targeting NPs. These targeting molecules include receptors for apolipoprotein E (APoE), glucagon-like transporter2 (GLP2), glutathione, tumor necrosis factor-alpha (TNF-α), transferrin, gamma-aminobutyric acid (GABAA), lactoferrin, melanotransferrin, angiopep, insulin, leptin, adenosine, tetanus toxin, diphtheria toxin, nicotinic acetyl choline, LDL, and G-protein. Also, brain endothelial transporters serve as effective tools for brain drug delivery which include transporters of glucose, vitamin C, vitamin B, lithium, glycoprotein P (P-gp), interlukin1, phosphorothiolate, and synthetic opioid peptide [18].

CDX peptide has been designed with a special affinity for nicotinic acetylcholine receptor (nAchR), a brain endothelial transporter, and can target the nanocarrier toward the brain [19]. GLP2 is a 33 amino acid antidepressant peptide [20] and low-density lipoprotein-related receptors (LRPs) are also present on BBB surface [18]. The polysorbate 80 coated NPs covered with APoE in the circulation and facilitates the attachment to LRPs receptor in the brain [21]. The P-gp transporter on BBB prevents the entrance of toxic substances such as alkaloids into the brain. Intrinsic analogous of P-gp ligand can be used for brain drug delivery [22]. Peptides obtained by phage display technique with specific tendency to brain cells receptors can be a targeting ligands. For example, the selective CAQR sequence prepared for targeting brain trauma can decorate NPs targeted brain trauma [23]. QSH and TGN are two peptides with high tendency to amyloid-beta (Aβ) and can therefore be functionalized on NPs intended for treatment of Alzheimer's diseases (AD) [24]. NPs for targeting the brain are listed in the **Table 1**.

Diseases/Drug	**NP**	**Passive/Active targeting**	**Effect of NP**	**Reference**
Stroke and spinal cord injury/ adenosine	Lipid squalene NP	Passive targeting of brain	Extend adenosine circulation and its interaction with the neurovascular unit in mouse models	[25]
Stroke/ tPA	Echogenic liposome, microspheres NP	Active targeting of fibrin in thrombus	Slight improvement of tPA delivery and facilitated thrombolysis in rats	[26]
Brain edema/ Tanshinone IIA	Tan IIA conjugated to albumin within PEG NP	Passive targeting of brain	Reduce side effect, improved functionality ischemia injury in rats	[27]
Alzheimer/ nerve growth factor (NGF)	Poly(butyl cyanoacrylate) (PBCA) NP coated with polysorbate 80	Active targeting of BBB and cholinergic neuron in basal forebrain	Increase drug concentration in mice brains	[28]
Alzheimer/ B6 peptide	PEG–PLA NP conjugated to transferrin	Active targeting and capillary endothelial and neurons	Higher accumulation in brain) to AD mouse models	[29]
Alzheimer/ coenzyme Q_{10}	Trimethylated chitosan-conjugated PLGA NP	Passive targeting of brain	Brain-targeted effects, improved memory impairment in mice models	[30]
Alzheimer/ Donepzil	PLGA-b-PEG NP	Passive targeting of brain	More penetration in BBB and reduced side effect in vitro	[31]
Alzheimer/curcumin	PLGA- curcumin NPs non-targeted and targeted with Tet-1 peptide	Active targeting of BBB and neuron in CNS	In vitro neuronal targeting efficiency	[32]

Diseases/Drug	NP	Passive/Active targeting	Effect of NP	Reference
Alzheimer/TGN and QSH peptide	PEG–PLA NP	Active targeting of BBB and Aβ in amyloid plaque	Enhanced, targeted and precise delivery toward Aβ in mice	[24]
Alzheimer/ nattokinase	PLGA NP covered by Tet1	Active targeting of BBB and neurons	Improves the pharmacokinetic properties, Decreased immunogenicity	[33]
Brain infection and other brain diseases/ Brain-derived neurotrophic factor (BDNF)	Poly(ethylene glycol)-b-poly(l-glutamic acid) (PEG-PLE) NP	Active targeting of olfactory bulb, hippocampus, and brainstem	Protects BDNF from nonspecific binding with serum proteins, controlled release intranasally in mice	[34]
Parkinson/ dopamine	PLGA NP	Passive targeting of brain	Increased levels of dopamine and reduced dopamine autoxidation-mediated toxicity in the striatum of parkinsonian rats	[35]
Parkinson/glial cell line-derived neurotrophic factor (GDNF)	PAMAM conjugated PEG NP functionalized with lactoferrin	Active targeting of BBB endothelial	Protection of GDNF from heparin displacement and DNase digestion. Enhance therapeutic efficacy in rats	[36]
Parkinson/gold NPs	Poly(allylamine hydrochloride) coated gold NP	Passive targeting of brain	Act as chaperones, preventing the misfolding of α-syn	[37]
Glioma/doxorubicin	Transferrin-conjugated PEGylated nanoscale graphene oxide (TPG)	Active targeting of BBB and glioma cells	Improve drug accumulation both in vitro and in vivo. Decrease side Effects and improve therapeutic effects in rats.	[38]
Glioma/Asiatic Acid	SLN	Passive targeting of brain	Higher cytotoxicity toward U87 MG cells and in vitro slow drug release	[39]
Glioma/Vincristine	Red blood cell membrane-coated SLN (RBCSLN)-based nanocarrier dual-modified with T7 and NGR peptide	Active targeting of BBB and BBTB (glioma cells)	Exhibited the most favorable antiglioma effects in vitro and in vivo by combining the dual-targeting delivery effect	[40]
Epilepsy/ Oxcarbazepine (OX)	Emulsome	Passive targeting of brain	Drug stability, reduced toxicity, prolonged releases and direct nose-to-brain transport in rats.	[41]

Diseases/Drug	NP	Passive/Active targeting	Effect of NP	Reference
Migraine/ Sumatriptan Succinate	Poly (butyl cyanoacrylate) (PBCA) and bovine serum albumin linked with apolipoprotein E3 (BSA-ApoE) NP.	Passive targeting of brain	High brain/plasma drug ratio in wistar rats and enhanced anti migraine potential on male Swiss albino mice	[42]
Migraine/Rizatriptan Benzoate (RB)	SLN	Passive targeting of brain	18.43-folds higher uptake compared to pure drug in adult male Swiss albino mice	[43]
MS/ Baclofen	NLC	Passive targeting of brain	Higher CNS concentration, sustained released and efficient drug delivery in in vitro and in vivo models.	[44]
Encephalomyelitis (EAE)/ Opioid Peptide DAMGO	Glutathione-PEGylated Liposomes	Active targeting of BBB endothelial	2-fold increased uptake in brain	[45]
Depression/ Glucagon-like peptide-2 (GLP-2)	Surfactant polyoxyethylene (25) lauryl ether (LAURETH-25) and β-cyclodextrin (b-CD) NPs.	Passive targeting brain	Protection of GLP-2 against DPP-4, facilitate transport across nasal mucosa, enhanced brain uptake in rats.	[20]
Depression/ Thymoquinone (TQ)	SLN	Passive targeting of brain	Improved the bio-efficacy of TQ in rats.	[46]
Organophosphate poisoning/ Pralidoxime and obidoxime	Chitosan	Passive targeting of brain	Improved efficacy and compatibility	[47]
NeuroAIDS/ antiretroviral drugs (ARV), latency reactivating agents (LRA) and drug abuse antagonist (AT)	Liposomal-magnetic nanoformulation conjugate to transferrin	Active targeting of BBB and astrocytes	Sustained drug release, reduced HIV-1 infectivity up to 40–50%, improved therapeutic adherence	[48]

Table 1.
NP for targeting the brain.

3. Drug delivery to musculoskeletal system

The general term arthritis is used to describe joint disorders which include one or more joint(s) of the musculoskeletal system. One of the prevalent forms of arthritis is osteoarthritis (OA). Other forms of musculoskeletal disorders currently pose global health issues include osteoporosis (OSP), rheumatoid arthritis (RA), infective arthritis, psoriasis, osteomyelitis (OM), and lupus. The specific structure associated with the cartilage and bone tissue complicates drug treatment related to aforesaid disorders [49]. Bone, the hardest organ of body belongs to connective tissue and is composed of basic substances such as collagen and carbonated hydroxyapatite. The bone hardness associated to the present of the inorganic salts, include calcium, phosphate, carbonate, and magnesium. The highly vascularized bone tissue increases capacity for treatment. Furthermore, bone has potential of bone-generation fixing minerals, particularly calcium. In general, three kinds of cells exist in bone tissue. Osteoblasts are bone-generating cells that synthesize inorganic mineral compounds known as osteoids which are mineralized and turn into bone. Osteocytes are produced by maturation of osteoblasts. Osteocytes are bone matrix-surrounded cells and the space they occupy called the lacunae. Osteocyte function is to assist bone formation, bone matrix retention, and calcium homeostasis regulation. Osteoclasts are responsible for bone resorption and reformation. They are huge multinucleated cells and exist near the bone surface. These cells are derived from monocytes and have phagocytic activity [50]. **Figure 2** shows the structure of typical long bone.

Cartilage is an elastic, flexible connective tissue encompassing the end of the bone. The cartilage consists of cells called chondrocytes. The chondrocyte matrix materials include water (70%), glycosaminoglycan (GAG) such as hyaluronic acid and chondroitin sulfate, glycoproteins such as aggrecan as well as proteins like elastin fibrils and collagen. This matrix can be reservoir for mediator, that is, chemokines and growth factors that are required for phenotype stability and protection of chondrocytes. Lack of vasculature in cartilage tissue is compensated by thick ECM that isolates chondrocytes and growth factors. Absence of blood vessels gives low repair capacity to cartilage, therefore events such as aging and damage, the decreased range of motion, gradual depletion of joints, pain and variety of joint diseases will occur. Synovial joint in the bones move against each other, surrounded by a membrane that is

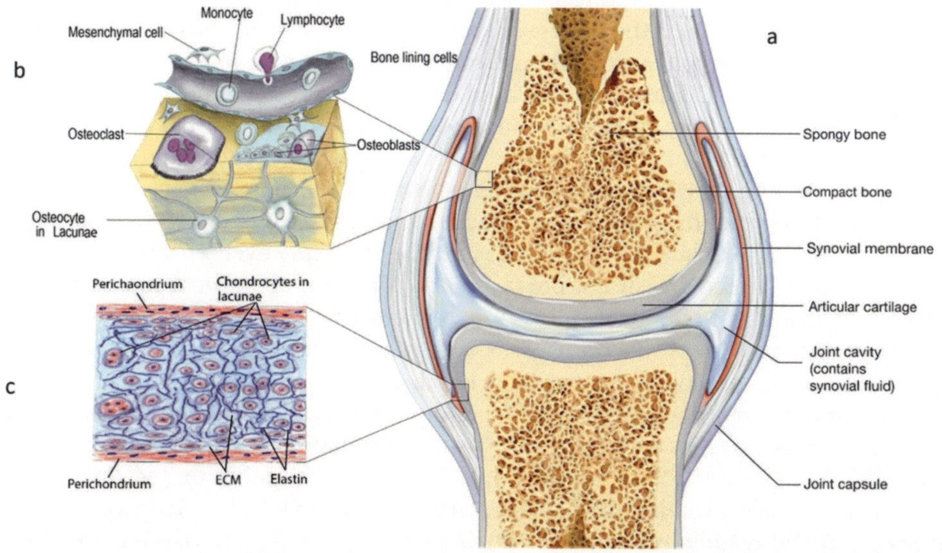

Figure 2.
Schematic illustration of (a) articular cartilage, long bone, and synovial cavity, (b) different types of cells in bone structure, (c) cartilage structure [51].

semipermeable and composed of a macrophages and fibroblast, regulating the material transfer in and out of the joints [52]. The cartilage structure is shown in **Figure 2**.

OA is a degenerative joint disorder in which chondrocytes are transformed from a cartilage-generating to a cartilage decomposing state or transfer from anabolic to catabolic state. In the catabolic mode, chondrocytes undergo autophagy accompanied by hypertrophy in which the volume of the cells increases [52]. RA is an autoimmune or chronic systemic inflammatory disease. In RA diseases, T-lymphocytes stimulate macrophage to overproduce inflammatory cytokines which have potential to induce receptor activator of NF-κβ ligand (RANKL). RANKL is osteoclastogenesis regulator which severe for generation of osteoclast and leading to resorption of calcium from the bone. Furthermore, synovial fibroblasts produce vesicular endothelial growth factor (VEGF) that stimulates angiogenesis and leads to retention of inflammation by recruitment of inflammatory leukocytes. The forgoing process plays a critical role in inflammation progress and degeneration of cartilage [53]. In addition to the aforementioned etiology, other factors involved in RA include, osteopontin (OPN) overproduction in synovial cavity, imbalance between tolerance and autoimmunity in joint inflammatory condition, activation of oncostatin M (OSM) cytokine and production of urokinase-type plasminogen activator (uPA) [49], as well as activation of notch 1 [54] and TREM-1 pathways [55]. In the OSP disease calcium and vitamin D deficiency due to hormonal changes creates sensitive and fragile bone [56]. Reduction in bone mineral density in OSP leads to bone strength reduction and makes it susceptible to fracture [57]. Dysregulation of homeostasis in bone, improves the osteoclast activity and leading to hasten bone turnover. Thereby, increase of pro-inflammatory molecules and cytokines causes resorption of bone and delays its formation [3].

3.1 Limitation of drug delivery to cartilage and bone

In musculoskeletal disorders, multiple factors or biochemical pathway is contributed. Systemic administration of drugs in polyarticular degenerative joint disorders such as hand OA is gone along with the limitations associated with delivery of insufficient doses to the target sites and increased risk of systemic toxicity. Common therapeutic approach in di-arthrodial joints; for example, the knee joint, involves intra-articular injection. This kind of injection increases drug concentration near the superficial layers of cartilage and reduces the total dose at the desired sites. The result of such administration is systemic toxicity whereas local administration of drugs in the form of ointment and hydrogel will increase drug bioavailability; however, suffers from fast clearance from the synovial cavity and lowers absorption of drug in cartilage. Sequential injections into the joint, however, are accompanied by the risk of infection and discomfort patient. Moreover, off-target accumulations of the drug result in its removal from lymphatic vessel in the synovial cavity due to the phagocytic activity of macrophages. Consequently, only the small amount of the therapeutic drug remains in the cartilage. Furthermore, presence of the dense collagen II network, absence of blood vessel, and the aggrecan negative electrical charge are main factors that prevent penetration of the drug molecules into the cartilage tissue [52, 58]. Therapeutic molecules larger than 100 kD exhibit limited clearance from cartilage, while smaller molecules such as non-steroidal anti-inflammatory drugs (NSAIDs) readily leak out from cartilage space. The aqueous composition of the synovial fluid presents a challenge for the hydrophobic drug delivery. Delivery of hydrophilic drugs into the synovial cavity is also limited by the concentration gradient of the fluid which is directed against the flow to the cavity. Intra-articular fluid is transported into the joint cavity by excessive filtration through capillaries and then flows out to the lymph node. Therefore, drug intra-articular injection is restricted by its short lifetime within the cartilage [58, 59]. Bone is the most important target tissue for drug action in OSP. Challenges in delivering drugs to bone include nonspecific bone formation, slow bone growth, and determination of the appropriate administered dose. Bone cement injection can cause toxicity problems. For example, Poly methyl methacrylate (PMMA) with high curie temperature can damage the surrounding tissue and subsequently post-injection polymerization. On the other hand, calcium phosphate cement presents the challenge of critical state of injection, poor mechanical strength, and rapid degradation [57]. In RA diseases, the most important limitation is considered to be the serious side effect is suppressing the immune system due to using NSAIDs and disease-modifying antirheumatic drugs (DMARDs) [49].

3.2 Nanotechnology for drug delivery to the bone and cartilage

The introduction of nanotechnology has partially addressed the obstacles of drug delivery to bone and cartilage. The small size, high retention capacity, and low possibility of phagocytosis of NPs facilitate drug delivery. Targeting NPs enables attachment to specific cells like chondrocytes and inflammatory agents. NPs designed for drug delivery to negatively charged cartilage must be positively charged for attachment, thus preventing filtration from cartilage pores. In OA, passive delivery is ineffective due to limited fenestration available in blood capillaries as a result of complete angiogenesis. The targeted NPs allow an increased reliability of drug supplement available in the cartilage ECM, a higher dose of chemical pathway inhibitors delivered to the arthritic joints, and reduces drug phagocytosis by macrophages. The fenestrated capillaries in RA lead to lymphatic leakage and produce enhanced permeability and retention (EPR) effect. Due to impaired angiogenesis in RA, blood vessels exhibit large fenestrations that aid in the passive delivery of therapeutic NPs. In the RA treatment, NPs smaller than 200 nm enable movement of drug molecules through porous capillaries. Coating the NPs with hydrophilic polymers helps slow down renal clearance and degradation of the NPs, enabling them to accumulate in arthritic patients' joints. The objectives of employing nanomedicine for treating RA are to attract inflammatory macrophages and inhibit lymphocyte proliferation. Therefore, surface markers of macrophages and lymphocytes are valuable for targeting NPs [52, 60]. **Table 2** lists nano-formulations for the delivery to bone and cartilage.

3.3 Targeted and non-targeted drug delivery

Common limitations associated with medications used to treat musculoskeletal diseases include reduced drug accumulation in joints, off-target effects, the need for painful procedures like injections, risk of systemic toxicity, and rapid removal from the joint cavity. These constraints have promoted the utilization of engineered NPs, like chitosan (CS), which are commonly employed for targeted delivery in arthritis. One issue with off-target delivery is the drug accumulation in the liver and spleen. Nevertheless, non-targeted drugs like curcumin and iron-saturated bovine lactoferrin (Fe-bLf) did not result in notable side effects in other tissues. On the other hand, special attention is required in arthritis for the use of targeted methotrexate (MTX) and methylprednisolone, which can have serious side effects [49]. While curcumin is effective in treating OSP, its efficacy is enhanced in nanoformulation because of its poor solubility, low bioavailability, rapid metabolism, poor kinetic, and physicochemical

Diseases	Drug in nano-formulation	Endpoint	Reference
OA	IGF-1 fused with heparin-binding domain (HpB)	Reduced cartilage loss in male Lewis rats	[61]
OA	Diacerein (DC) loaded lipid NPs modified with chondroitin sulfate (ChS)	Higher degree of cartilage regeneration in Charles foster rats	[62]
OA	Anti-Hif-2α siRNA condensed by PEI modified with CAP peptide (DWRVIIPPRPSA)	Significant reduction in cartilage degradation in joints of male Chinese Kun Ming mice	[63]
RA	Methotrexate and SPIONs into anti-CD64 antibody-conjugated PLGA NPs	NPs may potentiate the action of MTX without injuring healthy tissues and organs, simultaneously providing a non-invasive and specific imaging tool for RA	[64]
RA, OA, OM	Methotrexate in stealth Nanogels of Histinylated Poly Ethyleneimine	Sustained delivery of MTX and preferential accumulation of the nanogels in inflamed paw	[60]
RA	Methotrexate in Aspasome NP made of antioxidant, ascorbyl palmitate	Better disease modifications against RA than the free drug, improved penetration, reduced side effect and toxicity in Wistar rats.	[65]
RA	Lipase-labile fumagillin prodrug (Fum-PD) in αvβ3-integrin-targeted perfluorocarbon nanocarriers	Improve antiangiogenic therapies	[66]
OA	Iron saturated-bovine lactoferrin encapsulated in alginate-chitosan polymeric nanocarriers	Significantly induced disease modifying activity by affect gene expression.	[67]
OA	Berberine-loaded chitosan NPs	Increase berberine concentration and retention time in rates joint.	[68]
OA	Salmon calcitonin-hyaluronic acid nanocomplex	Reduced inflammation and potential to be a long acting I.A. injection with a more favorable risk–benefit profile than current options.	[69]
RA and other autoimmune disorders	TNF-related apoptosis inducing ligand (TRAIL) in PEG and HA	Good stability and sustained release of TRAIL in arthritic mice.	[70]
RA	Triggering receptor expressed on myeloid cells 1 (TREM-1) inhibitor i.e., GF9 peptide bound to macrophage-targeted NPs	Ameliorated CIA and protected against bone and cartilage damage and increased therapeutic efficacy.	[55]
OSP	RANK siRNA complexed with PEI entrapped in nanosized PLGA capsules	Suppression of osteoclast maturation and reduction of osteoclast activity	[71]

Table 2.
Application of nano-formulations for the delivery to bone and cartilage.

instability. Gold NP conjugated with curcumin-containing cyclodextrin (CD) can form a complex that inhibits osteoclast formation by bone marrow-derived macrophages. The mechanism of such drug delivery system is inhibiting the RANKL activator [72]. The surfaces of chondrocytes, osteoblasts, and osteoclasts cells feature integrin receptors that exhibit a strong attraction to the RGD-4 peptide. Research on the integrin and RGD-4 peptide interaction through docking and ab initio quantum mechanics has unveiled a robust receptor-binding affinity suitable for targeting applications [73].

Recently, NPs have been utilized for delivering calcium, bone cement, and growth factors like platelet-derived growth factor (PDGF), insulin-like growth factor (IGF), catabolic cartilage factor, genes, mRNA, and SiRNA molecules, and PTH for musculoskeletal treatment of diseases. For instance, in the OSP drug delivery, it allows for targeted delivery to bone tissue, preventing drug absorption into other organs. Additionally, NP-based delivery allows for sustained and slow release of medication. NPs improve calcium availability and help prevent the progression of OSP. The nanohydroxyapatite (nHA) and PMMA are other materials utilized in the treatment of OSP. The PMMA nanostructure is mechanically reinforced and its functionality provides the capacity for injection. Providing slow release and fewer injections, PTH was targeted by collagen-binding domains. CS NPs-incorporated PTH induces osteogenesis and decrease side effects on the stomach, due to absorption of H^+ in the by-amine groups of chitosan. PEG-coated CS-PTH improves the surface properties of NPs such as bioavailability, stability in the stomach, and facilitates drug transport. Also, the PEG-CS-PTH complex enhances mineralization of bone in the presence of intracellular Ca^{2+} and elimination of hemolytic activity [57]. Ex-vivo treatment of musculoskeletal diseases has prerequisites, that is, suitable scaffold, appropriate stem cells, and growth factors. In tissue engineering, a commonly used scaffold for bone and cartilage repair contains stem cells and growth factor-carrying NPs. NPs can enhance stem cell proliferation and differentiation stabilize growth factors, prevent their degradation, and provide their slow release [74, 75].

4. Drug delivery to the skin

Applying the drug topically enables more effective treatment with targeted dosing, minimized side effects, and improved patient compliance. It is also beneficial for addressing various skin conditions like vulgaris, alopecia, dermatitis, vitiligo, psoriasis, acne, and skin cancer [76]. The transdermal drug delivery can also be used to treat diseases like osteoporosis, rheumatoid arthritis, Parkinson's disease, Alzheimer's, and diabetes. In transdermal delivery, the drug crosses the skin layers, enters circulation, and reaches the target organ. The primary obstacle to penetrate the skin layers is the outermost skin layer known as the stratum corneum (SC). This layer consists of corneocytes or dead skin cells, which are embedded in lipid multilayers, often likened to a "brick and mortar" structure. Surmounting this barrier poses the greatest difficulty for researchers seeking to drug delivery systems and devices through the skin [76–78].

The skin is made up of three layers: the epidermis, dermis, and hypodermis. The dermal layer includes blood vessels and exhibits hydrophilic properties. Substances that penetrate the bloodstream from the skin's layers must pass through the epidermis. Corneocytes are linked together by desmosomes, enhancing adhesion. The SC's permeability is 1000 times lower than other membranes due to its distinctive lipid composition. Fatty acids, cholesterol, and ceramides align parallel to the skin's surface. In the SC lipids, the atypical length of the free fatty acid, the acyl chain of the ceramides, and the relatively small polar end of the ceramide result in a more stable arrangement in comparison to phospholipids. The corneocytes are rich in keratin. Unlike other cells, the hydrophobic and fibrous nature of corneocytes prevents the loss of body fluids and the entry of foreign substances. This unique structure is not present in sebaceous glands and hair follicles. The dermis is directly accessible from the hair follicle, but the number of hair follicles is insufficient for transdermal drug administration, just a little dose can be transported. However, utilizing hair follicles for drug delivery is logical if the aim is to deliver the drug to the hair roots [77–79]. **Figure 3** schematically illustrates the skin structure and the SC layer.

Only 5% of medications are appropriate for passing through the skin passively [78]. Those are low molecular weight (<500 kD) and moderate lipophilicity [81]. The dosage of the medication is also a restricting factor for transdermal use, where the maximum administered dose is capped at 10 mg/day and the absolute solubility must be over 1 mg/ml [82]. Hence, altering the medication formulation to address this limitation represents a novel approach to transdermal drug delivery.

4.1 Modification of the drug formulation using nano-carriers

The utilization of lipophilic NPs like liposomes and their derivatives, liquid crystals (LCs), SLNs, and nanoemulsions for drug delivery is commonly seen in the healthcare and cosmetic sectors and is effective for transdermal drug delivery. Nanoparticles are applied in the form of lotions, creams, gels, and solutions. The mechanism of NPs action involves disrupting the SC, tight junctions, cell membrane structure, and facilitating drug penetration. The advantages include protection against degradation by skin microbial flora, low cost, application over a large skin area, controlled release, and specific cell targeting [83, 84]. **Table 3** mentions NPs used for transdermal drug release.

4.1.1 Liposomes and their derivatives

Liposomes and their derivatives can transport hydrophilic drugs in the aqueous phase and lipophilic drugs in the liposome membrane bilayer. Cationic liposomes

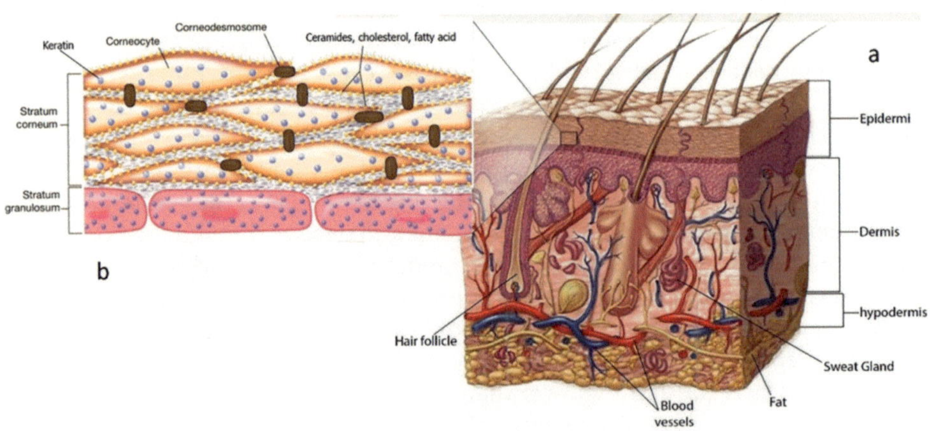

Figure 3.
Schematic illustration of (a) the three layers of skin and (b) stratum corneum [80].

Diseases/drug	Transdermal nanocarrier	Benefits	References
Diabetes/ glimepiride	Ethosome	Prevention of oral drug side effects, sustained release of drug, avoid the hepatic first pass metabolism.	[85]
Psoriasis/ Osthole	Transfersome and ethosome	Enhanced skin penetration, improve solubility, increased bioavailability	[86]
Hypertention/ Olmesartan medoxomil	Nano-invasome	Increace drug half-life and patient compliance	[87]
OA and RA/ Oxaprozin	Drug-cyclodextrin in liposome and NLC	Improve solubility and enhance penetration through skin	[88]
Skin cancer/ Epirubicin	Superparamagnetic Iron-Oxide NPs	Providing pH-sensitive release, better penetration and accumulation in tumor and reduce adverse effect.	[89]
Hormonal disturbances in pre- and postmenopausal women/ Progesterone	Liquid crystalline NPs (LCNPs)	Increased solubility and half-life of drug, prevent from first pass metabolism, decrease side effect and patient compliance	[90]
Atopic dermatitis/ Corticosteroids	Thermo-sensitive Poloxamer 407/ Carboxymethyl cellulose sodium (P407/CMCs) composite hydrogel	Skin hydration, reduce side effect, enhances bioadhesion and surface morphology.	[91]
Schizophrenia/ Risperidone	Nano soft lipid vesicle containing phospholipid, safranal and ethanol	Increase solubility and bioavailability, avoiding its first pass metabolism and produce stable plasma concentrations over a long period.	[92]
Rheumatic diseases/ Tenoxicam (TX)	Bilosome	Avoid unnecessary GI side effects associated with oral administration.	[93]
Rheumatism and neuralgia/ Paeonol	Transethosome	Increase solubility and bioavailability, decrease volatility	[94]
RA, psoriasis and cancer/Methotrexate (MTX)	NLC	Eliminate adverse effect of MTX	[95]
Skin diseases/ 8-methoxypsoraln (8-MOP)	Noisome	Eliminate gastrointestinal adverse effects and higher risk of severe complications e.g. glaucoma or carcinogenesis	[96]
OA and RA/ Meloxicam	Flexosomes	Deeper skin penetration, improved therapeutic effect compared with oral administration in rat paw	[97]
Dermatitis and eczema/ Triptolide	Nanoemulsion gels	Stable release of drug, maintaining effective drug concentration.	[98]
Skin cancer/ Curcumin and 5-flurouracil	Two copolymers: alginate coated aminated nanodextran (ALG@AND) and chitosan coated folate decorated aminated -CD nano particles (CS@FA-g-ACD).	Elute the drugs in a sustained manner, and could also act as penetration enhancers.	[99]

Diseases/drug	Transdermal nanocarrier	Benefits	References
RA, OA and ankylosing spondylitis/ Aceclofenac	NLC	Improved skin penetration and dermatokinetic, increase anti-inflammatory effect	[100]
RA/ Diflunisal (DIF)	Supramolecular nano-engineered lipidic carriers (SNLCs)	Decrease ear edema in mice and paw edema in CFA model. The levels of TNF-α were reduced in synovial fluid and serum.	[101]
Hemorrhage and pain/ Dencichine	Ionic liquid – microemulsions	10-fold increased penetration compared with drug solution, minor cell toxicity and skin irritation, significant hemostatic activity	[102]
Hypertension/ Lacidipine	Niosomal gel	Skin permeation enhancement of 2.15 times as compare to control gel, higher antihypertensive activity	[103]
Hypertension/ Eprosartan mesylate	Nano-transferosome	Higher and deeper penetration into the skin compared with liposome	[104]
Hypertention/ Amlodipine	NLCs	Enhanced bioavailability of amlodipine in the wistar rats	[105]
Gout/Febuxostat	Niosomal gel	Improved solubility and stability of drug	[106]
OSP/Raloxifene hydrochloride	Nano-transferosome	Provide controlled release and improve bioavailability	[107]

Table 3.
NPs used for transdermal drug release.

penetrate better because they interact with the negatively charged surface of skin cells. Penetration edge activators can be added to improve liposome capacity. Edge activators are surfactants that increase liposome elasticity, flowability, and deformability, allowing liposomes to squeeze through intercellular space and diffuse through skin layers. A liposome derivative contains edge activator is transferosome [76]. Another way to enhance liposome penetration is by adding absorption enhancers like ethanol or terpenes [92]. Ethanol boosts the fluidity of the liposome membrane, lowering the lipid multilayer density of the cell membrane. This leads to increased skin absorption of ethanol. An ethanol-containing liposome is referred to as an ethosome [85]. When stabilizing amphiphilic materials like nonionic, single-chain surfactants, and cholesterol are incorporated into the liposome structure, the chemical stability of the liposome is enhanced along with improved penetration. These liposomes, known as noisomes, show promise for formulation as an emulsion or cream due to their convenient storage and handling [76]. Bilosome referred to noisomes containing bile salts. Bilosomes increase absorption through the skin and can be administered orally because they tolerate digestive enzymes and bile [93]. When a combination of lysophosphatidylcholine (LPC), soy phosphatidylcholine, terpene, and ethanol is used, a liposome called an invasome is formed. Lysophosphatidycholine acts as a peripheral activator, while ethanol acts as an absorption and terpene permeation enhancer by disrupting SC lipid packaging [87]. SLN is another widely used NPs for transdermal drug delivery which belongs to the NLCs. Thus, SLN shows great potential for achieving the objective of controlled and site-specific drug delivery, garnering significant interest from scientists. These nanoparticles have potential for drug delivery commercialization and can also be utilized in the cosmetic and health sectors. Surfactants and alcohols can enhance the absorption and stability of SLNs [76, 108]. Nanoemulsions are a different type of effective drug delivery systems created by blending two immiscible liquids like water and oil. A surfactant can also be incorporated into nanoemulsions to enhance their stability by decreasing the interfacial tension through physical repulsion. Nanoemulsions have an optimal size that enables them to pass through hair follicles and sebaceous glands without causing skin irritation. Nanoemulsions can deliver drugs like minoxidil for hair growth or hair loss prevention [76, 84]. Liquid crystals (LCs) [109], solid-in-oil (S/O) dispersions [79], lyotropic liquid crystals [110], and cubosomes [90] are other nanostructures for transdermal drug delivery.

Microneedling provides an effective method to penetrate the skin barrier. Microneedle (MN) penetrates the SC, delivering the drug to the dermis layer and blood vessels. MNs do not penetrate deep into the skin, thus avoiding pain or bleeding. Nowadays, MNs in the skin patch form have been recognized as the most effective patch type and have gained wide commercial acceptance [111]. As MN is utilized for vaccine administration, immune cell presence in the skin patch application area is significantly increased, suggesting immune cell migration to lymph nodes to trigger an immune response [112]. Other benefits of MNs are capacity to transport large molecules, painlessness, simple administration, decline exposure to microbes compared to traditional injections, and swift drug delivery [113]. One of the issues with the use of MNs is related to solving lipophilic drugs in toxic solvents. The use of dissolving microneedle (DMN) permits solving the drug in the polymeric matrix of the DMN by decomposing the polymer so that the lipophilic drugs may be released from the matrix. The mentioned method circumvents the need to dissolve lipophilic drugs in toxic solvents [114]. The addition of NPs to dissolvable polymers enhances the mechanical properties of the patch without impacting the skin's dissolution rate. Nanostructures material like layered double hydroxide (LDH) can enhance

MN materials	Drug	Diseases	Reference
Titanium	Parathyroid hormone (Forteo)	Osteoporosis	[116]
PVP	Insulin	Diabetes	[117]
CMC, PVA, PVP	Capsaicin	RA	[114]
solid silicon	cholesterol-modified housekeeping gene (Gapdh) siRNA	Alopecia, allergic skin diseases, hyperpigmentation, psoriasis, skin cancer, pachyonychia Congenital	[118]
PVA and PVP in polymeric matrix	Memantine	AD	[119]
N-methyl 2-pyrrolidone or dimethyl sulfoxide	Diclofenac	Analgestic effect	[82]
PVP, PVA	Vitamin D3-PLGA	Vaccination goal	[120]

Table 4.
Microneedles used for drug delivery.

mechanical properties of MN and boost drug delivery efficiency [112]. However, integrating NPs carrying drug molecules to DMNs can provide slow and continuous drug release besides enhancing the mechanical properties of DMNs [115]. MN used for drug delivery is listed in **Table 4**.

5. Pulmonary drug delivery

In cases of pulmonary diseases, administering lung medicines is recommended. The key benefits of pulmonary administration include the lungs' large surface area, quick absorption through numerous blood vessels, and the ability to bypass first-pass metabolism in the liver [121]. According to statistics, chronic obstructive pulmonary disease (COPD), lower respiratory tract infections, and lung cancer are the third, fourth, and fifth most common diseases in the world [122]. Additionally, tuberculosis (TB) is among the top ten causes of death worldwide, caused by *Mycobacterium tuberculosis*. It primarily affects the lungs and spreads through the air from infected individuals to others [123]. Therefore, research and development on the treatment of pulmonary diseases is of particular significance.

The pulmonary system is well-suited for local drug delivery due to its properties. This is because it contains 280 billion blood vessels, 300 million alveoli, and a vast 70 m^2 area associated with the blood-gas interface [121]. The endothelium of the respiratory system comprises approximately 25% of the total blood vessel surface area in the body [124]. Alveolar gas exchange takes place at the interface of the capillary endothelium, alveolar epithelium, and intercellular layers. The alveoli are covered with surfactant, comprising phospholipids and proteins that decrease surface tension and lung tissue friction, thus being crucial for proper breathing. The existence of pulmonary surfactant (PS) provides various benefits for drug delivery. Specifically, it aids in the dissolution of poorly soluble drugs, effectively transports the medication through the pulmonary system via capillary diffusion, and protects the drug from extracellular barrier. The lower pulmonary pathway is supported by a thin layer of connective tissue which is surrounded by different cells including macrophages, fibroblasts, and nerves, as well as lymph vessels. Thus, the lower part of pulmonary route is ideal for drug delivery as it can reach both the pulmonary and lymph nodes. Despite the desirable properties of the pulmonary system for drug delivery, the defense mechanisms of the system must be considered to prevent the intrusion of foreign substances [121]. The pulmonary system comprises central and peripheral regions. In the central region, a mucus layer, respiratory cilia movement, and thick epithelium prevent foreign body entry. The mucous membrane eliminates foreign particles before reaching lower regions, leading to coughing and swallowing. In the peripheral lung regions, alveolar macrophages restrict absorption through phagocytosis [125]. These regions also contain high levels of lipids and proteins, forming a transport barrier. Along with alveolar defenses, epithelial cell tight junctions serve as the initial transport barrier [121]. To address these limitations, researchers have explored nano/microparticle drug delivery. **Figure 4** shows central and peripheral structures of the pulmonary system.

5.1 Characteristic of drug formulation for pulmonary drug delivery

Medicines delivered to the nasal cavity need to be in powder form to disperse as aerosols. Particle size is crucial here. Particles under 0.5 μm can exit the lungs, while

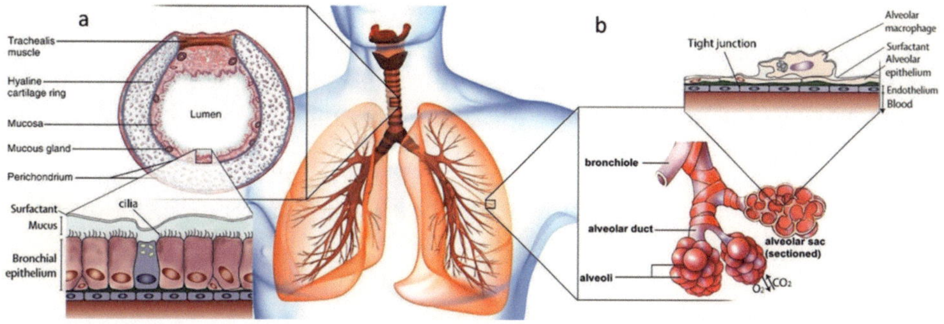

Figure 4.
Schematic illustration of (a) central pulmonary system and (b) peripheral pulmonary system [126].

those absorbed by alveolar macrophages range from 0.5–5 μm. Particles with a diameter less than 0.5 μm are ineffective for drug delivery as they may dislodge during exhalation due to their lightweight [121, 125]. On the other hand, decreasing particle size to nanometer values is linked to increased dissolution rate in the respiratory mucosa. To address the particle size issue, NPs can be engineered to aggregate into micrometer-sized formations upon aerosol separation, enabling them to settle due to their sufficient mass. The prolonged presence of these aggregates in the bronchi can achieve the intended therapeutic outcome [121]. Trojan particles, micrometer-sized porous particles designed with NPs, can also serve this purpose. These particles have sufficient weight to settle in the lung mucosal fluid, allowing them to break down into NPs and permeate the epithelium [125]. Another approach involves utilizing a proper matrix that includes NPs. For instance, NPs can be integrated into an excipient matrix, like a mannitol-based suspension, that is spray-dried to create a powder suitable for inhalation [127].

Another crucial aspect in the absorption and transportation of NPs in the pulmonary system is whether the particle is hydrophilic or not. NPs that enter the deeply in pulmonary system interact with PS. Lipids like phospholipids and cholesterol comprise 90% of PS and the remaining 10% composed of proteins. The PSs in contact with the NPs create a molecular shell around them which is known as corona. The structure of the PS-corona is influenced by the physical and chemical characteristics of the NP, like hydrophilicity/hydrophobicity and electric charge. This corona plays a crucial role in determining the destiny of the NP in the respiratory system. Studies indicate that the corona enveloping hydrophilic NPs facilitates easier absorption compared to hydrophobic NPs [128]. Furthermore, hydrophilic NPs coated with lipid molecules decorated with PS show enhanced interaction. This modified structure can merge with the plasma membrane to facilitate the transportation of hydrophilic NPs to secondary organs [129]. Another aspect to consider in the development of pulmonary medications is mucosal adhesion. Some natural polymers, like chitosan, exhibit strong mucosal adhesion. Apart from this property, chitosan can also swell upon contact with liquids, self-heal, accommodate both hydrophobic and hydrophilic drugs, and interact with cell membranes due to the amphiphilic nature of its polymer chains, thereby aiding in drug release [130, 131]. Hydrophobic drugs may not be readily encapsulated in chitosan and therefore require an aqueous coating. Key considerations in formulating drugs for pulmonary delivery involve prolonged residence, safeguarding against enzymatic breakdown or leakage, limited entry into the systemic circulation, targeting specific cells via ligands, and concealing odor or aftertaste [14].

Recently, various NPs have been developed for treating tuberculosis, like maleate-gellan gum-silk-sericin-chitosan nanocomposite loaded with pyrazinamide and rifampicin [132], alginate-chitosan NPs with ascorbic acid and rifampicin [133]. Other NPs like polymer NPs and microparticles (MPs), proliposomes, polymer NPs dry powder nanoaggregates, polymer-coated liposomes, polymer submicron particles, polymer self-assembled porous nanoaggregate particles (PNAP), polymer-coated lipopolymer NPs have been studied for the treatment of tuberculosis [123]. Some of the diseases treated by pulmonary drug delivery are listed in **Table 5**.

Diseases	Drug/NP complex	Effects	References
Pulmonary Arterial Hypertension (PAH)	Tacrolimus/Nanocomposite Microparticles (nCmP)	Provide targeted pulmonary delivery, improved solubility of tacrolimus, the potential of penetration through mucus barrier, and controlled drug release	[127]
Lung cancer	Paclitaxel/ DOPE and DPPC	No signs of interstitial pulmonary fibrosis, chronic inflammation and any other pulmonary toxicity. Improved fusogenicity and cytosolic drug release	[134]
Diarrhea	Loperamide/calcium carbonate particles modified with mucoadhesive biocompatible polymer, HA, poly-l-lysine as well as polysorbate 80	Bypassing the BBB	[16]
Asthma and COPD	Beclomethasone dipropionate/ PHEA-PEG2000-EDA-LA micelles	Protect drug from hydrolysis, controlled and prolonged release, enhanced mucosal penetration, more biocompatibility.	[135]
Pulmonary Arterial Hypertension (PAH)	Cinaciguat/ Chitosan	Adhesion to mucosa, controlled release by chitosan swelling, protection against esterase	[130]
Cystic Fibrosis	Ivacaftor/ PEGylated and Tat-decorated fluorescent NPs (FNPs)	Enhanced diffusion from pulmonary mucosal barrier and promoting ivacaftor lung cellular uptake	[136]
Pseudomonas aeruginosa Infections in Cystic Fibrosis	Tobramycin/, nano into micro formulations (NiMs) made of PVA, NAC, Arg, Cyst and helping materials	Facilitate diffusion of drug through the mucus and sustained delivery, pronounced antibacterial activity compared with TOBIPodhaler	[137]
Lung cancer	Doxorubicin/Nano-in-microparticles (NIMs) containing SPIONs and fluorescent nanospheres in a lactose matrix.	Better accumulation in lung using presence of magnetic field, maintain the therapeutic cytotoxicity of doxorubicin	[138]
HIV	SiRNA against Beclin1 gene /PEI	Direct delivery of the PEI-siRNA nanocomplex to the CNS	[139]

Diseases	Drug/NP complex	Effects	References
Lung cancer	Doxorubicin/PEGylated poly(amidoamine) dendrimer	Delivery of DOX to deep lungs, the modulation of DOX interaction with respiratory epithelium, and temporal/spatial control of DOX release from the dendrimer conjugates.	[140]
Lung cancer	AuNPs functionalized with oligo(2-oxazoline)-based optically stable fluorescent coatings, and conjugated with a laminin peptide (YIGSR) in chitosan matrix	Enhanced cellular uptake, sustained and controlled release of the embedded NPs.	[141]
Metastatic lung cancer	Doxorubicin and cisplatin in methoxy poly(ethylene glycol)-poly(ethylenimine)-poly(L-glutamate) (mPEG-OEI-PLG) copolymers	Higher accumulation and anti-tumor activity in comparison to doxorubicin and cisplatin alone in cancerous mice.	[142]
Lung infection in cystic fibrosis	Ciprofloxacin-loaded PLGA NP	Enhanced antibacterial activity, NPs' colloidal stability in mucus.	[143]
TB	Rifampicin and pyrazinamide in maleate gellan gum-silk sericin chitosan nanocopmosite	Higher antimycobacterial activity and rapid delivery of drugs at TB infected macrophages.	[132]
TB	Rifampicin and ascorbic acid in sodium alginate coated with chitosan and Tween 80 nanoparticle	Increasing the local drug concentrations, reducing the risk of systemic toxicity and hence improving the patient compliance,	[133]

Table 5.
Diseases treated by pulmonary drug delivery.

6. Drug delivery in diabetes

Diabetes is a group of metabolic disorders linked to high glucose levels (hyperglycemia). Type 1 diabetes (T1D), also known as juvenile diabetes, makes up 10% of all diabetes cases. It results from insufficient insulin production. Insulin regulates blood glucose by stimulating glucose consumption in liver and muscle cells. This malfunction is due to an autoimmune response in the patient, leading to destruction of pancreatic β-cells by T-lymphocytes. The insufficient insulin production results in an increase in blood glucose levels. Type 2 diabetes (T2D) is categorized as a lifestyle illness linked to obesity and insufficient physical activity. Individuals with T2D experience insulin resistance and high blood glucose levels because of the delayed reaction of body tissues to post-meal insulin [144].

The primary challenge in managing diabetes is not merely lowering blood sugar levels, but rather sustaining a typical, euglycemic glucose range of 40–170 mg/dl. Insulin replacement therapy is frequently used for Type 1 Diabetes (T1D) and advanced Type 2 Diabetes (T2D). Adequate blood insulin levels can be attained through whole pancreas or islets of Langerhans transplantation, genetically modified insulin-secreting cell transplantation, bioartificial pancreas implantation, and automatic insulin delivery [145]. In T1D, the aim is to administer insulin. Achieving a permanent treatment for T1D involves either replacing damaged pancreatic β-cells with healthy cells or delivering genes to damaged pancreatic cells [146]. Other treatments or medications mainly aim to manage diabetes and are not seen as permanent solutions. Cell therapy, on the other hand, focuses on replacing β cells to sustain insulin secretion in the bloodstream. In the method of cell therapy, a matrix is utilized to encapsulate replacement cells, shielding them from the immune response while enabling the diffusion of nutrients, oxygen, and glucose. Healthy β-cells, derived from induced pluripotent stem (iPS) cells and provided with glucose, oxygen, and nutrients, are encapsulated and transplanted [145]. Another method to address diabetes is through gene therapy. In this method, a gene that triggers insulin secretion in β-cells is transported using a carrier. The carrier needs to safeguard the gene from nuclease [146]. However, managing diabetes through glycemic control is a common approach, as definitive treatment of diabetes can incur significant costs, but can also result in immunosuppression, implant rejection, or lack of successful gene or cell delivery. Therefore, most individuals with T2D aim to lead a normal life by controlling their diet and using medications to manage their blood sugar levels [145, 146].

6.1 Nanotechnology in the treatment of diabetes

The use of nanotechnology in treating diabetes now focuses on maintaining normal glucose levels, shielding drugs from degradation, enhancing drug bioavailability in the bloodstream, and minimizing side effects. Insulin injections enable the controlled release of insulin based on glucose levels, thus avoiding hypoglycemia. Glucose-responsive polymers maintain a closed-loop system to prevent risky fluctuations in glucose levels [147]. A pH-sensitive polymer with the enzyme glucose oxidase (GOx) was used to design glucose concentration-responsive NPs. GOx catalyzes the conversion of glucose to gluconic acid, which causes the creation of acidic conditions in the environment surrounding the NP. A drop in pH causes the polymer to break down and release insulin. An increase in glucose concentration leads to a further lowering of pH and thus accelerates the degradation of the polymer and the release of insulin. Another system sensitive to glucose concentration was created using dextran and poly(α1,6-glucose) physically linked to CoA. When CoA collides with glucose in the environment, the glucose bond to the polymer is released and CoA binds the free glucose. In this way, the hydrogel breaks down [147]. Common diabetic drugs associated with NPs listed in **Table 6**.

The Self-regulating glucose-sensitive skin patches have also been constructed for insulin administration. These MNs contain a H_2O_2-labile amphiphilic copolymer that contains a positive charge and is used to form nanosized complex micelles (NCs). NC embedded in MN nucleus and delivered transcutaneously. The harmful effects of H_2O_2 on normal tissues have been reduced by the use of enzymes that remove H_2O_2. The oxygenated and acidic environment resulting from the oxidation of glucose enables the rapid release of insulin in a hyperglycemic state [160]. Recently, nanotechnology has enabled many targeted approaches in the treatment of diabetes. NPs protect trapped hypoglycemic drugs from decomposition in the high acidic environment of the gut. New formulations and devices to administer diabetes drugs also involve inconvenient daily injections. NPs for diabetes drugs optimize long-term blood glucose reduction, thus providing long-term improvement in euglycemic states. Recent nanotechnology research in diabetes treatment finds that blood glucose monitoring and simultaneous drug release depend on glucose levels, so they provide great control over glucose concentration.

Drugs	NPs	Effects	References
Liraglutide	Thermogelling PEG/polyester copolymers	Sustained and prolonged drug release, improved glucose tolerance of mice for one week.	[148]
Glibenclamide	Xanthan-grafted-C16 amphiphilic Copolymer	Enhanced water solubility, extended drug release in 8 h, provide pH-dependent release.	[149]
Insulin	PEG-PE micelle	Helping to renaturation of denatured insulin and prevent its aggregation.	[150]
Insulin	Con A anchored PEGylated PLGA diblock coplolymer	Provide insulin stability, improved absorption and enhanced oral bioavailability	[151]
γ-oryzanol	PLGA NP	Ameliorated fuel metabolism, decreased ER stress and inflammation in liver and adipose tissue	[152]
Insulin and gallic acid	PEG and Hydroxyapatite NP	Increased intestinal absorption	[153]
Rosiglitazone	Alendronic and undecylenic acid coated magnetic NP	Enhanced accumulation in adipose tissue	[154]
Insulin	Chitosan decorate with L-valine and PBA	Chemical stability in GI, pH and glucose responsive release.	[155]
Insulin	PLGA and folic acid modified chitosan	Provide stability in GI, improved therapeutic effect compared with injectable forms.	[156]
Bilirubin	Pluronic F127–Chitosan	Improve uptake by murine pancreatic islet cells and improve their viability following hypoxic stress	[157]
Insulin	Glycylglycine and alanyl-alanine conjugates of chitosan and trimethyl chitosan NP	Increase insulin permeability, reasonable increase in Serum insulin level and bioavailability.	[158]
Vildagliptin	Triangular DNA nanospheres coated with eudragit	Effectively bypasses the acidic pH of the stomach, enhanced therapeutic effect with no toxicity.	[159]

Table 6.
Common drugs used to treat diabetes.

7. Conclusion

Drug delivery represents one of the most challenging aspects of treatment. Attaining an optimal concentration at the site of the disease as well as controlled and continuous release of the drug are the most important goals in drug delivery. By modifying drug formulation using nanoparticles, the method of distribution and release as well as the usage of drugs can be optimized. Specifically, the size, surface charge, physicochemical characteristics, and shape of NPs are important optimization parameters. Manipulations of the formulation such as the targeting of the NPs, rendering the NP sensitive to changes in the ambient pH, increasing mucosal adhesion, enhancing drug solubility, utilization of NPs in new tools for drug delivery such as skin patches, and application of NPs in regenerative medicine are among the topics in the areas of nanomedicine and drug delivery discussed in this article. It is important to point out some of the limitations associated with the use of NPs. First, limitations such as toxicity, sensitization, immune reactions, accumulation of nanoparticles in the body, and creation of protein coronas in the body must be studied. Second, limitations such as costs, availability of the materials, and facilities required for a particular method of delivery must be considered. In spite of these limitations, applications of nanotechnology in the areas of drug delivery and regenerative medicine are growing rapidly. Utilization of peptide targeting agents, dissolvable skin patches, three-dimensional tissue engineering scaffolds, and multipurpose NPs in drug delivery represent promising results of research in nanomedicine and nanodrug delivery in recent years and future research will have an increasing concentration on these topics.

Acknowledgements

We acknowledge Professor Soheila Kashanian, who encourages us to write this special issue.

Conflict of interest

There is no conflict of interest between the authors.

Author details

Morteza Rabiei* and Seyedeh Sabereh Samavati
Faculty of Nanobiotechnology, Department of Innovative Science and Technology, Razi University, Kermanshah, Iran

*Address all correspondence to: mrabiei6768@gmail.com

References

[1] Nikalje AP. Nanotechnology and its applications in medicine. Medicinal Chemistry. 2015;**5**:81-89

[2] Ambesh P, Angeli DG. Nanotechnology in neurology: Genesis, current status, and future prospects. Annals of Indian Academy of Neurology. 2015;**18**:382

[3] Clayton ES, Hochberg MC. Osteoporosis and osteoarthritis, rheumatoid arthritis and spondylarthropathies. Current Osteoporosis Reports. 2013;**11**:257-262

[4] Dong X. Current strategies for brain drug delivery. Theranostics. 2018;**8**:1481

[5] Bajpayee AG, Grodzinsky AJ. Cartilage-targeting drug delivery: Can electrostatic interactions help? Nature Reviews Rheumatology. 2017;**13**:183

[6] Wang Q, Yan J, Yang J, Li B. Nanomaterials promise better bone repair. Materials Today. 2016;**19**:451-463

[7] Kesharwani P, Gorain B, Low SY, Tan SA, Ling ECS, Lim YK, et al. Nanotechnology based approaches for anti-diabetic drugs delivery. Diabetes Research and Clinical Practice. 2017;**136**:52-77

[8] Ramesh S, Velraj M. An overview on novel approach of transdermal drug delivery systems. Drug Invention Today. 2018;**10**:297

[9] Sousa MP, Neto AI, Correia TR, Miguel SP, Matsusaki M, Correia IJ, et al. Bioinspired multilayer membranes as potential adhesive patches for skin wound healing. Biomaterials Science. 2018;**6**:1962-1975

[10] Omlor AJ, Nguyen J, Bals R, Dinh QT. Nanotechnology in respiratory medicine. Respiratory Research. 2015;**16**:64

[11] Saeedi M, Eslamifar M, Khezri K, Dizaj SM. Applications of nanotechnology in drug delivery to the central nervous system. Biomedicine & Pharmacotherapy. 2019;**111**:666-675

[12] Rabiei M, Kashanian S, Samavati SS, Jamasb S, McInnes SJ. Active targeting towards and inside the brain based on nanoparticles: A review. Current Pharmaceutical Biotechnology. 2020;**21**:374-383

[13] Banks WA. From blood–brain barrier to blood–brain interface: New opportunities for CNS drug delivery. Nature Reviews Drug Discovery. 2016;**15**:275

[14] Katare YK, Piazza JE, Bhandari J, Daya RP, Akilan K, Simpson MJ, et al. Intranasal delivery of antipsychotic drugs. Schizophrenia Research. 2017;**184**:2-13

[15] Gao H. Progress and perspectives on targeting nanoparticles for brain drug delivery. Acta Pharmaceutica Sinica B. 2016;**6**:268-286

[16] Borodina T, Trushina D, Marchenko I, Bukreeva T. Calcium carbonate-based mucoadhesive microcontainers for intranasal delivery of drugs bypassing the blood–brain barrier. BioNanoScience. 2016;**6**:261-268

[17] Hirschberg H, Madsen SJ. Cell mediated photothermal therapy of brain tumors. Journal of Neuroimmune Pharmacology. 2017;**12**:99-106

[18] Georgieva JV, Hoekstra D, Zuhorn IS. Smuggling drugs into the brain: An overview of ligands targeting transcytosis for drug delivery across the blood–brain barrier. Pharmaceutics. 2014;**6**:557-583

[19] Dai T, Jiang K, Lu W. Liposomes and lipid disks traverse the BBB and BBTB as intact forms as revealed by two-step Förster resonance energy transfer imaging. Acta Pharmaceutica Sinica B. 2018;**8**:261-271

[20] Nakao Y, Horiguchi M, Nakamura R, Sasaki-Hamada S, Ozawa C, Funane T, et al. LARETH-25 and β-CD improve central transitivity and central pharmacological effect of the GLP-2 peptide. International Journal of Pharmaceutics. 2016;**515**:37-45

[21] Neves AR, Queiroz JF, Reis S. Brain-targeted delivery of resveratrol using solid lipid nanoparticles functionalized with apolipoprotein E. Journal of Nanobiotechnology. 2016;**14**:27

[22] Gomes MJ, Fernandes C, Martins S, Borges F, Sarmento B. Tailoring lipid and polymeric nanoparticles as siRNA carriers towards the blood-brain barrier–from targeting to safe administration. Journal of Neuroimmune Pharmacology. 2017;**12**:107-119

[23] Mann AP, Scodeller P, Hussain S, Joo J, Kwon E, Braun GB, et al. A peptide for targeted, systemic delivery of imaging and therapeutic compounds into acute brain injuries. Nature Communications. 2016;**7**:11980

[24] Zhang C, Wan X, Zheng X, Shao X, Liu Q, Zhang Q, et al. Dual-functional nanoparticles targeting amyloid plaques in the brains of Alzheimer's disease mice. Biomaterials. 2014;**35**:456-465

[25] Gaudin A, Yemisci M, Eroglu H, Lepetre-Mouelhi S, Turkoglu OF, Dönmez-Demir B, et al. Squalenoyl adenosine nanoparticles provide neuroprotection after stroke and spinal cord injury. Nature Nanotechnology. 2014;**9**:1054

[26] Zamanlu M, Farhoudi M, Eskandani M, Mahmoudi J, Barar J, Rafi M, et al. Recent advances in targeted delivery of tissue plasminogen activator for enhanced thrombolysis in ischaemic stroke. Journal of Drug Targeting. 2018;**26**:95-109

[27] Tang C, Xue H, Bai C, Fu R, Wu A. The effects of Tanshinone IIA on blood–brain barrier and brain edema after transient middle cerebral artery occlusion in rats. Phytomedicine. 2010;**17**:1145-1149

[28] Kurakhmaeva KB, Djindjikhashvili IA, Petrov VE, Balabanyan VU, Voronina TA, Trofimov SS, et al. Brain targeting of nerve growth factor using poly (butyl cyanoacrylate) nanoparticles. Journal of Drug Targeting. 2009;**17**:564-574

[29] Liu Z, Gao X, Kang T, Jiang M, Miao D, Gu G, et al. B6 peptide-modified PEG-PLA nanoparticles for enhanced brain delivery of neuroprotective peptide. Bioconjugate Chemistry. 2013;**24**:997-1007

[30] Wang ZH, Wang ZY, Sun CS, Wang CY, Jiang TY, Wang SL. Trimethylated chitosan-conjugated PLGA nanoparticles for the delivery of drugs to the brain. Biomaterials. 2010;**31**:908-915

[31] Baysal I, Ucar G, Gultekinoglu M, Ulubayram K, Yabanoglu-Ciftci S. Donepezil loaded PLGA-b-PEG nanoparticles: Their ability to induce destabilization of amyloid fibrils and to cross blood brain barrier *in vitro*. Journal of Neural Transmission. 2017;**124**:33-45

[32] Mathew A, Fukuda T, Nagaoka Y, Hasumura T, Morimoto H, Yoshida Y, et al. Curcumin loaded-PLGA nanoparticles conjugated with Tet-1 peptide for potential use in Alzheimer's disease. PLoS One. 2012;**7**:e32616

[33] Bhatt PC, Verma A, Al-Abbasi FA, Anwar F, Kumar V, Panda BP. Development of surface-engineered PLGA nanoparticulate-delivery system of Tet1-conjugated nattokinase enzyme for inhibition of Aβ40 plaques in Alzheimer's disease. International Journal of Nanomedicine. 2017;**12**:8749

[34] Jiang Y, Fay JM, Poon CD, Vinod N, Zhao Y, Bullock K, et al. Nanoformulation of brain-derived neurotrophic factor with target receptor-triggered-release in the central nervous system. Advanced Functional Materials. 2018;**28**:1703982

[35] Pahuja R, Seth K, Shukla A, Shukla RK, Bhatnagar P, Chauhan LKS, et al. Trans-blood brain barrier delivery of dopamine-loaded nanoparticles reverses functional deficits in parkinsonian rats. ACS Nano. 2015;**9**:4850-4871

[36] Huang R, Han L, Li J, Ren F, Ke W, Jiang C, et al. Neuroprotection in a 6-hydroxydopamine-lesioned Parkinson model using lactoferrin-modified nanoparticles. The Journal of Gene Medicine. 2009;**11**:754-763

[37] Yang JA, Lin W, Woods WS, George JM, Murphy CJ. α-Synuclein's adsorption, conformation, and orientation on cationic gold nanoparticle surfaces seeds global conformation change. The Journal of Physical Chemistry B. 2014;**118**:3559-3571

[38] Dong H, Jin M, Liu Z, Xiong H, Qiu X, Zhang W, et al. *In vitro* and in vivo brain-targeting chemo-photothermal therapy using graphene oxide conjugated with transferrin for gliomas. Lasers in Medical Science. 2016;**31**:1123-1131

[39] Garanti T, Stasik A, Burrow AJ, Alhnan MA, Wan K-W. Anti-glioma activity and the mechanism of cellular uptake of asiatic acid-loaded solid lipid nanoparticles. International Journal of Pharmaceutics. 2016;**500**:305-315

[40] Fu S, Liang M, Wang Y, Cui L, Gao C, Chu X, et al. Dual-modified novel biomimetic nanocarriers improve targeting and therapeutic efficacy in glioma. ACS Applied Materials & Interfaces. 2018;**11**:1841-1854

[41] El-Zaafarany GM, Soliman ME, Mansour S, Awad GA. Identifying lipidic emulsomes for improved oxcarbazepine brain targeting: *In vitro* and rat *in vivo* studies. International Journal of Pharmaceutics. 2016;**503**:127-140

[42] Girotra P, Singh SK. A comparative study of orally delivered PBCA and ApoE coupled BSA nanoparticles for brain targeting of sumatriptan succinate in therapeutic management of migraine. Pharmaceutical Research. 2016;**33**:1682-1695

[43] Girotra P, Singh SK. Multivariate optimization of rizatriptan benzoate-loaded solid lipid nanoparticles for brain targeting and migraine management. AAPS PharmSciTech. 2017;**18**:517-528

[44] Ghasemian E, Vatanara A, Navidi N, Rouini MR. Brain delivery of baclofen as a hydrophilic drug by nanolipid carriers: Characteristics and pharmacokinetics evaluation. Journal of Drug Delivery Science and Technology. 2017;**37**:67-73

[45] Lindqvist A, Rip J, van Kregten J, Gaillard PJ, Hammarlund-Udenaes M. *In vivo* functional evaluation of increased brain delivery of the opioid peptide DAMGO by glutathione-PEGylated liposomes. Pharmaceutical Research. 2016;**33**:177-185

[46] Alam M, Najmi AK, Ahmad I, Ahmad FJ, Akhtar MJ, Imam SS, et al.

Formulation and evaluation of nano lipid formulation containing CNS acting drug: Molecular docking, *in-vitro* assessment and bioactivity detail in rats. Artificial Cells, Nanomedicine, and Biotechnology. 2018;**46**:1-12

[47] Krishnan JK, Arun P, Appu AP, Vijayakumar N, Figueiredo TH, Braga MF, et al. Intranasal delivery of obidoxime to the brain prevents mortality and CNS damage from organophosphate poisoning. Neurotoxicology. 2016;**53**:64-73

[48] Jayant RD, Tiwari S, Atluri V, Kaushik A, Tomitaka A, Yndart A, et al. Multifunctional nanotherapeutics for the treatment of neuroAIDS in drug abusers. Scientific Reports. 2018;**8**:12991

[49] Roy K, Kanwar RK, Kanwar JR. Molecular targets in arthritis and recent trends in nanotherapy. International Journal of Nanomedicine. 2015;**10**:5407

[50] D'Mello S, Atluri K, Geary SM, Hong L, Elangovan S, Salem AK. Bone regeneration using gene-activated matrices. The AAPS Journal. 2017;**19**:43-53

[51] Rabiei M, Kashanian S, Samavati SS, Derakhshankhah H, Jamasb S, McInnes SJ. Nanotechnology application in drug deliverytoosteoarthritis(OA),rheumatoid arthritis (RA), and osteoporosis (OSP). Journal of Drug Delivery Science and Technology. 2021;**61**:102011

[52] Bottini M, Bhattacharya K, Fadeel B, Magrini A, Bottini N, Rosato N. Nanodrugs to target articular cartilage: An emerging platform for osteoarthritis therapy. Nanomedicine: Nanotechnology Biology and Medicine. 2016;**12**:255-268

[53] Dolati S, Sadreddini S, Rostamzadeh D, Ahmadi M, Jadidi-Niaragh F, Yousefi M. Utilization of nanoparticle technology in rheumatoid arthritis treatment. Biomedicine & Pharmacotherapy. 2016;**80**:30-41

[54] Kim MJ, Park J-S, Lee SJ, Jang J, Park JS, Back SH, et al. Notch1 targeting siRNA delivery nanoparticles for rheumatoid arthritis therapy. Journal of Controlled Release. 2015;**216**:140-148

[55] Shen ZT, Sigalov AB. Rationally designed ligand-independent peptide inhibitors of TREM-1 ameliorate collagen-induced arthritis. Journal of Cellular and Molecular Medicine. 2017;**21**:2524-2534

[56] Dubey KA, Chaudhari CV, Bhardwaj YK, Varshney L. Polymers, blends and nanocomposites for implants, scaffolds and controlled drug release applications. Advances in Biomaterials for Biomedical Applications. 2017:1-44

[57] Wei D, Jung J, Yang H, Stout DA, Yang L. Nanotechnology treatment options for osteoporosis and its corresponding consequences. Current Osteoporosis Reports. 2016;**14**:239-247

[58] Holyoak DT, Tian YF, van der Meulen MC, Singh A. Osteoarthritis: Pathology, mouse models, and nanoparticle injectable systems for targeted treatment. Annals of Biomedical Engineering. 2016;**44**:2062-2075

[59] Kavanaugh TE, Werfel TA, Cho H, Hasty KA, Duvall CL. Particle-based technologies for osteoarthritis detection and therapy. Drug Delivery and Translational Research. 2016;**6**:132-147

[60] Abolmaali S, Tamaddon A, Kamali-Sarvestani E, Ashraf M, Dinarvand R. Stealth nanogels of histinylated poly ethyleneimine for sustained delivery of methotrexate

in collagen-induced arthritis model. Pharmaceutical Research. 2015;**32**:3309-3323

[61] Loffredo FS, Pancoast JR, Cai L, Vannelli T, Dong JZ, Lee RT, et al. Targeted delivery to cartilage is critical for *in vivo* efficacy of insulin-like growth factor 1 in a rat model of osteoarthritis. Arthritis and Rheumatology. 2014;**66**:1247-1255

[62] Jain A, Mishra SK, Vuddanda PR, Singh SK, Singh R, Singh S. Targeting of diacerein loaded lipid nanoparticles to intra-articular cartilage using chondroitin sulfate as homing carrier for treatment of osteoarthritis in rats. Nanomedicine: Nanotechnology, Biology and Medicine. 2014;**10**:e1031-e1040

[63] Pi Y, Zhang X, Shao Z, Zhao F, Hu X, Ao Y. Intra-articular delivery of anti-Hif-2α siRNA by chondrocyte-homing nanoparticles to prevent cartilage degeneration in arthritic mice. Gene Therapy. 2015;**22**:439

[64] Moura CC, Segundo MA, das Neves JS, Sarmento RB. Co-association of methotrexate and SPIONs into anti-CD64 antibody-conjugated PLGA nanoparticles for theranostic application. International Journal of Nanomedicine. 2014;**9**:4911

[65] Ghosh S, Mukherjee B, Chaudhuri S, RoyT,MukherjeeA,SenguptaS.Methotrexate aspasomes against rheumatoid arthritis: Optimized hydrogel loaded liposomal formulation with *in vivo* evaluation in Wistar rats. AAPS PharmSciTech. 2018;**19**:1320-1336

[66] Zhou H-F, Yan H, Hu Y, Springer LE, Yang X, Wickline SA, et al. Fumagillin prodrug nanotherapy suppresses macrophage inflammatory response via endothelial nitric oxide. ACS Nano. 2014;**8**:7305-7317

[67] Samarasinghe RM, Kanwar RK, Kanwar JR. The effect of oral administration of iron saturated-bovine lactoferrin encapsulated chitosan-nanocarriers on osteoarthritis. Biomaterials. 2014;**35**:7522-7534

[68] Zhou Y, Liu S-Q, Peng H, Yu L, He B, Zhao Q. In vivo anti-apoptosis activity of novel berberine-loaded chitosan nanoparticles effectively ameliorates osteoarthritis. International Immunopharmacology. 2015;**28**:34-43

[69] Ryan SM, McMorrow J, Umerska A, Patel HB, Kornerup KN, Tajber L, et al. An intra-articular salmon calcitonin-based nanocomplex reduces experimental inflammatory arthritis. Journal of Controlled Release. 2013;**167**:120-129

[70] Kim Y-J, Chae SY, Jin C-H, Sivasubramanian M, Son S, Choi KY, et al. Ionic complex systems based on hyaluronic acid and PEGylated TNF-related apoptosis-inducing ligand for treatment of rheumatoid arthritis. Biomaterials. 2010;**31**:9057-9064

[71] Sezlev Bilecen D, Uludag H, Hasirci V. Development of PEI-RANK siRNA complex loaded PLGA nanocapsules for the treatment of osteoporosis. Tissue Engineering Part A. 2018;**25**:1-2

[72] Yallapu MM, Nagesh PKB, Jaggi M, Chauhan SC. Therapeutic applications of curcumin nanoformulations. The AAPS Journal. 2015;**17**:1341-1356

[73] Adhikari P, Wen AM, French RH, Parsegian VA, Steinmetz NF, Podgornik R, et al. Electronic structure, dielectric response, and surface charge distribution of RGD (1FUV) peptide. Scientific Reports. 2014;**4**:5605

[74] Jeon OH, Elisseeff J. Orthopedic tissue regeneration: Cells, scaffolds,

and small molecules. Drug Delivery and Translational Research. 2016;**6**:105-120

[75] Monteiro N, Martins A, Reis RL, Neves NM. Nanoparticle-based bioactive agent release systems for bone and cartilage tissue engineering. Regenerative Therapy. 2015;**1**:109-118

[76] Desmet E, Van Gele M, Lambert J. Topically applied lipid-and surfactant-based nanoparticles in the treatment of skin disorders. Expert Opinion on Drug Delivery. 2017;**14**:109-122

[77] Amamoto T, Hirakawa S, Santa T, Funatsu T, Kato M. Surface modification of silica nanoparticles using 4-aryloxy boron dipyrromethene (BODIPY) enhances skin permeation. Journal of Materials Chemistry B. 2016;**4**:7676-7680

[78] Jampilek J, Brychtova K. Azone analogues: Classification, design, and transdermal penetration principles. Medicinal Research Reviews. 2012;**32**:907-947

[79] Kitaoka M, Wakabayashi R, Kamiya N, Goto M. Solid-in-oil nanodispersions for transdermal drug delivery systems. Biotechnology Journal. 2016;**11**:1375-1385

[80] Rabiei M, Kashanian S, Samavati SS, Jamasb S, McInnes SJ. Nanomaterial and advanced technologies in transdermal drug delivery. Journal of Drug Targeting. 2020;**28**:356-367

[81] Monti D, Egiziano E, Burgalassi S, Chetoni P, Chiappe C, Sanzone A, et al. Ionic liquids as potential enhancers for transdermal drug delivery. International Journal of Pharmaceutics. 2017;**516**:45-51

[82] Ramezanli T, Karry K, Zhang Z, Shah K, Michniak-Kohn B. Transdermal delivery of drugs using patches and patchless delivery systems. Drug Delivery: Principles and Applications. 2016:207-226

[83] Zakrewsky M, Kumar S, Mitragotri S. Nucleic acid delivery into skin for the treatment of skin disease: Proofs-of-concept, potential impact, and remaining challenges. Journal of Controlled Release. 2015;**219**:445-456

[84] Sivaram AJ, Rajitha P, Maya S, Jayakumar R, Sabitha M. Nanogels for delivery, imaging and therapy. Wiley Interdisciplinary Reviews: Nanomedicine and Nanobiotechnology. 2015;**7**:509-533

[85] Ahmed TA, Khalid M, Aljaeid BM, Fahmy UA, Abd-Allah FI. Transdermal glimepiride delivery system based on optimized ethosomal nano-vesicles: Preparation, characterization, *in vitro*, *ex vivo* and clinical evaluation. International Journal of Pharmaceutics. 2016;**500**:245-254

[86] Meng S, Zhang C, Shi W, Zhang XW, Liu DH, Wang P, et al. Preparation of osthole-loaded nano-vesicles for skin delivery: Characterization, *in vitro* skin permeation and preliminary *in vivo* pharmacokinetic studies. European Journal of Pharmaceutical Sciences. 2016;**92**:49-54

[87] Kamran M, Ahad A, Aqil M, Imam SS, Sultana Y, Ali A. Design, formulation and optimization of novel soft nano-carriers for transdermal olmesartan medoxomil delivery: *In vitro* characterization and *in vivo* pharmacokinetic assessment. International Journal of Pharmaceutics. 2016;**505**:147-158

[88] Mennini N, Cirri M, Maestrelli F, Mura P. Comparison of liposomal and NLC (nanostructured lipid carrier) formulations for improving the transdermal delivery of oxaprozin: Effect of cyclodextrin complexation.

International Journal of Pharmaceutics. 2016;**515**:684-691

[89] Rao YF, Chen W, Liang XG, Huang YZ, Miao J, Liu L, et al. Epirubicin-loaded superparamagnetic iron-oxide nanoparticles for transdermal delivery: Cancer therapy by circumventing the skin barrier. Small. 2015;**11**:239-247

[90] Elgindy NA, Mehanna MM, Mohyeldin SM. Self-assembled nano-architecture liquid crystalline particles as a promising carrier for progesterone transdermal delivery. International Journal of Pharmaceutics. 2016;**501**:167-179

[91] Wang W, Wat E, Hui PC, Chan B, Ng FS, Kan C-W, et al. Dual-functional transdermal drug delivery system with controllable drug loading based on thermosensitive poloxamer hydrogel for atopic dermatitis treatment. Scientific Reports. 2016;**6**:24112

[92] Imam SS, Ahad A, Aqil M, Akhtar M, Sultana Y, Ali A. Formulation by design based risperidone nano soft lipid vesicle as a new strategy for enhanced transdermal drug delivery: *in-vitro* characterization, and *in-vivo* appraisal. Materials Science and Engineering: C. 2017;**75**:1198-1205

[93] Al-mahallawi AM, Abdelbary AA, Aburahma MH. Investigating the potential of employing bilosomes as a novel vesicular carrier for transdermal delivery of tenoxicam. International Journal of Pharmaceutics. 2015;**485**:329-340

[94] Chen Z, Li B, Liu T, Wang X, Zhu Y, Wang L, et al. Evaluation of paeonol-loaded transethosomes as transdermal delivery carriers. European Journal of Pharmaceutical Sciences. 2017;**99**:240-245

[95] Garg NK, Tyagi RK, Singh B, Sharma G, Nirbhavane P, Kushwah V, et al. Nanostructured lipid carrier mediates effective delivery of methotrexate to induce apoptosis of rheumatoid arthritis via NF-κB and FOXO1. International Journal of Pharmaceutics. 2016;**499**:301-320

[96] Kassem AA, El-Alim SHA, Asfour MH. Enhancement of 8-methoxypsoralen topical delivery via nanosized niosomal vesicles: Formulation development, *in vitro* and *in vivo* evaluation of skin deposition. International Journal of Pharmaceutics. 2017;**517**:256-268

[97] Alomrani AH, Badran MM. Flexosomes for transdermal delivery of meloxicam: Characterization and antiinflammatory activity. Artificial Cells, Nanomedicine, and Biotechnology. 2017;**45**:305-312

[98] Yang M, Gu Y, Yang D, Tang X, Liu J. Development of triptolide-nanoemulsion gels for percutaneous administration: Physicochemical, transport, pharmacokinetic and pharmacodynamic characteristics. Journal of Nanobiotechnology. 2017;**15**:88

[99] Anirudhan T, Nair AS, Bino SJ. Nanoparticle assisted solvent selective transdermal combination therapy of curcumin and 5-flurouracil for efficient cancer treatment. Carbohydrate Polymers. 2017;**173**:131-142

[100] Garg NK, Sharma G, Singh B, Nirbhavane P, Tyagi RK, Shukla R, et al. Quality by design (QbD)-enabled development of aceclofenac loaded-nano structured lipid carriers (NLCs): An improved dermatokinetic profile for inflammatory disorder (s). International Journal of Pharmaceutics. 2017;**517**:413-431

[101] Kaur A, Bhoop BS, Chhibber S, Sharma G, Gondil VS, Katare OP. Supramolecular nano-engineered lipidic carriers based on diflunisal-phospholipid complex for transdermal delivery: QbD based optimization, characterization and preclinical investigations for management of rheumatoid arthritis. International Journal of Pharmaceutics. 2017;**533**:206-224

[102] Wang C, Zhu J, Zhang D, Yang Y, Zheng L, Qu Y, et al. Ionic liquid–microemulsions assisting in the transdermal delivery of dencichine: Preparation, *in-vitro* and *in-vivo* evaluations, and investigation of the permeation mechanism. International Journal of Pharmaceutics. 2018;**535**:120-131

[103] Qumbar M, Imam SS, Ali J, Ahmad J, Ali A. Formulation and optimization of lacidipine loaded niosomal gel for transdermal delivery: *In-vitro* characterization and *in-vivo* activity. Biomedicine & Pharmacotherapy. 2017;**93**:255-266

[104] Ahad A, Al-Saleh AA, Al-Mohizea AM, Al-Jenoobi FI, Raish M, Yassin AEB, et al. Formulation and characterization of novel soft nanovesicles for enhanced transdermal delivery of eprosartan mesylate. Saudi Pharmaceutical Journal. 2017;**25**:1040-1046

[105] Kapoor H, Aqil M, Imam SS, Sultana Y, Ali A. Formulation of amlodipine nano lipid carrier: Formulation design, physicochemical and transdermal absorption investigation. Journal of Drug Delivery Science and Technology. 2019;**49**:209-218

[106] Singh S, Parashar P, Kanoujia J, Singh I, Saha S, Saraf SA. Transdermal potential and anti-gout efficacy of febuxostat from niosomal gel. Journal of Drug Delivery Science and Technology. 2017;**39**:348-361

[107] Joshi A, Kaur J, Kulkarni R, Chaudhari R. *In-vitro* and *ex-vivo* evaluation of raloxifene hydrochloride delivery using nano-transfersome based formulations. Journal of Drug Delivery Science and Technology. 2018;**45**:151-158

[108] Rostami E, Kashanian S, Azandaryani AH, Faramarzi H, Dolatabadi JEN, Omidfar K. Drug targeting using solid lipid nanoparticles. Chemistry and Physics of Lipids. 2014;**181**:56-61

[109] Takeuchi I, Shimamura Y, Kakami Y, Kameda T, Hattori K, Miura S, et al. Transdermal delivery of 40-nm silk fibroin nanoparticles. Colloids and Surfaces B: Biointerfaces. 2019;**175**:564-568

[110] Rajabalaya R, Musa MN, Kifli N, David SR. Oral and transdermal drug delivery systems: Role of lipid-based lyotropic liquid crystals. Drug Design, Development and Therapy. 2017;**11**:393

[111] Zelikin AN, Ehrhardt C, Healy AM. Materials and methods for delivery of biological drugs. Nature Chemistry. 2016;**8**:997

[112] Yan L, Yang Y, Zhang W, Chen X. Advanced materials and nanotechnology for drug delivery. Advanced Materials. 2014;**26**:5533-5540

[113] Bariya SH, Gohel MC, Mehta TA, Sharma OP. Microneedles: An emerging transdermal drug delivery system. Journal of Pharmacy and Pharmacology. 2012;**64**:11-29

[114] Dangol M, Yang H, Li CG, Lahiji SF, Kim S, Ma Y, et al. Innovative polymeric system (IPS) for solvent-free lipophilic

drug transdermal delivery via dissolving microneedles. Journal of Controlled Release. 2016;**223**:118-125

[115] Rabiei M, Kashanian S, Bahrami G, Derakhshankhah H, Barzegari E, Samavati SS, et al. Dissolving microneedle-assisted long-acting liraglutide delivery to control type 2 diabetes and obesity. European Journal of Pharmaceutical Sciences. 2021;**167**:106040

[116] Daddona PE, Matriano JA, Mandema J, Maa Y-F. Parathyroid hormone (1-34)-coated microneedle patch system: Clinical pharmacokinetics and pharmacodynamics for treatment of osteoporosis. Pharmaceutical Research. 2011;**28**:159-165

[117] Lee I-C, Wu Y-C, Tsai S-W, Chen C-H, Wu M-H. Fabrication of two-layer dissolving polyvinylpyrrolidone microneedles with different molecular weights for in vivo insulin transdermal delivery. RSC Advances. 2017;**7**:5067-5075

[118] Deng Y, Chen J, Zhao Y, Yan X, Zhang L, Choy K, et al. Transdermal delivery of siRNA through microneedle array. Scientific Reports. 2016;**6**:21422

[119] del Río-Sancho S, Serna-Jimenez C, Sebastián-Morelló M, Calatayud-Pascual M, Balaguer-Fernández C, Femenía-Font A, et al. Transdermal therapeutic systems for memantine delivery. Comparison of passive and iontophoretic transport. International Journal of Pharmaceutics. 2017;**517**:104-111

[120] Vora LK, Donnelly RF, Larrañeta E, González-Vázquez P, Thakur RRS, Vavia PR. Novel bilayer dissolving microneedle arrays with concentrated PLGA nano-microparticles for targeted intradermal delivery: Proof of concept. Journal of Controlled Release. 2017;**265**:93-101

[121] Paranjpe M, Müller-Goymann CC. Nanoparticle-mediated pulmonary drug delivery: A review. International Journal of Molecular Sciences. 2014;**15**:5852-5873

[122] De Backer L, Cerrada A, Pérez-Gil J, De Smedt SC, Raemdonck K. Bio-inspired materials in drug delivery: Exploring the role of pulmonary surfactant in siRNA inhalation therapy. Journal of Controlled Release. 2015;**220**:642-650

[123] Patil TS, Deshpande AS, Deshpande S, Shende P. Targeting pulmonary tuberculosis using nanocarrier-based dry powder inhalation: Current status and futuristic need. Journal of Drug Targeting. 2019;**27**:12-27

[124] Brenner JS, Kiseleva RY, Glassman PM, Parhiz H, Greineder CF, Hood ED, et al. The new frontiers of the targeted interventions in the pulmonary vasculature: Precision and safety (2017 Grover conference series). Pulmonary Circulation. 2018;**8**:2045893217752329

[125] Ruge CA, Kirch J, Lehr C-M. Pulmonary drug delivery: From generating aerosols to overcoming biological barriers—Therapeutic possibilities and technological challenges. The Lancet Respiratory Medicine. 2013;**1**:402-413

[126] Rabiei M, Kashanian S, Samavati SS, Derakhshankhah H, Jamasb S, McInnes SJ. Characteristics of SARS-CoV2 that may be useful for nanoparticle pulmonary drug delivery. Journal of Drug Targeting. 2022;**30**:233-243

[127] Wang Z, Cuddigan JL, Gupta SK, Meenach SA. Nanocomposite microparticles (nCmP) for the delivery of tacrolimus in the treatment of pulmonary arterial hypertension.

International Journal of Pharmaceutics. 2016;**512**:305-313

[128] Hu Q, Bai X, Hu G, Zuo YY. Unveiling the molecular structure of pulmonary surfactant corona on nanoparticles. ACS Nano. 2017;**11**:6832-6842

[129] Xu Y, Deng L, Ren H, Zhang X, Huang F, Yue T. Transport of nanoparticles across pulmonary surfactant monolayer: A molecular dynamics study. Physical Chemistry Chemical Physics. 2017;**19**:17568-17576

[130] Ni R, Zhao J, Liu Q, Liang Z, Muenster U, Mao S. Nanocrystals embedded in chitosan-based respirable swellable microparticles as dry powder for sustained pulmonary drug delivery. European Journal of Pharmaceutical Sciences. 2017;**99**:137-146

[131] Motiei M, Kashanian S, Lucia LA, Khazaei M. Intrinsic parameters for the synthesis and tuned properties of amphiphilic chitosan drug delivery nanocarriers. Journal of Controlled Release. 2017;**260**:213-225

[132] Mehnath S, Sithika MAA, Arjama M, Rajan M, Praphakar RA, Jeyaraj M. Sericin-chitosan doped maleate gellan gum nanocomposites for effective cell damage in *Mycobacterium tuberculosis*. International Journal of Biological Macromolecules. 2019;**122**:174-184

[133] Scolari IR, Páez PL, Sánchez-Borzone ME, Granero GE. Promising chitosan-coated alginate-tween 80 nanoparticles as rifampicin coadministered ascorbic acid delivery carrier against *Mycobacterium tuberculosis*. AAPS PharmSciTech. 2019;**20**:67

[134] Joshi N, Shirsath N, Singh A, Joshi KS, Banerjee R. Endogenous lung surfactant inspired pH responsive nanovesicle aerosols: Pulmonary compatible and site-specific drug delivery in lung metastases. Scientific Reports. 2014;**4**:7085

[135] Triolo D, Craparo E, Porsio B, Fiorica C, Giammona G, Cavallaro G. Polymeric drug delivery micelle-like nanocarriersforpulmonaryadministration of beclomethasone dipropionate. Colloids and Surfaces B: Biointerfaces. 2017;**151**:206-214

[136] Porsio B, Craparo EF, Mauro N, Giammona G, Cavallaro G. Mucus and cell-penetrating nanoparticles embedded in nano-into-micro formulations for pulmonary delivery of ivacaftor in patients with cystic fibrosis. ACS Applied Materials & Interfaces. 2017;**10**:165-181

[137] Porsio B, Cusimano MG, Schillaci D, Craparo EF, Giammona G, Cavallaro G. Nano into micro formulations of tobramycin for the treatment of *Pseudomonas aeruginosa* infections in cystic fibrosis. Biomacromolecules. 2017;**18**:3924-3935

[138] Price DN, Stromberg LR, Kunda NK, Muttil P. In vivo pulmonary delivery and magnetic-targeting of dry powder nano-in-microparticles. Molecular Pharmaceutics. 2017;**14**:4741-4750

[139] Rodriguez M, Lapierre J, Ojha CR, Kaushik A, Batrakova E, Kashanchi F, et al. Intranasal drug delivery of small interfering RNA targeting Beclin1 encapsulated with polyethylenimine (PEI) in mouse brain to achieve HIV attenuation. Scientific Reports. 2017;**7**:1862

[140] Zhong Q, Humia BV, Punjabi AR, Padilha FF, da Rocha SR. The interaction of dendrimer-doxorubicin conjugates with a model pulmonary epithelium

and their cosolvent-free, pseudo-solution formulations in pressurized metered-dose inhalers. European Journal of Pharmaceutical Sciences. 2017;**109**:86-95

[141] Silva AS, Sousa AM, Cabral RP, Silva MC, Costa C, Miguel SP, et al. Aerosolizable gold nano-in-micro dry powder formulations for theragnosis and lung delivery. International Journal of Pharmaceutics. 2017;**519**:240-249

[142] Xu C, Wang Y, Guo Z, Chen J, Lin L, Wu J, et al. Pulmonary delivery by exploiting doxorubicin and cisplatin co-loaded nanoparticles for metastatic lung cancer therapy. Journal of Controlled Release. 2019;**295**:153-163

[143] Türeli NG, Torge A, Juntke J, Schwarz BC, Schneider-Daum N, Türeli AE, et al. Ciprofloxacin-loaded PLGA nanoparticles against cystic fibrosis *P. aeruginosa* lung infections. European Journal of Pharmaceutics and Biopharmaceutics. 2017;**117**:363-371

[144] Veiseh O, Tang BC, Whitehead KA, Anderson DG, Langer R. Managing diabetes with nanomedicine: Challenges and opportunities. Nature Reviews Drug Discovery. 2015;**14**:45

[145] Zamboni F, Collins MN. Cell based therapeutics in type 1 diabetes mellitus. International Journal of Pharmaceutics. 2017;**521**:346-356

[146] Yamada Y, Tabata M, Yasuzaki Y, Nomura M, Shibata A, Ibayashi Y, et al. A nanocarrier system for the delivery of nucleic acids targeted to a pancreatic beta cell line. Biomaterials. 2014;**35**:6430-6438

[147] Sharma G, Sharma AR, Nam J-S, Doss GPC, Lee S-S, Chakraborty C. Nanoparticle based insulin delivery system: The next generation efficient therapy for type 1 diabetes. Journal of Nanobiotechnology. 2015;**13**:74

[148] Chen Y, Li Y, Shen W, Li K, Yu L, Chen Q, et al. Controlled release of liraglutide using thermogelling polymers in treatment of diabetes. Scientific Reports. 2016;**6**:31593

[149] Maiti S, Mukherjee S, Datta R. Core–shell nano-biomaterials for controlled oral delivery and pharmacodynamic activity of glibenclamide. International Journal of Biological Macromolecules. 2014;**70**:20-25

[150] Fang X, Yang T, Wang L, Yu J, Wei X, Zhou Y, et al. Nano-cage-mediated refolding of insulin by PEG-PE micelle. Biomaterials. 2016;**77**:139-148

[151] Sharma R, Gupta U, Garg NK, Tyagi RK, Jain N. Surface engineered and ligand anchored nanobioconjugate: An effective therapeutic approach for oral insulin delivery in experimental diabetic rats. Colloids and Surfaces B: Biointerfaces. 2015;**127**:172-181

[152] Kozuka C, Shimizu-Okabe C, Takayama C, Nakano K, Morinaga H, Kinjo A, et al. Marked augmentation of PLGA nanoparticle-induced metabolically beneficial impact of γ-oryzanol on fuel dyshomeostasis in genetically obese-diabetic ob/ob mice. Drug Delivery. 2017;**24**:558-568

[153] Zhang Y, Zhang L, Ban Q, Li J, Li C-H, Guan Y-Q. Preparation and characterization of hydroxyapatite nanoparticles carrying insulin and gallic acid for insulin oral delivery. Nanomedicine: Nanotechnology Biology and Medicine. 2018;**14**:353-364

[154] Saatchi K, Tod SE, Leung D, Nicholson KE, Andreu I, Buchwalder C, et al. Characterization of alendronic- and undecylenic acid coated magnetic

nanoparticles for the targeted delivery of rosiglitazone to subcutaneous adipose tissue. Nanomedicine: Nanotechnology, Biology and Medicine. 2017;**13**:559-568

[155] Li L, Jiang G, Yu W, Liu D, Chen H, Liu Y, et al. Preparation of chitosan-based multifunctional nanocarriers overcoming multiple barriers for oral delivery of insulin. Materials Science and Engineering: C. 2017;**70**:278-286

[156] Xu B, Jiang G, Yu W, Liu D, Liu Y, Kong X, et al. Preparation of poly (lactic-co-glycolic acid) and chitosan composite nanocarriers via electrostatic self assembly for oral delivery of insulin. Materials Science and Engineering: C. 2017;**78**:420-428

[157] Fullagar B, Rao W, Gilor C, Xu F, He X, Adin CA. Nano-encapsulation of bilirubin in pluronic F127–chitosan improves uptake in β cells and increases islet viability and function after hypoxic stress. Cell Transplantation. 2017;**26**:1703-1715

[158] Omid NJ, Javan NB, Dehpour A-R, Partoazar A, Tehrani MR, Dorkoosh F. *In-vitro* and *in-vivo* cytotoxicity and efficacy evaluation of novel glycyl-glycine and alanyl-alanine conjugates of chitosan and trimethyl chitosan nano-particles as carriers for oral insulin delivery. International Journal of Pharmaceutics. 2018;**535**:293-307

[159] Baig MMFA, Khan S, Naeem MA, Khan GJ, Ansari MT. Vildagliptin loaded triangular DNA nanospheres coated with eudragit for oral delivery and better glycemic control in type 2 diabetes mellitus. Biomedicine & Pharmacotherapy. 2018;**97**:1250-1258

[160] Zhang Y, Wang J, Yu J, Wen D, Kahkoska AR, Lu Y, et al. Bioresponsive microneedles with a sheath structure for H_2O_2 and pH cascade-triggered insulin delivery. Small. 2018;**14**:1704181

Section 5

Fabricated Drug Delivery System

Chapter 9

Smart Drug Delivery for Targeted Therapeutics via Remotely Controlled Microdevices

Negar Fouladvari, Roberto Bernasconi and Luca Magagnin

Abstract

Remotely controlled smart drug delivery systems represent a remarkable integration of materials science, physics, and biology. They offer precise control over drug delivery through tailored adjustments in shape, size, and material composition. Microdevices for targeted delivery can be manufactured using a wealth of techniques, like 3D printing or lithography, enabling accurate control at the microscale. Smart materials sensitive to external stimuli like temperature, pH and electric or magnetic field variations can be exploited to enable targeted drug delivery. This interdisciplinary approach aims at refining drug administration precision, minimizing side effects and maximizing therapeutic impact. The impact of these technologies is potentially groundbreaking, envisioning a future where medical treatments are not only more effective but also finely tuned to individual patient needs. This chapter aims to discuss the current literature on drug delivery microrobots, emphasizing the strategies employable to integrate smart delivery functionalities on remotely actuated microcarriers.

Keywords: targeted drug delivery, microrobots, microdevices, remote control, healthcare innovation

1. Introduction

Drug delivery systems (DDSs) transport therapeutic drugs to achieve desired effects on well-defined target organs inside the human body [1]. They aim at enhancing drug solubility, stability, and pharmacological activity while minimizing side effects [2]. One of the most interesting examples of advanced DDSs is the so-called biomedical microrobots. Indeed, miniaturized untethered medical robots, driven by advancements in microtechnology, promise to revolutionize minimally invasive therapeutic procedures. These tiny devices, equipped with micro-actuators and in some cases sensors, are able to navigate intricate paths within the body and carry out complex tasks. Utilizing precise movements and real-time data feedback, they enhance accessibility and reduce invasiveness for what concerns drug delivery duties. Their potential to improve patient outcomes marks a significant advancement in medical technology [3].

IntechOpen

Microdevices will potentially play a crucial role in modern DDSs by offering precise, controlled, and targeted delivery of therapeutic agents [4]. In general, they encompass specific tools, which allow them to work with minimal solution volumes in order to enable a wide range of tasks, including target immobilization, detection, laboratory testing, transport, etc. [5]. In the specific case, these miniature devices can be engineered to release drugs at specific rates, locations and times, enhancing the efficacy and reducing the side effects of treatments. For example, implantable microdevices can deliver medication directly to a target area, such as a tumor, minimizing systemic exposure and side effects [4]. Untethered microdevices can also borrow some of the functionalities typical of microfluidic devices, facilitating diagnostic and monitoring functions by detecting biomarkers within various body fluids or analyte-containing solutions [6]. Progress in fabrication strategies and miniaturization technologies has facilitated the development of biomedical microdevices aimed at assisting in the diagnosis, monitoring, and treatment of a range of chronic and non-chronic illnesses [7].

Microdevices can also be integrated with smart technologies, allowing for real-time monitoring and adjustment of drug delivery based on the patient's needs. This approach not only improves the precision of treatment but also enables personalized medicine, where the therapy is tailored to the individual patient's condition and response [8]. From this point of view, the effectiveness of biomedical microrobots can be further improved by implementing them with materials able to release drugs only in correspondence with specific external stimulation. Indeed, stimuli-responsive delivery stands out as a leading strategy in drug delivery, aiming for specific disease delivery and controlled release. Endogenous triggers such as diffusion, ROS (reactive oxygen species), pH, enzymes or temperature may potentially target release on specific disease sites like tumors. Exogenous stimuli like light or temperature can also trigger responses, and magnetic or electric fields are utilized as well. In addition, even ultrasounds offer the possibility to carry out remote control by delivering localized heat for precise release within the body, enhancing site-specific control [9]. DDSs employing microdevices may utilize several mechanisms to achieve targeted and controlled release of drugs, but their functioning at the microscale experiences completely different physical interactions with the surrounding environment compared to their macro counterparts [10]. This aspect must be carefully considered during their design.

In this chapter, some key mechanisms for drug loading and release that can be implemented in microrobotic devices are discussed. These include, for example, advanced drug loading technologies or the use of responsive materials that react to external stimuli (for example, pH, light, or heat) to trigger the drug release. In addition, remote control mechanisms such as wireless control or magnetic actuation are discussed [11]. The primary objective of the chapter is to provide a comprehensive review on drug-releasing microdevices and to investigate the various release mechanisms they employ for accurate and controlled drug delivery. By exploring the complex world of microrobots, this chapter aims to clarify the interaction between miniature devices and the precise release of therapeutic agents. Through explanations and examples, readers will gain a general understanding of how microdevices work and of the mechanisms they utilize to achieve controlled drug release. Readers will be equipped with the knowledge necessary to appreciate the complexity and potential of untethered microdevices in the realm of targeted drug delivery, opening the path for advancements in precision medicine and improved patient outcomes.

2. Microrobots

2.1 Base concepts

"Micro robotics is not simply about making traditional robots smaller" [10].

Microdevices can enhance drug therapy by enabling precise and complex dosing, reducing pain, and improving patient compliance. Historically, microneedles have been tested on humans and other drug-delivery devices have demonstrated promise in both in vitro and in vivo studies [12]. In the late twentieth century, the introduction of microrobotics revolutionized our scientific outlook, offering vast potential across diverse fields. From micromanipulation, environmental remediation and precision sampling to drug delivery, point-of-care clinical diagnostics and sensitive bioanalytical systems, their applications span the spectrum of scientific and biomedical domains, reshaping our understanding and capabilities [13]. In the case of the topic treated in the present chapter, transitioning to microrobotics demands a shift in engineering intuition and the cultivation of novel perspectives. Microrobotics extends beyond conventional robotics, requiring expertise in physics, material science, and biology [10]. Furthermore, as the possibility of utilizing microdevices in mass production increases, there is a critical need to advance analytical models to determine flow and transport phenomena, optimize design and control methodologies, and enhance sensing and monitoring performances [14].

The concept of "medical microrobots" is to non-invasively in-vivo navigate the body and enhance healthcare outcomes. This can be done by providing real-time diagnosis, monitoring diseases like Alzheimer's, measuring glucose levels in individuals with diabetes, sending robotic swarms to deliver precise therapies to tumors or performing minimally invasive surgery perhaps in the eye or even in the brain [15]. In general, microrobots offer the promise of reaching inaccessible body regions through natural pathways. Their wireless connectivity can potentially mitigate many limitations associated with systemic treatments and facilitate innovative minimally invasive procedures [16].

As already mentioned, microrobots experience different physical interactions with respect to macroscopic machines. Certainly, the laws of physics remain constant at the microscale, but their relative influence on the behavior of microfluidic devices can vary significantly due to the unique characteristics of microscale phenomena. At the microscale, various physical principles such as surface tension, viscosity, and capillary forces become more pronounced and dominant compared to macroscale systems. Micromachines typically operate within the low Reynolds number (*Re*) regime, which is characterized by the dominance of viscous forces over inertial forces. The Reynolds number (*Re*) is a dimensionless quantity used to predict fluid flow patterns and transitions between different flow regimes. It is defined by Eq. (1).

$$\mathrm{Re} = \frac{\rho.v.L}{\mu} \tag{1}$$

Where ρ is the fluid density, v is the characteristic velocity of the flow (in this case, of the microdevice), L is the characteristic length scale (such as the largest dimension of the microdevice), and μ is the dynamic viscosity of the fluid. *Re* represents the ratio between inertial (F_i) and viscous (F_v) forces acting on the system (Eq. (2)).

$$\mathrm{Re} = \frac{F_i}{F_v} \tag{2}$$

Purcell's work on low Reynolds number flows in 1977 is fundamental to understand the behavior of fluids at small scales, where viscous forces dominate over inertial forces. At low Reynolds numbers ($Re \ll 1$), which typically occur in microfluidic systems and biological environments, fluid dynamics are primarily governed by viscosity rather than inertia. Volume-related forces tend to become negligible with respect to surface-related forces. Under these conditions, the fluid dynamics of the system is characterized by instantaneous and time-reversible flows. Indeed, these highly reversible flows around objects swimming at the microscale make reciprocal motion impossible and the dynamics are dominated by viscosity rather than inertia. The "Scallop Theorem" in physics states that in a highly viscous fluid environment characterized by low Reynolds numbers, a swimmer or an object undergoing reciprocal motion cannot achieve net displacement. This means that if a swimmer moves back and forth in a symmetrical manner, the fluid forces generated will cancel each other out over a complete cycle, resulting in no overall movement [17].

Consequently, microrobots can only be actuated with non-reciprocating actuation strategies and this basically translates into four possibilities. The most obvious is

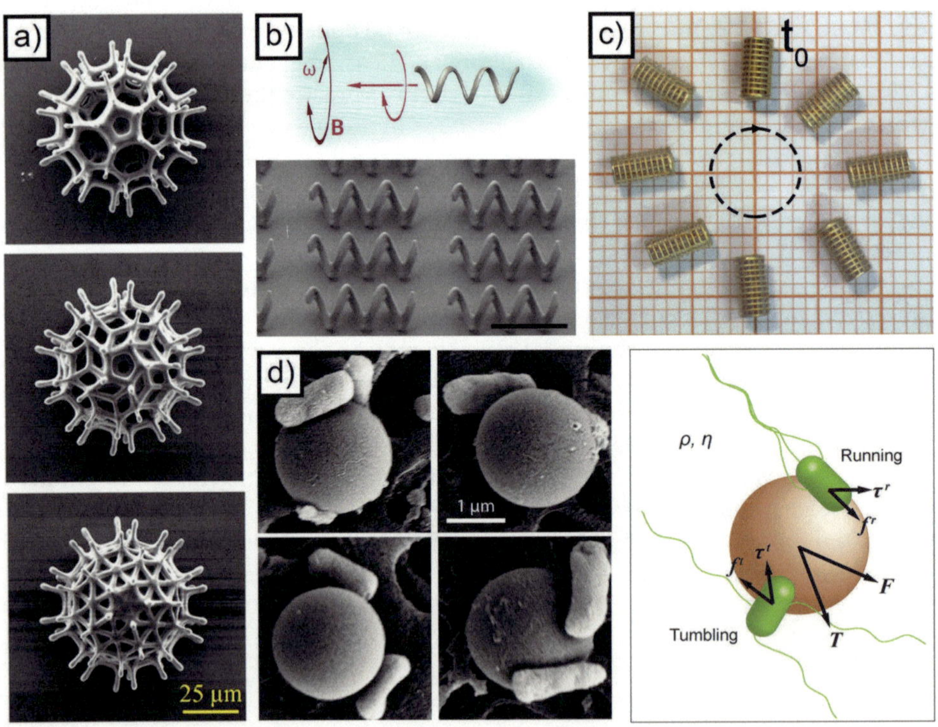

Figure 1.
Complex shaped microrobots propelled by the direct application of a magnetic force (a); base concept behind helical microdevices propelled by a rotating magnetic field and SEM image of a 3D printed array on a glass substrate (b, scale bar 10 µm); circular pattern actuation of a microdevice in contact with a glass surface (c); base concept and SEM images of bacteria-driven micro swimmers with a spherical body (d). Reprinted with permission from [18–21].

direct propulsion, where the device is directly pulled or pushed by a force (**Figure 1a**) [18]. The second possibility is the swimming motion, which is inspired by the cilia and flagella used by many procaryotic cells. In this case, the device swims into the fluid with a corkscrewing motion (**Figure 1b**) [19]. Non-reciprocating movements can be obtained also by exploiting the presence of solid surfaces or external bodies. For example, microrobots can be placed in contact with a solid surface and use friction to convert a rotative movement into a linear one (**Figure 1c**) [20]. Finally, a smart way to propel devices at the microscale is represented by the use of naturally occurring "micromotors", like prokaryotic cells. These can be connected to the microdevices and propel them using natural cilia and flagella (**Figure 1d**) [21].

2.2 Microrobots actuation

Keeping in mind the challenges connected to their reduced dimensions and the necessity of non-reciprocating motions, scientists have developed different methods to propel and guide microrobots toward their targets that can be inscribed into the four categories previously discussed [22]. For microrobot actuation, traditional motors cannot be used as power sources due to their size mismatch with the devices. Consequently, researchers have developed various alternative actuation methods, including the use of magnetic fields, electromagnetic fields, light, acoustic actuation or chemical propulsion [23]. Thanks to these tailored actuation approaches, untethered devices hold promise for revolutionary applications in medicine, biotechnology, environmental remediation, and beyond [22, 24]. Actuation mechanisms in microdevices are crucial for the manipulation and control of microscale components in a variety of applications such as biomedical purpose microrobots. These mechanisms convert various forms of energy into mechanical motion at the microscale. It is possible to use only one mechanism at a time or a combination of more than one mechanism, such as a temperature and electric field dual-stimulus.

The first form of propulsion historically adopted for microdevices propulsion is the chemical one. Chemically actuated microrobots exploit chemical reactions to induce and control their movements or functionalities at the microscale (**Figure 2a**) [25]. Microactuators driven by chemical reactions typically comprise two regions: one able to catalyze a chemical reaction or to work as an anode, the second inert or able to work as a cathode. The most typical example is the decomposition of hydrogen peroxide into water and oxygen. A device that uses this chemical fuel for its propulsion is composed of a bimetallic structure, which translates into an anodic and a cathodic region. The resulting self-electrophoresis effect (the spontaneous generation of a chemical gradient around the device able to move it) propels the device. Chemically propelled devices can also rely on the direct chemical degradation of a suitable species or on self-diffusiophoresis [29]. Beside the two regions present on the surface, the device can be composed of additional layers, which act as a supportive substrate that facilitates actuation [30].

The most common and promising (from the applicative point of view) actuation route is, however, magnetic actuation (**Figure 2b**) [26]. In this method, a magnetic field is applied to a device that is composed for a certain fraction of its mass of ferromagnetic or superparamagnetic material. Such magnetic material responds to the application of an external field with a force F_m or a torque T_m, which are expressed by Eqs. (3) and (4), respectively.

$$\overrightarrow{F_m} = \int_V \left(\vec{M} \cdot \nabla\right) \vec{B} dV \tag{3}$$

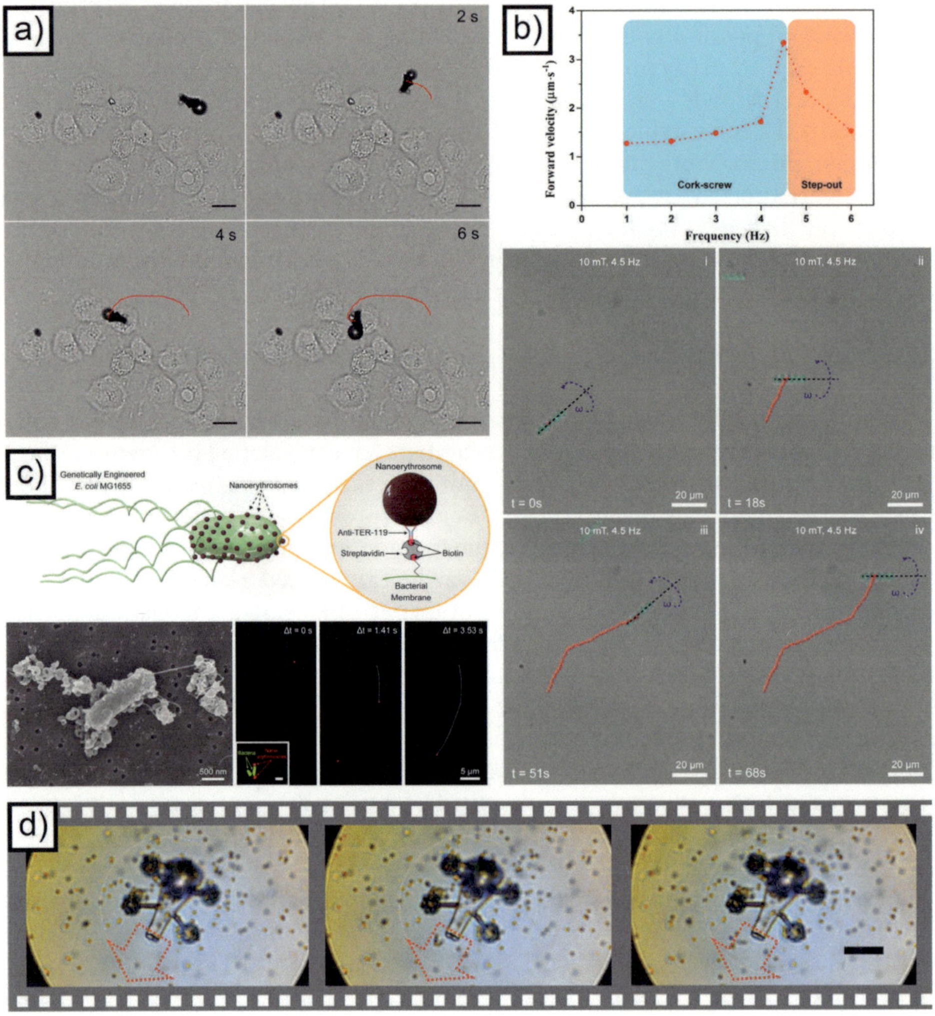

Figure 2.
Time-lapse images of the movement of hydrogen peroxide chemically propelled microrockets toward sheets of Hela cells (a; scale bar = 20 μm); actuation and steering of ABFs microswimmers using a rotating magnetic field (b); base concept and SEM images of biohybrid bacterial microswimmers functionalized with red blood cells (c); light-driven micro-tool equipped with a syringe function (d). Reprinted with permission from [25–28].

$$\overrightarrow{T_m} = \int_V \vec{M} \times \vec{B} dV \quad (4)$$

Where V is the volume of magnetic material, B is the external magnetic field and M is the magnetization. As a consequence, the device can be moved in a very precise way by applying gradients, oscillating or rotating magnetic fields. In addition to the great precision achievable during actuation, magnetic field is not harmful to the human body and it represents the most interesting strategy to actuate drug-releasing devices that must operate in-vivo.

Typically, in order to get non-reciprocating motion, magnetic microrobots are controlled within a workspace using two primary methods: utilizing a rotating magnetic field for swimming motion, or directly propelling them with a magnetic gradient. In the case of rotational motion, a magnetic torque spins an asymmetric structure like a helix to generate forward thrust (**Figure 1b** and **2b**). Such structures, due to their similarity with naturally occurring prokaryotic flagella, are named artificial bacteria flagella (ABF). For translational movement, a magnetic gradient directly applies a propulsive force on microrobots (**Figure 1a**), enabling precise control over their desired translational degrees of freedom (DOF) [31, 32]. A special type of magnetic actuation is the so-called rolling motion, which exploits the contact with a solid surface and can be assimilated to a wheel that rotates under the influence of a magnetic torque (**Figure 1c**). The linear speed is proportional to the radius of the microdevice and to the rotation frequency [33]. The actuability of this kind of device was demonstrated by applying rotating magnetic fields on devices containing a semi-hard magnetic material like CoNiP [34]. Finally, also more complex magnetic actuation strategies based on the use of oscillating fields and complex magnetic patterns have been implemented [35].

Magnetic actuation generally requires the generation of highly controlled fields and gradients. This can be achieved, for example, by means of the so-called electromagnetic field actuation (EMA), which involves the use of electromagnets to induce and control the motion at the microscale. This method relies on the interaction between an external magnetic field generated by current-carrying coils and the magnetic materials present in the devices to achieve movement and manipulation. To control untethered microrobots effectively, the electromagnetic actuation (EMA) system must be carefully designed to ensure adequate propulsion aligned with specific application goals. It is crucial to develop an EMA setup that is efficient, provides sufficient degrees of freedom (DOF), and avoids singularities [36].

Optically actuated microrobots use electromagnetic radiation to induce mechanical motion, either through photothermal effects or through optoelectronic mechanisms [24]. Such actuators are based, for example, on polymers modified with chromophores that can be employed for photomechanical actuation. Suitably designed optical actuators can be therefore integrated into microdevices, allowing reproducible and controlled actuation [37].

Another interesting approach to move devices at the microscale is the use of acoustic waves. Combining acoustic actuation with microrobots significantly broadens their application areas, thanks to its flexibility, biocompatibility, and controllability. Acoustically actuated microrobots can be classified into three common types based on their working principle: bubble propulsion, sharp-edge propulsion, and in-situ microrotors. Despite many examples available in literature, this category of microrobots is still in its early development stage and many challenges lie ahead [38].

Finally, microrobots can be propelled also by employing temperature gradients (**Figure 2d**) [39] or by integrating them with biological entities like bacteria or protozoans, resulting into the so-called bio-hybrid propulsion (**Figure 2c**) [27].

2.3 Microrobots production

Besides actuation, also the fabrication of micrometric-sized entities like microrobots is non-trivial. By employing a wide variety of materials (metals, polymers or ceramics), researchers fabricated remotely actuated devices using 3D printing, photolithography [40], bio-templating [41], sputtering deposition [42], wet deposition [43] or combinations of these techniques [44]. **Figure 3** schematizes the working principles of the most common fabrication techniques applicable to the manufacturing of microrobots.

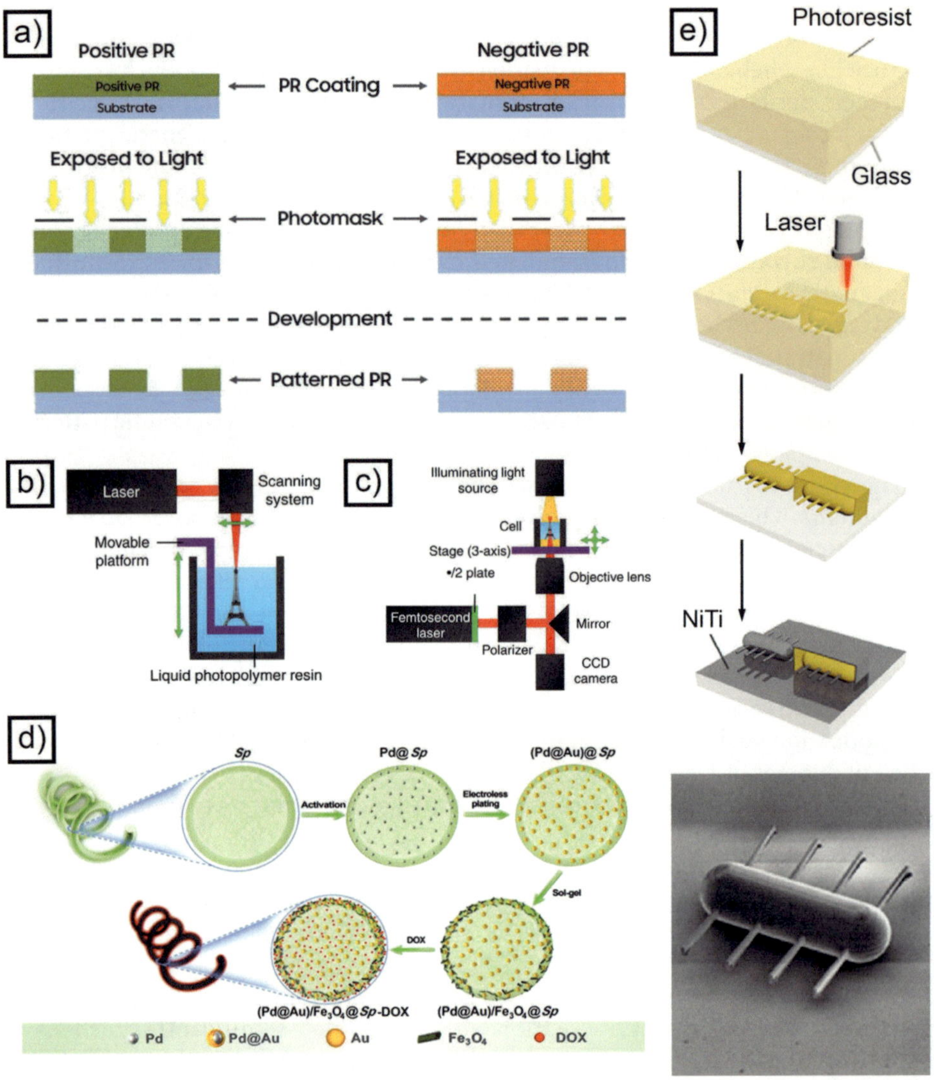

Figure 3.
Schematic representation of the lithography process (a); schematic representation of a stereolithography setup (b); schematic representation of a direct laser writing setup (c); manufacturing procedure for ABFs obtained by adsorbing magnetite nanoparticles on the surface of the cyanobacterium Arthrospira Platensis (d); microwalkers production by sputtering metal on DLW templates (e). Reprinted with permission from [45–47].

Most of the technologies employed to transfer patterns during microrobots fabrication are based on light. Photolithography stands out as a primary method for transferring intricate patterns onto substrates, forming the foundation of many fabrication processes (**Figure 3a**). The photolithographic process begins with the application of a photosensitive coating, often called photoresist (PR), onto the surface of the substrate. This coating is sensitive to light and undergoes a chemical change upon exposure. A mask, containing a precise image of the desired pattern, is then placed over the coated substrate. When exposed to light, the pattern on the mask is transferred onto the photoresist-coated substrate [48].

Also 3D printing stands as a powerful manufacturing technique [49], facilitating the production of biomedical devices and systems whose production would pose challenges with conventional methods like machining or molding. A variety of 3D printing technologies are available, prominently light-based approaches due to their superior resolution. Indeed, each modality presents distinct advantages and limitations [50], but light-based approaches like stereolithography (SLA, **Figure 3b**) and direct laser writing (DLW, **Figure 3c**) are the most used for the fabrication of micrometric structures like microrobots. SLA works by solidifying a photocurable liquid resin in 2D patterns by means of a laser. The resist absorbs single photons and the resulting 2D patterns constitute the single layers of the final object, which is therefore fabricated in a layer-by-layer fashion. DLW, and multi-photon polymerization (MPP), work in a similar way, but in this case the material absorbs more than one photon of light (allowing resolutions down to 100 nm). Moreover, DLW does not necessarily work in layer-by-layer way, allowing a higher flexibility in terms of printable shapes.

Besides pattern transferring, microrobots production strongly relies on a variety of post-processing techniques like sputtering or wet deposition. These are fundamental, for example, to deposit the metallic layers used in some magnetic devices fabricated via polymer-based 3D printing. For example, sputtering deposition can be used to deposit metallic layers on templates obtained by DLW (**Figure 3e**). Nanoparticle deposition or self-assembly approaches, finally, are fundamental for the vast majority of bio-templating fabrication routes. As a representative example, it is worth mentioning the deposition of magnetite nanoparticles on the Spirulina cyanobacterium (*Arthrospira platensis*). This micrometric living being is naturally characterized by a spiral structure and, by depositing some magnetic material on its surface, it is possible to obtain fully working ABFs (**Figure 3d**).

The production of microrobots is an intrinsically multidisciplinary field and it is not possible to enumerate all the different approaches described in the literature in a concise way. The cases reported are the most common and straightforward. In addition to these, a wealth of smart strategies have been proposed, like self-folding [51], inkjet assisted electroforming [52] or microfluidic gelation [53].

3. Drug loading on microdevices

Efficiently loading drugs on microrobots is a crucial part of their development and the strategy selected strongly depends on the working environment of the device and on its delivery profile. In general, the oral route for drug administration is highly preferred due to its convenience, affordability, and high patient compliance. However, despite these advantages, many small-molecule drugs and biotherapeutics face challenges when administered orally due to various physiological barriers, and as a result, drugs suffer from issues like low solubility, low permeability, and degradation following oral administration [54]. These limitations basically apply also to microrobots that navigate the human body through the digestive apparatus. Devices that travel into blood vessels, on the contrary, experience slightly different challenges connected to the presence of immune cells in the bloodstream and to the clearance action operated by the liver and the kidneys. Finally, all the types of drug-releasing devices potentially suffer from the same issue: off-target administration. This happens when a certain fraction of the drug released reaches non-target organs, potentially resulting in side effects and medical complications.

To overcome these challenges, pharmaceutical scientists employ various strategies to enhance the delivery of drugs. These include formulation approaches such as nanotechnology-based delivery systems, lipid-based formulations, prodrugs, mesoporous silica nanoparticles, and pH-sensitive coatings to protect drugs from degradation and enhance their absorption [55, 56]. In addition, many newly developed biotherapeutics, encompassing peptides, proteins, DNA, RNA, and other macromolecules, often exhibit optimal oral bioavailability [57]. Indeed, the development of permeation enhancers and transporter-targeted delivery systems can improve drug uptake across the intestinal epithelium [56].

The discovery of nanotechnologies, including nanoparticles, nanofibers, nanogels, micelles, and microspheres, has led to the development of innovative DDSs, which have become a promising tool in the pharmaceutical field [58]. There are several parameters to consider when designing microdevices, including drug-loading capacity, particle size and size distribution, biocompatibility, and thermodynamic and kinetic stability. Methods for drug loading on biomedical microdevices include a range of techniques tailored to suit specific device designs and drug types. Some common methods are discussed in the following sections with the support of some relevant examples.

3.1 Physical entrapment

Physical entrapment is widely used in DDSs to improve the stability, bioavailability, and controlled release of therapeutic agents. Drugs are physically entrapped within a continuous matrix or a porous structure without forming covalent bonds between the drug and the carrier. The positive points are that this method is simple and preserves drug activity. Another advantage is that it allows a controlled release through diffusion or matrix degradation. For example, the anticancer drug Adriamycin (ADR) can be incorporated into polymeric micelles formed from a poly(ethylene glycol)-poly(aspartic acid) block copolymer through physical entrapment [59]. Regarding the field of microrobotics, a notable example can be seen in the works shown in **Figure 4a** and **b**. In both papers [60, 61], the authors loaded rhodamine B (RhB) into various types of alginate hydrogels, which were applied on the surface of magnetically actuated microdevices. RhB did not interact significantly with the hydrogel chains and it was physically entrapped into the mesh of the swollen polymeric network.

3.2 Chemical conjugation

Chemical conjugation is a sophisticated method used to attach drugs to microdevices through the formation of stable covalent bonds. This technique enhances the stability and control over drug release, making it particularly useful for applications requiring precise drug delivery with a strong and stable attachment. This approach reduces the risk of drug strain and it is suitable for applications requiring long-term stability [63]. Moreover, the chemical bonds present between the matrix and the drug can be selectively broken by external stimuli, allowing smart drug release. Obviously, tuning the strength and type of bond formed between the drug and the matrix is fundamental to tune it release and avoid drug degradation. Applications can be found in biosensors, implantable devices and systems requiring prolonged drug retention [64]. For what concerns microrobots, a few examples of chemically conjugated

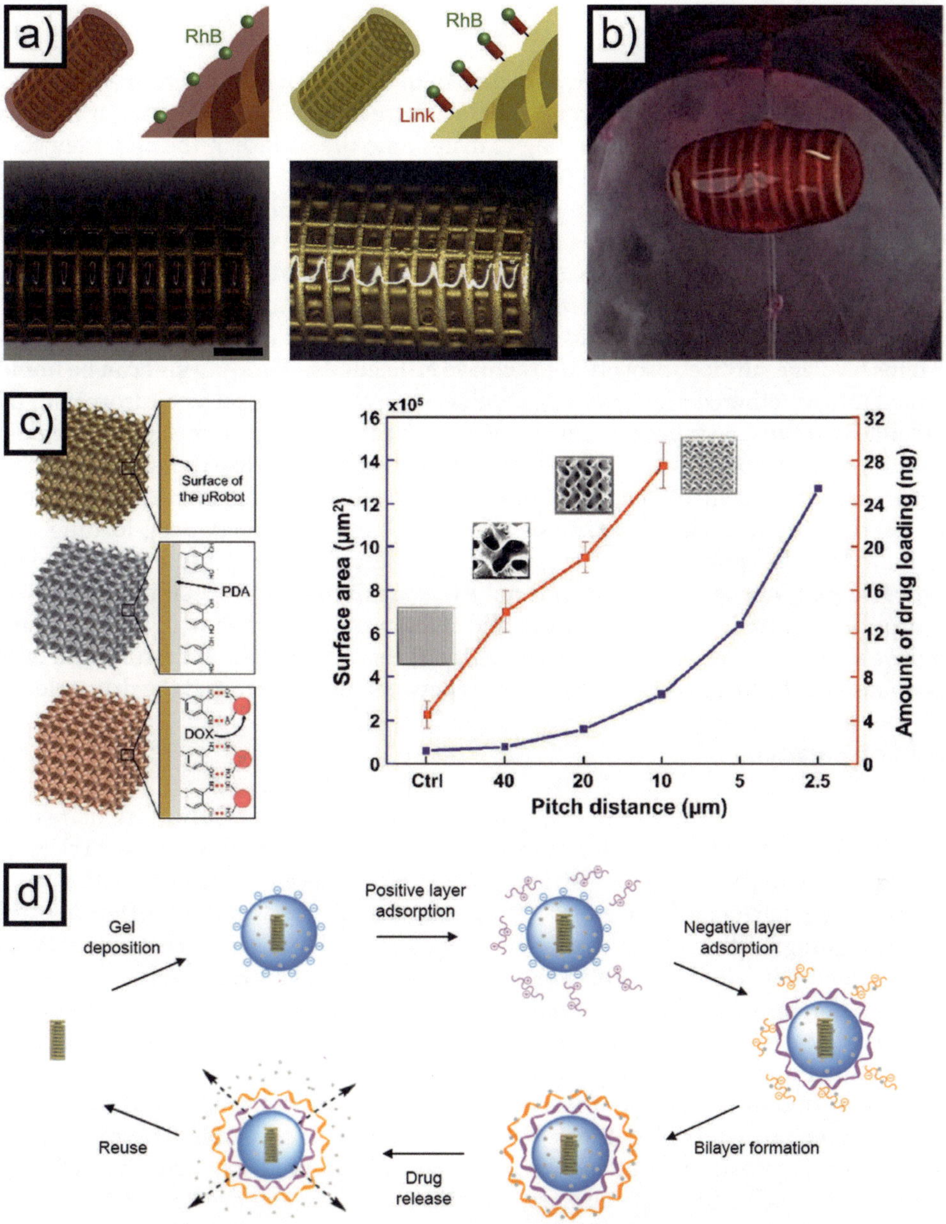

Figure 4.
Physically trapped drug and pH-cleavable drug-hydrogel conjugates applied on magnetically actuated rolling microdevices (a); visual appearance of a magnetically steerable microdevice coated with a reticulated hydrogel physically entrapping a drug (b); schematic of the gyroid surface ABFs drug loading mechanism and the correlated dependence of drug loading on specific surface (c); layer-by-layer hydrogel coating procedure for a magnetically controlled drug releasing device. Reprinted with permission from [33, 60–62].

drug-releasing devices are available. One of the most notable is reported in **Figure 4a** [60]. The authors not only loaded RhB via physical entrapment on their devices, but they also created RhB-alginate conjugates. These structures, created via click chemistry, could release RhB under the influence of a pH variation.

3.3 Surface adsorption

Surface absorption in drug delivery refers to the process where drugs or active pharmaceutical ingredients (APIs) reversibly adhere to the surface of a carrier material. This method involves the weak binding of drugs onto the surface of the microdevices. These interactions can be physical (e.g., van der Waals forces, electrostatic interactions) or chemical (e.g., hydrogen bonding) in nature. This mechanism plays a vital role in DDSs, allowing for controlled drug release and targeted delivery [65]. This method is simple and cost effective, suitable for a variety of drugs and materials. Examples of DDSs utilizing surface absorption include lipid-based nanoparticles [66], polymeric nanoparticles [67] and mesoporous silica nanoparticles [68] among others. These systems leverage surface absorption to achieve efficient drug loading and can be implemented into untethered microdevices. Obviously, in the case of surface adsorption, the guideline that must be followed to increase drug loading is specific surface area maximization. In addition, it is also important to properly functionalize the surface of the devices in order to control the type of bond formed with the drug and tune its adsorption/release kinetics. A notable example of microrobot that bases its drug-loading capability on adsorption and that is very useful to describe these aspects is reported in **Figure 4c** [62]. Zheng et al. manufactured ABFs maximizing the specific area for drug adsorption by introducing a complex gyroid structure and by applying gold nanostars on the surface. In addition, they functionalized the surface with polydopamine in order to enhance the formation of hydrogen bonds between the surface and the drug selected.

3.4 Encapsulation

Nanocarriers can be used to encapsulate and deliver pharmaceuticals that are too toxic, insoluble, rapidly cleared, or unstable as free molecules. These nanocarriers utilize passive or active targeting strategies, depending on the final formulation, to enhance drug delivery effectiveness [69]. The encapsulation technique offers versatility in designing DDSs tailored to specific drugs and applications. Microencapsulation of drug microparticles is indeed a valuable technique for achieving prolonged release of drugs. This approach involves enclosing drug molecules within microspheres or microparticles, typically composed of polymers or liposomes, to control drug release kinetics and improve therapeutic efficacy [70]. From the production point of view, microfabricated fluidic devices that can produce emulsified droplets of uniform size with precisely controlled dimensions and contents are available. These droplets can encapsulate a variety of biological and chemical components, including cells, microgels, beads, hydrogel precursors, polymer initiators, and even other droplets. Encapsulated emulsions are highly desirable for numerous applications because the droplets may serve as miniature reaction vessels, enabling high-throughput reactions at rapid rates while minimizing the use of samples and solvents due to their small size (in the few microns range). The ease of mixing and droplet coalescence facilitates a wide range of on-chip assays with adjustable parameters [71]. The advantage of this method is mainly the protection of the drugs from degradation, enabling controlled and sustained release. Encapsulation is suitable for both hydrophilic and hydrophobic drugs. Some notable examples of microrobots able to carry encapsulated drugs are available in literature. For example, Qiu et al. functionalized the surface of ABFs with temperature sensitive liposomes containing a specific drug [62]. Akolpoglu et al. loaded doxorubicin encapsulated into liposomes on an *Escherichia coli* bacterium, which was guided into complex 3D biological matrices [72].

DOI: http://dx.doi.org/10.5772/intechopen.1008761

3.5 Layer-by-layer assembly

The layer-by-layer (LbL) self-assembly technique, developed in the 1990s, is a versatile method for coating nanometer-thick films on various surfaces. This technique relies on the sequential adsorption of oppositely charged components, typically polymers or polyelectrolytes, onto a substrate surface to build up multi-layered thin films [73]. In the case of microdevices, alternating layers of oppositely charged polymers or molecules are deposited onto the surface of the device itself, with drugs incorporated within the layers or released from the assembled structure. In this way, layers characterized by different diffusivities can be superimposed, tuning the release rate of the drug. A representative example is reported in **Figure 4d**. The authors sequentially coated the surface of 3D-printed magnetically steerable devices with layers of chitosan and alginate or poly(allylamine) hydrochloride and alginate [33]. In this way, they successfully confined the drug inside the device and tuned its release.

3.6 Electrospinning

The popularity of electrospinning rose at the end of the twentieth century, as numerous publications began to emerge. This trend continues today, with ongoing research into various applications for electrospun fibers, including drug delivery [74], wound healing [75], tissue engineering [76], textiles and sensors [77]. In recent years, electrospun nanofibers have gained increasing attention due to their unique features, such as biocompatibility and versatility. Incorporating active compounds into nanofibrous meshes has proven to be an efficient method for *in situ* delivery of a wide range of drugs, thereby expanding the potential and applicability of these devices [78]. Electrospinning is a technique where a polymer solution containing the drug is subjected to a high electric field, resulting in the formation of drug-loaded nanofibers that can be deposited onto a microdevice [79]. Pharmacological applications are connected to the use of antibiotics, antitumoral drugs, wound healing, cardiovascular diseases and ocular disease. The vast potential of electrospinning offers an exceptional platform for developing innovative DDS that maximize therapeutic benefits while minimizing undesired side effects. The choice of drug and polymer can be easily tailored to specific applications or precise requirements. By adjusting the mechanical properties or the release kinetics, electrospun scaffolds represent a promising new frontier in personalized medicine [78]. For what concerns microrobots, an interesting example of electrospun devices is represented by the work published by Su et al. [80]. They used melt electrospinning writing (MEW) to build magnetically actuated microdevices.

3.7 In situ synthesis

Drugs can also be synthesized directly onto the surface of the microdevice. This approach can enhance drug stability, control release profiles, and improve the efficiency of DDSs. Methods of in-situ synthesis are chemical reactions (polymerization or cross-linking), bioconjugation techniques and surface functionalization. Metal-organic frameworks (MOFs) can be a good example of drug loading at room temperature. Applications of this method are targeted drug delivery, implantable devices, diagnostic devices, and personalized medicine [81].

4. Drug release mechanisms

The term "release mechanism" has been defined in various ways. It is often used to describe the method by which drug molecules are transported or released [82]. Over the past few decades, it has become evident that the method of drug delivery significantly influences its therapeutic effectiveness, impacting various factors such as pharmacokinetics, distribution, pharmacodynamics, metabolism, and toxicity [83]. The most common state-of-the-art methods of drug administration include pills, injections, lotions, and suppositories. Oral dosage forms are typically preferred, as they are simple, painless and can be self-administered. However, drugs administered orally are often degraded in the gastrointestinal tract or not absorbed in sufficient quantities to be effective [84].

One of the biggest challenges in drug delivery for liposomes or other drug carriers like microrobots is to initiate and produce the release of the encapsulated drug specifically at the diseased site. This often involves using external power sources such as ultrasound or radio frequency waves to target areas like solid tumors, allowing for controlled local hyperthermia and phase transitions that increase the release rates precisely where needed [85]. As previously mentioned, external stimuli (ultrasounds, light, heat, etc.) can also be employed to trigger the release from specifically tailored materials able to change their physical or chemical state in response to such stimuli [86].

Controlled release can be defined as a technique by which active compounds are delivered to a target at a specific rate and duration to achieve the desired effect. Various types of mass transport processes can influence the control of drug release from a dosage form [87]. Tunable drug release from microdevices involves various processes that control the rate and extent of drug delivery to the target site. These mechanisms are designed to ensure optimal therapeutic effects while minimizing side effects [88, 89]. It is essential to understand the release mechanisms and physicochemical processes that affect the release rate in order to develop controlled release DDSs.

Numerous processes and events influence the rate of drug diffusion and degradation kinetics, such as polymer-drug interactions [90], drug-drug interactions [91], water absorption [92], and pore closure [93]. Understanding these detailed processes is essential to thoroughly comprehend drug release and control the release rate. Drug release often involves a sequence of processes, including water absorption, hydrolysis, and erosion, all of which are influenced by various factors, adding to the complexity of drug release. The term "release mechanism" is used indifferently in the literature, further complicating the understanding. Various techniques have been employed to study release mechanisms, and the findings vary, which is not surprising given the complexity of drug release [94]. A mechanistic and realistic mathematical description of mass transport in controlled DDSs can be highly beneficial [95]. The most common techniques employed to achieve controlled drug release are discussed in the following sections.

4.1 Diffusion

Release from a device can be considered diffusion controlled when the molecular diffusion of the active agent through any part of the device controls the release rate. The two most relevant types of diffusion-controlled architectures are reservoir and monolithic devices [87]. The solubility of the drug and the geometry of the device determine the type of mathematical equation that must be applied to describe the release. From this point of view, a clear road map for diffusion controlled release modeling has been provided by Siepmann et al., which explained how to identify the appropriate equations for a specific type of DDS. Their treatise covers reservoir and matrix systems, whether they exhibit an initial excess of the drug or not, and includes different geometries such as slabs, spheres, and cylinders. The assumptions underlying the models and their limitations are also discussed [96].

In general, Fick's laws of diffusion (Eqs. (5) and (6)) are the principles that describe the flux of particles in a medium due to diffusion.

$$J = -D\nabla C \tag{5}$$

$$\frac{\partial C}{\partial t} = D\,\nabla^2 C \tag{6}$$

The molar flux J due to diffusion is proportional to the concentration C gradient multiplied by the diffusion coefficient D. In addition, the evolution over time of the concentration profile can be correlated to the Laplacian of the spatial concentration profile again through the diffusion coefficient. Overall, mass transfer within individual particles typically adheres to the straightforward principles of Fick's diffusion. Even in complex systems, the diffusion coefficient remains a well-defined quantity, rendering qualifiers like "effective," "seeming," or "apparent" unnecessary and potentially misleading [97]. Diffusion-controlled release technologies based on the use of polymeric barriers offer a viable alternative to conventional delivery systems. The two important applications of this technology are complex reservoir systems and monolithic matrix systems [98].

4.1.1 Reservoir devices

In reservoir systems, the drug is contained within a core surrounded by a polymer membrane. The drug diffuses through the membrane at a controlled rate. The thickness and permeability of the membrane are critical factors that determine the rate of drug diffusion. Reservoir-based systems, a subset of microfabricated DDSs, offer unique advantages. These reservoirs, whether external or implanted, create a well-controlled environment for drug formulations, enhancing drug stability and allowing prolonged delivery times. They are versatile, supporting various delivery schemes such as zero-order, pulsatile, and on-demand dosing, unlike the standard sustained release profile. Additionally, the development of reservoir-based systems for targeted delivery in challenging applications (e.g., ocular treatments) has led to promising platforms for patient therapy [99]. From the microrobotics point of view, a good example of reservoir device are the devices obtained through the layer-by-layer process represented in **Figure 4d**. The superimposition of layers able to tune diffusion of chemicals from the hydrogel layers to the external environment optimized drug release and avoided the phenomenon of burst release.

4.1.2 Monolithic devices

As an alternative to reservoir systems, the use of environmentally interactive monolithic devices made with hydrophilic polymers has been proposed and extensively investigated. In these systems, when a solvent enters the drug-entrapping matrix, the polymer swells, allowing the active ingredient to diffuse from the swollen region [100]. The relaxation-controlled desorption is governed by the solvent concentration at the interface separating the swollen from the unpenetrated polymer. The polymer at this interface relaxes and swells at a constant rate as long as the penetrant concentration at the moving boundary remains constant. Achieving controlled release from this type of device requires a constant surface area and a constant swelling rate of the polymer matrix, as well as a high diffusivity of the entrapped species. These conditions are generally difficult to maintain for extended-release times, as they strongly depend on the evolving interactions among the polymer, the penetrant solvent, and the solute [101]. As an example of the materials employed, polyethylene oxide (PEO) is used for monolithic devices for drug release [98]. As microrobotic examples, the devices represented in **Figure 4a** and **b** can be considered highly significant. In addition, a peculiar example is the device visible in **Figure 5a**, manufactured by Ye et al. [102]. In this case, the drug doxorubicin (DOX) is simply loaded and released by diffusion, but the microdevices are functionalized with folic acid in order to mediate endocytosis (strongly enhancing drug bioavailability).

4.2 Temperature

These systems often incorporate temperature-sensitive materials and temperature-dependent mechanisms to achieve precise, controlled, and responsive drug release. Biodegradable polymer matrixes such as polyesters and poly(ortho esters) are used in *T*-controlled drug release delivery systems. They degrade geometrically from the surface without inner degradation, since drug release can be controlled by the degradation of the matrix [105, 106]. Thermal-sensitive liposomes for cancer treatment utilize dipalmitoyl-sn-glycero-3-phosphocholine (DPPC), whose transition temperature of 41.5°C is just above body temperature, making it ideal for temperature-triggered drug-release technology. After demonstrating enhanced permeability at the phase transition, this property has been applied in liposomes for drug delivery, in conjunction with hyperthermia (a condition that occurs when the body absorbs or generates more heat than it can release) and as an adjunct to radiation therapy [107, 108]. A good example of untethered microdevices that exploit temperature-sensitive materials to guide drug release is represented by the ABFs realized by Zhou et al. They employed a temperature sensitive hydrogel that increased its swelling rate with increasing temperatures (**Figure 5b**) [103]. Another interesting example is represented by the devices produced by Chen et al. [109]. They manufactured fillable microrobots able to release a drug thanks to a temperature variation.

4.3 pH

Drug pharmacokinetics can be pH-sensitive. For this reason, variations in disease state and drug plasma concentration must be considered when developing DDSs to ensure appropriate dosing for effective treatment. However, pH variations can also be exploited in pH-sensitive drug delivery systems (PSDDS), which are becoming important as they release drugs at specific times according to the pathophysiological needs of the disease. This capability results in improved therapeutic efficacy and patient compliance. PSDDS show promise in treating diseases such as asthma, peptic ulcers, cardiovascular diseases, cancer, and hypertension [110]. Tumors, for example, induce localized acidification of the cellular tissues, which can be exploited as a trigger for pH-sensitive materials.

As representative example, it is useful to discuss state-of-the-art gastrointestinal smart drug delivery. It is obtained by coating a core tablet of the gastric fluid-sensitive drug with a combination of an intestinal fluid-insoluble polymer, like ethyl cellulose,

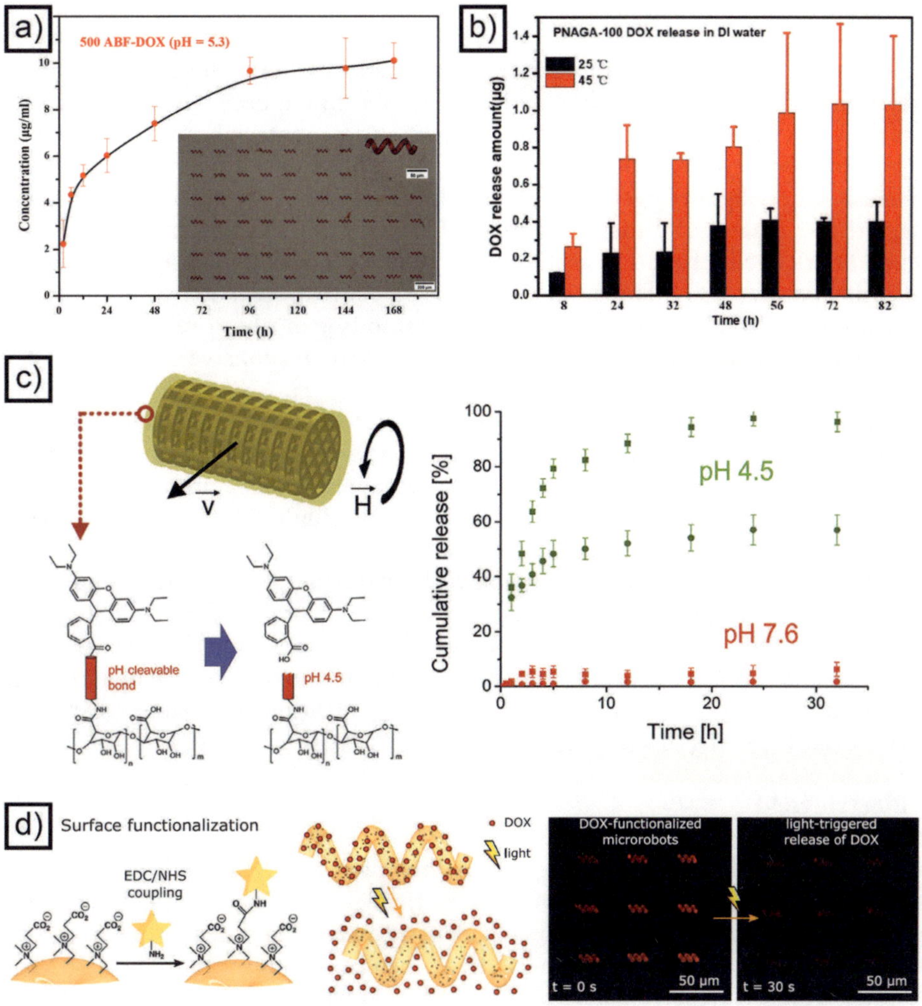

Figure 5.
Drug release curve of magnetic ABFs with folate targeting for drug delivery (a); temperature triggered drug release from hydrogel based microrobots at 25°C and 45°C (b); pH responsive drug-hydrogel conjugates applied on magnetically driven microdevices (c); surface functionalization of microrobots through carboxybetaine functional groups and consequent UV light triggered drug release (d). Reprinted with permission from [60, 102–104].

and an intestinal fluid-soluble polymer, like hydroxylmethyl cellulose phthalate. In the stomach, the coating membrane resists the degrading action of gastric fluid (pH < 3) and the drug molecules are thus protected from the acidic degradation. After gastric emptying, the tablet travels to the small intestine and the intestinal fluid-soluble component in the coating membrane is dissolved away by the intestinal fluid (pH > 7.5), releasing the drug [111]. As representative microrobotic example, the devices loaded with the pH-dependent conjugates reported in **Figure 4a** can be considered. Thanks to the presence of cleavable bonds between the drug and the alginate hydrogel chains, RhB release rate was virtually 0 at pH 7.6. On the contrary, the molecule was efficiently released when the pH fell at 4.5 (**Figure 5c**). Another interesting example has been proposed by Cao et al. [112]. The swarming devices proposed are MOF-based and can release a specific drug as a consequence of pH variations.

4.4 Light

Light-responsiveness is gaining increasing attention due to the potential to develop materials that are sensitive to harmless electromagnetic radiations (primarily in the UV, visible, and near-infrared ranges). These materials can be applied on demand to specific sites in the body. Some light-responsive DDSs are designed for single use, where light triggers an irreversible structural change, releasing the entire dose. Others, capable of undergoing reversible structural changes in response to light and dark cycles, function as multi-switchable carriers, releasing the drug in a pulsatile manner [113]. The development of biocompatible materials for *in vivo* applications, coupled with an improved understanding of photo-regulated solute transport, has expanded the prospects for using photo-responsive materials in drug delivery [114].

As an example, 3D-printed multifunctional zwitterionic microrobots with embedded superparamagnetic iron oxide nanoparticles have been developed, enabling magnetic torque-based swimming locomotion at low Reynolds numbers (**Figure 5d**). Biomolecules were encapsulated in the devices with a single 3D printing step, allowing for the simultaneous incorporation of three fluorescent biomolecules in the microstructure. Surface functionalization with carboxybetaine functional groups enabled UV light-triggered drug release, showcasing controlled drug release capabilities [104]. Another interesting example is the case study reported by Lee et al., who bound gemcitabine (GEM) and doxorubicin (DOX) to the surface of ABFs with light-cleavable bonds. Upon irradiation with infrared light, the devices efficiently released the two cancer treating drugs [115].

4.5 Electric field

Drugs electric field triggered release possibly involves a synergistic process of electrochemical reduction/oxidation and electric-field-driven movement of charged molecules [116]. For example, nanoparticles of a conducting polymer like polypyrrole, loaded with therapeutic pharmaceuticals, can be subcutaneously localized *in vivo* using a temperature-sensitive hydrogel. Subsequently, drug release from the conductive nanoparticles can be controlled by the application of a weak, external DC electric field [116].

4.6 Magnetic field

Effective drug delivery strategies must achieve therapeutic drug concentrations in the specific target area, such as a tumor, while minimizing delivery to off-target tissues [117]. Delivery of drugs to non-target tissues can lead to a range of complications, from mild discomfort to life-threatening side effects [118]. Because biological tissues are minimally responsive to magnetic fields, there has been significant interest in using magnetic nanoparticles in conjunction with applied magnetic fields to selectively control the accumulation and release of drugs in target tissues, thereby minimizing the impact on surrounding tissues [119]. In addition, magnetic actuation is also the preferable propulsion strategy in case of *in-vivo* applications and it can be proficiently coupled with controlled magnetic-induced release.

For example, magnetic fields can be used to induce a highly localized hyperthermia effect at a polymersome membrane, enhancing drug release. This method offers new possibilities for developing smart delivery systems capable of releasing drugs on demand, thereby improving treatment control [120]. Several inorganic magnetic cores are currently available for potential use in magnetically induced drug delivery [121].

5. Conclusions and outlooks

In the last few decades, extensive experimentation has been conducted by researchers on biomedical microrobots for targeted drug delivery. The results clearly demonstrate the potential of the basic concept behind this family of untethered microdevices: bringing the drug exactly in correspondence with the organ that requires it, avoiding overdosage and side effects for all the remaining organs. The task of building, actuating and controlling drug release of micrometric entities moving at the microscale proved challenging. Nevertheless, many smart approaches have been developed in order to address the issues encountered along the experimental path. Despite these efforts, however, virtually all the models of drug-releasing microrobots currently existing are still in their early stage of preclinical validation. Most of the experiments have been carried out *in-vitro*, with only a few examples of experimentation on animals. Still, the complex environment found in living organisms prevents the research from safely moving to real *in-vivo* tests for active delivery. In particular, untethered microdevices face problems with feedback control over speed and position and from uncertainties on their effective recoverability from the body (or biodegradability in the case of disposable devices). Beyond clinical challenges, also the industrialization of biomedical untethered microrobots offers serious challenges. Most of the available devices have been manufactured only at the lab scale, often using relatively complex and semi-artisanal techniques. Scale-up issues and difficulties in large-scale production may therefore constitute additional barriers to the wide-scale clinical use of untethered biomedical devices. In conclusion, the way toward the adoption of remotely controlled drug delivery devices is still long and full of difficulties. Nevertheless, the potential impact of this technology is so profound that it is still catalyzing research efforts. The possibility of dramatically enhancing drug delivery, especially in critical applications like cancer therapy, will realistically lead, one day, to the successful transfer of drug-releasing microrobots from the laboratory practice to *in-vivo* clinical applications.

Author details

Negar Fouladvari, Roberto Bernasconi and Luca Magagnin*
Dipartimento di Chimica, Materiali e Ingegneria Chimica "Giulio Natta", Politecnico di Milano, Milano, Italy

*Address all correspondence to: luca.magagnin@polimi.it

References

[1] Ezike TC, Okpala US, Onoja UL, Nwike CP, Ezeako EC, Okpara OJ, et al. Advances in drug delivery systems, challenges and future directions. Heliyon. 2023;**9**(6):e17488. Available from: https://www.sciencedirect.com/science/article/pii/S2405844023046960

[2] Park K. Controlled drug delivery systems: Past forward and future back. Journal of Controlled Release. 2014;**190**:3-8

[3] Vikram Singh A, Sitti M. Targeted drug delivery and imaging using mobile milli/microrobots: A promising future towards theranostic pharmaceutical design. Current Pharmaceutical Design. 2016;**22**(11):1418-1428

[4] Chirra HD, Desai TA. Emerging microtechnologies for the development of oral drug delivery devices. Advanced Drug Delivery Reviews. 2012;**64**(14):1569-1578. Available from: https://www.sciencedirect.com/science/article/pii/S0169409X12002578

[5] Pusta A, Casian M, Hosu O, Tertis M, Cristea C. 16 - Microdevice-based aptamer sensors. In: Kesharwani P, editor. Aptamers Engineered Nanocarriers for Cancer Therapy. Cambridge, US: Woodhead Publishing; 2023. pp. 367-402. Available from: https://www.sciencedirect.com/science/article/pii/B9780323858816000063

[6] Kar A, Rout SR, Giri L, Sahebkar A, Kesharwani P, Dandela R. 8 - Aptamer-functionalized nanoparticles for targeted cancer therapy. In: Kesharwani P, editor. Aptamers Engineered Nanocarriers for Cancer Therapy. Cambridge, US: Woodhead Publishing; 2023. pp. 191-218. Available from: https://www.sciencedirect.com/science/article/pii/B9780323858816000208

[7] Elman NM, Patta Y, Scott AW, Masi B, Ho Duc HL, Cima MJ. The next generation of drug-delivery microdevices. Clinical Pharmacology and Therapeutics. 2009;**85**(5):544-547

[8] Varadan VK, Varadan VV. Microsensors, microelectromechanical systems (MEMS), and electronics for smart structures and systems. Smart Materials and Structures. 2000;**9**(6):953

[9] Pusta A, Casian M, Hosu O, Tertis M, Cristea C. Microdevice-based aptamer sensors. In: Aptamers Engineered Nanocarriers for Cancer Therapy. Cambridge, US: Elsevier; 2023. pp. 367-402

[10] Abbott JJ, Nagy Z, Beyeler F, Nelson BJ. Robotics in the small, part I: Microbotics. IEEE Robotics and Automation Magazine. 2007;**14**(2):92-103

[11] Li C, Wang J, Wang Y, Gao H, Wei G, Huang Y, et al. Recent progress in drug delivery. Acta Pharmaceutica Sinica B. 2019;**9**(6):1145-1162. Available from: https://www.sciencedirect.com/science/article/pii/S2211383519306008

[12] Shawgo RS, Richards Grayson AC, Li Y, Cima MJ. BioMEMS for drug delivery. Current Opinion in Solid State and Materials Science. 2002;**6**(4):329-334. Available from: https://www.sciencedirect.com/science/article/pii/S1359028602000323

[13] Singh TRR, Mcmillan H, Mooney K, Alkilani AZ, Donnelly RF. 6 - Microneedles for drug delivery and monitoring. In: Li X(J), Zhou Y, editors. Microfluidic Devices for Biomedical

Applications. Kidlington, UK: Woodhead Publishing; 2013. pp. 185-230. Available from: https://www.sciencedirect.com/science/article/pii/B9780857096975500062

[14] Tonomura O, Maenaka K, Hasebe S. Simplified model-based design of plate-fin microdevices with uniform flow distribution at high flow rates. In: Montastruc L, Negny S, editors. Computer Aided Chemical Engineering. Kyoto, Japan: Elsevier; 2022. pp. 319-324. Available from: https://www.sciencedirect.com/science/article/pii/B9780323958790500540

[15] Ornes S. Medical microrobots have potential in surgery, therapy, imaging, and diagnostics. National Academy of Sciences of the United States of America. 2017;**114**(47):12356-12358

[16] Iacovacci V, Diller E, Ahmed D, Menciassi A. Medical microrobots. Annual Review of Biomedical Engineering. 2024;**26**:561-591

[17] Purcell EM. Life at low Reynolds number. In: Physics and our World: Reissue of the Proceedings of a Symposium in Honor of Victor F Weisskopf. Croydon, UK: World Scientific; 2014. pp. 47-67

[18] Wei T, Li J, Zheng L, Wang C, Li F, Tian H, et al. Development of a cell-loading microrobot with simultaneously improved degradability and mechanical strength for performing In vivo delivery tasks. Advanced Intelligent Systems. 2021;**3**(11):2100052

[19] Ding Y, Qiu F, Casadevall I, Solvas X, Chiu FWY, Nelson BJ, et al. Microfluidic-based droplet and cell manipulations using artificial bacterial flagella. Micromachines (Basel). 2016;**7**(2):25

[20] Bernasconi R, Cuneo F, Carrara E, Chatzipirpiridis G, Hoop M, Chen X, et al. Hard-magnetic cell microscaffolds from electroless coated 3D printed architectures. Materials Horizons. 2018;**5**(4):699-707

[21] Zhuang J, Park B, Sitti M. Propulsion and chemotaxis in bacteria-driven microswimmers. Advanced Science. 2017;**4**(9):1700109

[22] Sitti M. Mobile Microrobotics. Cham, Switzerland: MIT Press; 2017

[23] Halder A, Sun Y. Biocompatible propulsion for biomedical micro/nano robotics. Biosensors & Bioelectronics. 2019;**139**:111334

[24] Sitti M, Wiersma DS. Pros and cons: Magnetic versus optical microrobots. Advanced Materials. 2020;**32**(20):1906766

[25] Wu Z, Lin X, Zou X, Sun J, He Q. Biodegradable protein-based rockets for drug transportation and light-triggered release. ACS Applied Materials & Interfaces. 2015;**7**(1):250-255

[26] Bozuyuk U, Yasa O, Yasa IC, Ceylan H, Kizilel S, Sitti M. Light-triggered drug release from 3D-printed magnetic chitosan microswimmers. ACS Nano. 2018;**12**(9):9617-9625

[27] Buss N, Yasa O, Alapan Y, Akolpoglu MB, Sitti M. Nanoerythrosome-functionalized biohybrid microswimmers. APL Bioengineering. 2020;**4**(2)

[28] Villangca MJ, Palima D, Banas AR, Glückstad J. Light-driven micro-tool equipped with a syringe function. Light: Science & Applications. 2016;**5**(9):e16148-e16148

[29] Puigmartí-Luis J, Pellicer E, Jang B, Chatzipirpiridis G, Sevim S, Chen XZ, et al. Magnetically and chemically propelled nanowire-based

swimmers. In: Magnetic Nano-and Microwires. Cambridge, UK: Elsevier; 2020. pp. 777-799

[30] Reynolds MF, Miskin MZ. Materials for electronically controllable microactuators. MRS Bulletin. 2024;**49**:107-114

[31] Honda T, Arai KI, Ishiyama K. Micro swimming mechanisms propelled by external magnetic fields. IEEE Transactions on Magnetics. 1996;**32**(5):5085-5087

[32] Jeong S, Choi H, Choi J, Yu C, Oh PJ, Park S. Novel electromagnetic actuation (EMA) method for 3-dimensional locomotion of intravascular microrobot. Sensors and Actuators A: Physical. 2010;**157**(1):118-125

[33] Bernasconi R, Pizzetti F, Rossetti A, Butler B, Levi M, Pané S, et al. Layer-by-layer fabrication of hydrogel microsystems for controlled drug delivery from untethered microrobots. Frontiers in Bioengineering and Biotechnology. 2021;**9**:692648

[34] Bernasconi R, Favara N, Fouladvari N, Invernizzi M, Levi M, Pané S, et al. Nanostructured polypyrrole layers implementation on magnetically navigable 3D printed microdevices for targeted gastrointestinal drug delivery. Multifunctional Materials. 2020;**3**(4):045003

[35] Xu R, Xu Q. A survey of recent developments in magnetic microrobots for micro-/nano-manipulation. Micromachines (Basel). 2024;**15**(4):468

[36] Chen R, Folio D. Electromagnetic actuation microrobotic systems. Current Robotics Reports. 2022;**3**(3):119-126

[37] Nocentini S, Parmeggiani C, Martella D, Wiersma DS. Optically driven soft micro robotics. Advanced Optical Materials. 2018;**6**(14):1800207

[38] Xiao Y, Zhang J, Fang B, Zhao X, Hao N. Acoustics-actuated microrobots. Micromachines (Basel). 2022;**13**(3):481

[39] Mourran A, Zhang H, Vinokur R, Möller M. Soft Microrobots Employing Nonequilibrium Actuation Via Plasmonic Heating. Germany; 2017

[40] Rajabasadi F, Schwarz L, Medina-Sánchez M, Schmidt OG. 3D and 4D lithography of untethered microrobots. Progress in Materials Science. 2021;**120**:100808

[41] Chen T, Cai Y, Ren B, Sánchez BJ, Dong R. Intelligent micro/nanorobots based on biotemplate. Materials Horizons. 2024

[42] Wang Z, Mu X, Tan L, Zhong Y, Cheang UK. A rolled-up-based fabrication method of 3D helical microrobots. Front Robot AI. 2022;**9**:1063987

[43] Alcântara C, CJ, Kim S, Lee S, Jang B, Thakolkaran P, Kim J-Y, et al. 3D fabrication of fully iron magnetic microrobots. Small. 2019;(16):**15**:1805006

[44] Bernasconi R, Pané S, Magagnin L. Chapter one - soft microrobotics. In: Magagnin L, Rossi F, editors. Advances in Chemical Engineering. Cambridge, UK: Academic Press; 2021. pp. 1-44. Available from: https://www.sciencedirect.com/science/article/pii/S0065237721000065

[45] Kim S, Lee S, Lee J, Nelson BJ, Zhang L, Choi H. Fabrication and manipulation of ciliary microrobots with non-reciprocal magnetic actuation. Scientific Reports. 2016;**6**(1):30713

[46] Wang X, Cai J, Sun L, Zhang S, Gong D, Li X, et al. Facile fabrication of

magnetic microrobots based on spirulina templates for targeted delivery and synergistic chemo-photothermal therapy. ACS Applied Materials & Interfaces. 2019;**11**(5):4745-4756

[47] Low ZX, Chua YT, Ray BM, Mattia D, Metcalfe IS, Patterson DA. Perspective on 3D printing of separation membranes and comparison to related unconventional fabrication techniques. Journal of Membrane Science. 2017;**523**:596-613. Available from: https://www.sciencedirect.com/science/article/pii/S0376738816304215

[48] Zafar Razzacki S, Thwar PK, Yang M, Ugaz VM, Burns MA. Integrated microsystems for controlled drug delivery. Advanced Drug Delivery Reviews. 2004;**56**(2):185-198. Available from: https://www.sciencedirect.com/science/article/pii/S0169409X03001935

[49] Li J, Pumera M. 3D printing of functional microrobots. Chemical Society Reviews. 2021;**50**(4):2794-2838

[50] Hwang HH, Zhu W, Victorine G, Lawrence N, Chen S. 3D-printing of functional biomedical microdevices via light-and extrusion-based approaches. Small Methods. 2018;**2**(2):1700277

[51] Darmawan BA, Lee SB, Du NV, Go G, Nguyen KT, Lee HS, et al. Self-folded microrobot for active drug delivery and rapid ultrasound-triggered drug release. Sensors and Actuators B: Chemical. 2020;**324**:128752. Available from: https://www.sciencedirect.com/science/article/pii/S0925400520310996

[52] Bernasconi R, Nova A, Aktas B, Pané S, Magagnin L. Inkjet assisted electroforming and collective actuation of disk-shaped magnetic micromotors. Applied Materials Today. 2024;**40**:102365

[53] Qiao S, Ouyang H, Zheng X, Qi C, Ma L. Magnetically actuated hydrogel-based capsule microrobots for intravascular targeted drug delivery. Journal of Materials Chemistry B. 2023;**11**(26):6095-6105

[54] Fox CB, Kim J, Le LV, Nemeth CL, Chirra HD, Desai TA. Micro/nanofabricated platforms for oral drug delivery. Journal of Controlled Release. 2015;**219**:431-444. Available from: https://www.sciencedirect.com/science/article/pii/S0168365915300456

[55] Albayati TM, Alardhi SM, Khalbas AH, Humdi ZJ, Ali NS, Salih IK, et al. Comprehensive review of mesoporous silica nanoparticles: Drug loading, release, and applications as hemostatic agents. ChemistrySelect. 2024;**9**(23):e202400450

[56] Plaza-Oliver M, Santander-Ortega MJ, Lozano MV. Current approaches in lipid-based nanocarriers for oral drug delivery. Drug Delivery and Translational Research. 2021;**11**:471-497

[57] Goldberg M, Gomez-Orellana I. Challenges for the oral delivery of macromolecules. Nature Reviews. Drug Discovery. 2003;**2**(4):289-295

[58] Pant B, Park M, Park SJ. Drug delivery applications of core-sheath nanofibers prepared by coaxial electrospinning: A review. Pharmaceutics. 2019;**11**(7):305

[59] Yokoyama M, Fukushima S, Uehara R, Okamoto K, Kataoka K, Sakurai Y, et al. Characterization of physical entrapment and chemical conjugation of adriamycin in polymeric micelles and their design for in vivo delivery to a solid tumor. Journal of Controlled Release. 1998;**50**(1):79-92. Available from: https://www.sciencedirect.com/science/article/pii/S0168365997001156

[60] Bernasconi R, Mauri E, Rossetti A, Rimondo S, Suriano R, Levi M, et al.

3D integration of pH-cleavable drug-hydrogel conjugates on magnetically driven smart microtransporters. Materials and Design. 2021;**197**:109212

[61] Bernasconi R, Pizzetti F, Rossetti A, Perugini R, Nova A, Levi M, et al. Effect of different physical cross-linkers on drug release from hydrogel layers coated on magnetically steerable 3D-printed microdevices. Technologies (Basel). 2021;**9**(2):43

[62] Zheng S, Hoang MC, Du NV, Go G, Nan M, Darmawan BA, et al. Microrobot with gyroid surface and gold nanostar for high drug loading and near-infrared-triggered chemo-photothermal therapy. Pharmaceutics. 2022;**14**(11):2393

[63] Ke X, Ng VWL, Ono RJ, Chan JMW, Krishnamurthy S, Wang Y, et al. Role of non-covalent and covalent interactions in cargo loading capacity and stability of polymeric micelles. Journal of Controlled Release. 2014;**193**:9-26

[64] Joung YH. Development of implantable medical devices: From an engineering perspective. International Neurourology Journal. 2013;**17**(3):98

[65] Hill TL. Theory of physical adsorption. In: Frankenburg WG, Komarewsky VI, Rideal EK, editors. Advances in Catalysis. Cambridge, UK: Academic Press; 1952. pp. 211-258. Available from: https://www.sciencedirect.com/science/article/pii/S036005640860615X

[66] Chakraborty S, Shukla D, Vuddanda PR, Mishra B, Singh S. Utilization of adsorption technique in the development of oral delivery system of lipid based nanoparticles. Colloids and Surfaces B: Biointerfaces. 2010;**81**(2):563-569. Available from: https://www.sciencedirect.com/science/article/pii/S0927776510004388

[67] He C, Yin L, Tang C, Yin C. Size-dependent absorption mechanism of polymeric nanoparticles for oral delivery of protein drugs. Biomaterials. 2012;**33**(33):8569-8578. Available from: https://www.sciencedirect.com/science/article/pii/S0142961212008587

[68] Vallet-Regí M, Schüth F, Lozano D, Colilla M, Manzano M. Engineering mesoporous silica nanoparticles for drug delivery: Where are we after two decades? Chemical Society Reviews. 2022;**51**(13):5365-5451

[69] Sykes EA, Chen J, Zheng G, Chan WCW. Investigating the impact of nanoparticle size on active and passive tumor targeting efficiency. ACS Nano. 2014;**8**(6):5696-5706

[70] Leong KW, Brott BC, Langer R. Bioerodible polyanhydrides as drug-carrier matrices. I: Characterization, degradation, and release characteristics. Journal of Biomedical Materials Research. 1985;**19**(8):941-955

[71] Desmarais SM, Haagsman HP, Barron AE. Microfabricated devices for biomolecule encapsulation. Electrophoresis. 2012;**33**(17):2639-2649

[72] Akolpoglu MB, Alapan Y, Dogan NO, Baltaci SF, Yasa O, Aybar Tural G, et al. Magnetically steerable bacterial microrobots moving in 3D biological matrices for stimuli-responsive cargo delivery. Science Advances. 2022;**8**(28):eabo6163

[73] Lvov Y, Decher G, Moehwald H. Assembly, structural characterization, and thermal behavior of layer-by-layer deposited ultrathin films of poly (vinyl sulfate) and poly (allylamine). Langmuir. 1993;**9**(2):481-486

[74] Zelkó R, Lamprou DA, Sebe I. Recent Development of Electrospinning for

Drug Delivery, Pharmaceutics. Vol. 12. Basel, Switzerland: MDPI; 2019. p. 5

[75] Sandri G, Rossi S, Bonferoni MC, Caramella C, Ferrari F. Electrospinning technologies in wound dressing applications. In: Boateng J, editor. Therapeutic Dressings and Wound Healing Applications. US: John Wiley and Sons Ltd; 2020. pp. 315-336

[76] Tan GZ, Zhou Y. Electrospinning of biomimetic fibrous scaffolds for tissue engineering: A review. International Journal of Polymeric Materials and Polymeric Biomaterials. 2020;**69**(15):947-960

[77] Mirjalili M, Zohoori S. Review for application of electrospinning and electrospun nanofibers technology in textile industry. Journal of Nanostructure in Chemistry. 2016;**6**:207-213

[78] Luraghi A, Peri F, Moroni L. Electrospinning for drug delivery applications: A review. Journal of Controlled Release. 2021;**334**:463-484. Available from: https://www.sciencedirect.com/science/article/pii/S0168365921001449

[79] Afshari M. Electrospun nanofibers. Cambridge, UK: Woodhead Publishing; 2016

[80] Su Y, Qiu T, Song W, Han X, Sun M, Wang Z, et al. Melt electrospinning writing of magnetic microrobots. Advanced Science. 2021;**8**(3):2003177

[81] Motakef-Kazemi N, Shojaosadati SA, Morsali A. In situ synthesis of a drug-loaded MOF at room temperature. Microporous and Mesoporous Materials. 2014;**186**:73-79. Available from: https://www.sciencedirect.com/science/article/pii/S1387181113005933

[82] Sansdrap P, Moës AJ. In vitro evaluation of the hydrolytic degradation of dispersed and aggregated poly (DL-lactide-co-glycolide) microspheres. Journal of Controlled Release. 1997;**43**(1):47-58

[83] Fenton OS, Olafson KN, Pillai PS, Mitchell MJ, Langer R. Advances in biomaterials for drug delivery. Advanced Materials. 2018;**30**(29):1705328

[84] Ding C, Li Z. A review of drug release mechanisms from nanocarrier systems. Materials Science and Engineering: C. 2017;**76**:1440-1453. Available from: https://www.sciencedirect.com/science/article/pii/S0928493117307282

[85] Needham D, Dewhirst MW. The development and testing of a new temperature-sensitive drug delivery system for the treatment of solid tumors. Advanced Drug Delivery Reviews. 2001;**53**(3):285-305. Available from: https://www.sciencedirect.com/science/article/pii/S0169409X01002332

[86] Sun J, Cai S, Yang W, Leng H, Ge Z, Liu T. Microrobots based on smart materials with their manufacturing methods and applications. Inventions. 2024;**9**(3):67

[87] Fan L, tseng, Singh SK. Controlled Release: A Quantitative Treatment. Vol. 13. Berlin, Germany: Springer Science & Business Media; 2012

[88] Liu D, Wang T, Lu Y. Untethered microrobots for active drug delivery: From rational design to clinical settings. Advanced Healthcare Materials. 2022;**11**(3):2102253

[89] Schmidt CK, Medina-Sánchez M, Edmondson RJ, Schmidt OG. Engineering microrobots for targeted cancer therapies from a medical perspective. Nature Communications. 2020;**11**(1):5618

[90] Blanco MD, Alonso MJ. Development and characterization of protein-loaded poly (lactide-co-glycolide) nanospheres. European Journal of Pharmaceutics and Biopharmaceutics. 1997;**43**(3):287-294

[91] Kang J, Lambert O, Ausborn M, Schwendeman SP. Stability of proteins encapsulated in injectable and biodegradable poly (lactide-co-glycolide)-glucose millicylinders. International Journal of Pharmaceutics. 2008;**357**(1-2):235-243

[92] Desai KGH, Olsen KF, Mallery SR, Stoner GD, Schwendeman SP. Formulation and in vitro-in vivo evaluation of black raspberry extract-loaded PLGA/PLA injectable millicylindrical implants for sustained delivery of chemopreventive anthocyanins. Pharmaceutical Research. 2010;**27**:628-643

[93] Kang J, Schwendeman SP. Pore closing and opening in biodegradable polymers and their effect on the controlled release of proteins. Molecular Pharmaceutics. 2007;**4**(1):104-118

[94] Fredenberg S, Wahlgren M, Reslow M, Axelsson A. The mechanisms of drug release in poly(lactic-co-glycolic acid)-based drug delivery systems—A review. International Journal of Pharmaceutics. 2011;**415**(1):34-52. Available from: https://www.sciencedirect.com/science/article/pii/S0378517311004807

[95] Baker RW. Controlled Release of Biologically Active Agents. New York, US: John Wiley & Sons; 1987

[96] Siepmann J, Siepmann F. Modeling of diffusion controlled drug delivery. Journal of Controlled Release. 2012;**161**(2):351-362. Available from: https://www.sciencedirect.com/science/article/pii/S0168365911009588

[97] Titze T, Lauerer A, Heinke L, Chmelik C, Zimmermann NER, Keil FJ, et al. Transport in nanoporous materials including MOFs: The applicability of Fick's laws. Angewandte Chemie International Edition. 2015;**54**(48):14580-14583

[98] Apicella A, Cappello B, Del Nobile MA, La Rotonda MI, Mensitieri G, Nicolais L. Poly(Ethylene oxide) (PEO) and different molecular weight PEO blends monolithic devices for drug release. Biomaterials. 1993;**14**(2):83-90. Available from: https://www.sciencedirect.com/science/article/pii/014296129390215N

[99] Stevenson CL, Santini JT, Langer R. Reservoir-based drug delivery systems utilizing microtechnology. Advanced Drug Delivery Reviews. 2012;**64**(14):1590-1602. Available from: https://www.sciencedirect.com/science/article/pii/S0169409X12000282

[100] Hopfenberg HB, Apicella A, Saleeby DE. Factors affecting water sorption in and solute release from glassy ethylene—Vinyl alcohol copolymers. Journal of Membrane Science. 1981;**8**(3):273-282. Available from: https://www.sciencedirect.com/science/article/pii/S0376738800823157

[101] Korsmeyer RW, Peppas NA. Solute and penetrant diffusion in swellable polymers. III. Drug release from glassy poly(HEMA-co-NVP) copolymers. Journal of Controlled Release. 1984;**1**(2):89-98. Available from: https://www.sciencedirect.com/science/article/pii/0168365984900014

[102] Ye M, Zhou Y, Zhao H, Wang X. Magnetic microrobots with folate targeting for drug delivery. Cyborg and Bionic Systems. 2023;**4**:0019

[103] Zhou Y, Ye M, Zhao H, Wang X. 3D-printed PNAGA thermosensitive

hydrogelbased microrobots: An effective cancer therapy by temperature-triggered drug release. International Journal of Bioprinting. 2023;**9**(3):709

[104] Cabanach P, Pena-Francesch A, Sheehan D, Bozuyuk U, Yasa O, Borros S, et al. Zwitterionic 3D-printed non-immunogenic stealth microrobots. Advanced Materials. 2020;**32**(42):2003013

[105] Heller J. Controlled drug release from poly (ortho esters)—A surface eroding polymer. Journal of Controlled Release. 1985;**2**:167-177

[106] Aso Y, Yoshioka S, Po ALW, Terao T. Effect of temperature on mechanisms of drug release and matrix degradation of poly (d, l-lactide) microspheres. Journal of Controlled Release. 1994;**31**(1):33-39

[107] Yatvin MB, Weinstein JN, Dennis WH, Blumenthal R. Design of liposomes for enhanced local release of drugs by hyperthermia. Science. 1979;**202**(4374):1290-1293

[108] Herman TS. Temperature dependence of adriamycin, cis-diamminedichloroplatinum, bleomycin, and 1, 3-bis (2-chloroethyl)-1-nitrosourea cytotoxicity in vitro. Cancer Research. 1983;**43**(2):517-520

[109] Chen MS, Sun R, Wang R, Zuo Y, Zhou K, Kim J, et al. Fillable magnetic microrobots for drug delivery to cardiac tissues in vitro. Advanced Healthcare Materials. 2024;**13**:2400419

[110] Balamuralidhara V, Pramodkumar TM, Srujana N, Venkatesh MP, Gupta NV, Krishna KL, et al. pH sensitive drug delivery systems: A review. American Journal of Drug Discovery and Development. 2011;**1**(1):24-48

[111] Chien WY. Potential development and new approaches in oral controlled-release drug delivery systems. Drug Development and Industrial Pharmacy. 1983;**9**(7):1291-1330

[112] Cao Q, Zhang Y, Tang Y, Wu C, Wang J, Li D. MOF-based magnetic microrobot swarms for pH-responsive targeted drug delivery. Science China. Chemistry. 2024;**67**(4):1216-1223

[113] Alvarez-Lorenzo C, Bromberg L, Concheiro A. Light-sensitive intelligent drug delivery systems. Photochemistry and Photobiology. 2009;**85**(4):848-860

[114] Lohmann D, Petrak K. Photoactivation and photocontrolled release of bioactive materials. Critical Reviews in Therapeutic Drug Carrier Systems. 1989;**5**(4):263-320

[115] Lee H, Park S. Magnetically actuated helical microrobot with magnetic nanoparticle retrieval and sequential dual-drug release abilities. ACS Applied Materials & Interfaces. 2023;**15**(23):27471-27485

[116] Ge J, Neofytou E, Cahill TJ III, Beygui RE, Zare RN. Drug release from electric-field-responsive nanoparticles. ACS Nano. 2012;**6**(1):227-233

[117] Bae YH, Park K. Targeted drug delivery to tumors: Myths, reality and possibility. Journal of Controlled Release. 2011;**153**:198-205

[118] Kim W, Kim HH, Han SU, Kim MC, Hyung WJ, Ryu SW, et al. Decreased morbidity of laparoscopic distal gastrectomy compared with open distal gastrectomy for stage I gastric cancer: Short-term outcomes from a multicenter randomized controlled trial (KLASS-01). Boston, MA, US: LWW; 2016

[119] Liu JF, Jang B, Issadore D, Tsourkas A. Use of magnetic fields and nanoparticles to trigger drug release and improve tumor targeting. Wiley Interdisciplinary Reviews. Nanomedicine and Nanobiotechnology. 2019;**11**(6):e1571

[120] Oliveira H, Pérez-Andrés E, Thevenot J, Sandre O, Berra E, Lecommandoux S. Magnetic field triggered drug release from polymersomes for cancer therapeutics. Journal of Controlled Release. 2013;**169**(3):165-170. Available from: https://www.sciencedirect.com/science/article/pii/S0168365913000308

[121] Shubayev VI, Pisanic TR II, Jin S. Magnetic nanoparticles for theragnostics. Advanced Drug Delivery Reviews. 2009;**61**(6):467-477